# SOMATIZATION
Physical Symptoms and
Psychological Illness

FOR HELENA,
HUGO AND THEO

# SOMATIZATION

## Physical Symptoms and Psychological Illness

*Edited by*

## CHRISTOPHER M. BASS

MA, MD, MRCPsych
Consultant Psychiatrist
and Senior Lecturer,
Academic Department of
Psychological Medicine,
King's College Hospital,
London

*Foreword by*

## R.H. CAWLEY

Emeritus Professor of
Psychological Medicine
in the University of London
at King's College
School of Medicine and Dentistry
and the
Institute of Psychiatry

OXFORD

## BLACKWELL SCIENTIFIC PUBLICATIONS

LONDON EDINBURGH BOSTON

MELBOURNE PARIS BERLIN VIENNA

© 1990 by
Blackwell Scientific Publications
Editorial Offices:
Osney Mead, Oxford OX2 0EL
25 John Street, London WC1N 2BL
23 Ainslie Place, Edinburgh EH3 6AJ
3 Cambridge Center, Suite 208
  Cambridge, Massachusetts 02142, USA
54 University Street, Carlton
  Victoria 3053, Australia

First published 1990

Set by Best-set Typesetter Ltd, Hong Kong
Printed and bound in Great Britain
by Hartnolls Ltd, Bodmin, Cornwall

DISTRIBUTORS

Marston Book Services Ltd
PO Box 87
Oxford OX2 0DT
(*Orders*:  Tel: 0865 791155
             Fax: 0865 791927
             Telex: 837515)

USA
Mosby-Year Book, Inc.
200 North LaSalle Street
Chicago, Illinois 60601
(*Orders*:  Tel: (312) 726-9733)

Canada
Mosby-Year Book, Inc.
5240 Finch Avenue East
Scarborough, Ontario
(*Orders*:  Tel: (416) 298-1588)

Australia
Blackwell Scientific Publications
(Australia) Pty Ltd
54 University Street
Carlton, Victoria 3053
(*Orders*:  Tel: (03) 347-0300)

British Library
Cataloguing in Publication Data

Somatization.
  1. Man. Somatopsychic diseases
  I. Bass, Christopher
  616.89

  ISBN 0-632-02839-4

# Contents

# List of Contributors

C. M. BASS MA, MD, MRCPsych, *Senior Lecturer and Honorary Consultant in Psychological Medicine, King's College School of Medicine and Dentistry and Institute of Psychiatry, London SE5 9RS*

R. W. BEARD MD, FRCOG, *Professor of Obstetrics and Gynaecology, St Mary's Hospital Medical School, London W2 1PG*

A. P. BOARDMAN Bsc MB BS MRCPsych, *Lecturer in Psychiatry, United Medical and Dental School of Guy's and St Thomas' Hospitals, London Bridge, London SE1 7EH*

T. K. J. CRAIG MB, BS, MRCPsych, *Senior Lecturer and Honorary Consultant, United Medical and Dental School of Guy's and St Thomas's Hospitals, London Bridge, London SE1 7EH*

F. H. CREED MA, MD, MRCP, MRCPsych, *Senior Lecturer and Honorary Consultant Psychiatrist, University of Manchester, Department of Psychiatry, Manchester Royal Infirmary, Manchester M13 9WL*

M. HUNTER PhD, CPsychol, *Principal Clinical Psychologist, King's College Hospital, Denmark Hill, London SE5 9RS*

M. R. MURPHY MRCP, MRCPsych, *Lecturer in Psychological Medicine, King's College School of Medicine and Dentistry and Institute of Psychiatry, London SE5 9RS*

S. PEARCE BA, MPhil, PhD, CPsychol, *Lecturer in Psychology, Department of Psychology, University College London, Gower Street, London WC1E 6BT*

B. K. TOONE MB, BS, MPhil, FRCP, FRCPsych, *Consultant Psychiatrist, King's College Hospital; Honorary Consultant Psychiatrist, The Bethlem Royal Hospital and the Maudsley Hospital; Honorary Senior Lecturer, Institute of Psychiatry, Denmark Hill, London SE5 9RS*

S. C. WESSELY MA, MSc, MRCP, MRCPsych, *Wellcome Training Fellow in Epidemiology, Institute of Psychiatry, De Crespigny Park, London SE5 8AF*

P. D. WHITE BSc, MRCP, MRCPsych, *Senior Lecturer and Honorary Consultant in Psychological Medicine, St Bartholomew's Hospital Medical College, London EC1A 7BE*

# Foreword

This book addresses an aspect of clinical science, for historical reasons sadly neglected, which is now of growing concern to the day-to-day practice of physicians, general practitioners, psychiatrists and psychologists. Symptoms in the body are commonly attributable, in whole or in part, to emotional disturbance. Mental symptoms commonly accompany organic illness and its management. Competent medical practice calls for skills in unscrambling these sequences of cause and effect to make correct diagnoses and devise appropriate treatment plans. Such clinical skills will be sharpened by the study of reviews and inquiries such as those lucidly exemplified by Dr Bass and his colleagues.

Nature, said Bacon, is more infinite in her manifestations than man in his conceptions, and nowhere is this better shown than in the story of mind–body dualism, a human artefact. This notion took root in Plato's day, and was encouraged over the centuries for religious purposes before being brought into scientific thinking in the 17th century by Descartes and his pupils. There it has remained despite, and because of, the best efforts of modern philosophy and psychology. Persistence of raw dualism as a basis for thought and action has been rife in medical practice and distorted the advancement of medical science. Although psychiatrists have long recognized no sharp boundaries between psychopathology and organic pathology, we are only slowly finding ways to overcome this compartmentalizing of the mental and the physical, in concept and practice. Organic, psychological and social processes and events always interact in varying modes and degrees to produce symptoms and signs and illness behaviour. These interactions are amenable to rigorous study. That is a central theme in this book.

There is no shortage of chapters and manuals on liaison psychiatry. The best of these provide a liaison psychiatrist's vade-mecum, but few, if any, are based even in part on collaborative research effort systematically undertaken by psychiatrists and other clinicians. In this corner of clinical science, now ripe for development, Dr Bass and his collaborators have by this compilation established their leadership. The book is most welcome, and deserves to be read widely.

R.H. CAWLEY

*Emeritus Professor of Psychological Medicine*
*in the University of London at King's College*
*School of Medicine and Dentistry*
*and the Institute of Psychiatry*

# Preface

Somatic manifestations of psychological distress are among the commonest problems encountered in primary care and general medical settings. In spite of this they have attracted little attention in medical textbooks, and family doctors, physicians and psychiatrists receive little instruction in the detection and management of patients with this type of ill health.

In recent years this phenomenon has come to be known as somatization, a term which essentially refers to the presentation of psychological disorders with somatic symptoms which are attributed by the patient to organic disease. It is a term that subsumes many psychiatric disorders, notably conversion hysteria, hypochondriasis and factitious illness, but also includes the more common somatic manifestations of anxiety and depression.

These so-called 'functional illnesses' inhabit a borderland between psychiatry and medicine, and are often overlooked by both. Certainly the failure of psychiatrists to develop a satisfactory classification of this subject matter, or even to agree on the principles on which that classification should be based, has proved a barrier to useful research in this field.

The purpose of this book is to describe some of the more common somatoform syndromes. A special chapter on taxonomy compares and contrasts ICD-10 and DSM-III classifications, and proposes a multiaxial system of assessment of these disorders. Many aspects of somatization are covered, from the more transient acute and subacute forms seen in primary care to the more chronic and enduring syndromes seen by hospital specialists.

There are certain omissions in the book, in particular those disorders affecting the face and the back. The reader can find reference to these elsewhere. Each contributor has considerable experience of managing the patients he or she has written about. In addition, each has conducted original clinical research in their area. The book is therefore aimed at both clinicians and researchers.

The book has been written primarily for the psychiatrist in training, but physicians and general practitioners will find much to interest them. The reader who approaches the subject from general medicine or gynaecology should find the sections on management of particular help.

It is hoped that this book will stimulate further enquiry into what remains a neglected field of scientific endeavour. Patients with so-called functional disorders are likely to be investigated by both physicians and psychiatrists, and a further aim of this book is to stimulate more collaborative research into this unexplored area of medical practice.

I would like to thank all those who have helped in the preparation of this book. In particular Robert Cawley, Michael Murphy, Brian Toone, Paul Robinson, Simon Wessely, John Chambers and Bill Gardner for stimulating discussions and suggesting amendments. I am grateful to my secretary, Jackie Robinson, for her efficiency and patience.

CHRISTOPHER BASS
1989

# 1

# Introduction

C.M. BASS

Psychiatric nosology has never readily accommodated patients with physical symptoms that lack an organic basis and in whom psychological factors are thought to be aetiologically relevant. The terms hysteria, hypochondriasis and 'functional' have been used more or less interchangeably, since the end of the 18th century, to describe such disorders. But any historical account of these disorders has to consider the term 'neurosis', introduced in 1769 by Cullen. He insisted that the neuroses never resulted from local but from 'general alterations of the nervous system' (Lopez Pinero, 1983). They included diverse conditions such as epilepsy, chorea and diabetes, but as organic causes of more and more diseases became understood, the concept became restricted. Furthermore, Cullen's definition was to clash, in the fullness of time, with the anatomoclinical view and its single principle, namely that all disease can be reduced to an anatomical lesion.

As medicine became more technologically and anatomically orientated in the mid-19th century, the concept of neurosis came under attack. These developments can be traced to a number of factors. First, the formulation by Virchow of the cellular theory of disease; second, discovery of microorganisms by Pasteur; and third, the description by Koch of the germ theory of disease. These advances led to a reductionist view, based on localization and a reduction to the anatomical level, that was in conflict with the concept of neurosis.

But supporters of the term 'neurosis' attempted to retain it without forfeiting this principle of anatomoclinical localization. For example, Foville (1834) wrote that 'I believe that it is better to define the neuroses as diseases that, to judge by their symptoms, must be localized in the nervous system, but that show no observable alteration'. This view gave rise to the period of 'functional localization', a term which reflected the fact that brain function was disordered but not detectable.

During the latter part of the 19th century neurasthenia was regarded as the quintessential 'functional disorder'. It was also the most common neurosis, and patients with this disorder were managed by neurologists (reflecting the reluctance of patients to go to mental hospitals). As Sicherman (1977) has remarked, neurasthenia '... provided the most respectable label for distressing, but not life-threatening, complaints, one that conferred many of the benefits — and fewest of the liabilities — associated with illness. Certainly it was preferable to its nearest alternatives — hypochondria, hysteria, and insanity, not to mention malingering.' However, towards the latter part of the 19th century the organic cause of neurasthenia became difficult to sustain. Together with other influences, such as the rise of neurology as a medical specialty and Freud's attempt to detach 'anxiety attacks' from the main group of neurasthenic disorders, interest in neurasthenia began to wane. From being regarded as an authentic organically determined illness managed by neurologists, neurasthenia came to be viewed as a psychiatric disorder connoting vulnerability or constitutional deficiency. The word 'functional' also became equated with 'psychologically determined' and this use of the word has continued to the present day (Wessely, 1990).

Moreover, throughout this century, the term 'functional' has been used in a pejorative sense to denote illnesses that do not have an ascertainable organic basis. As Trimble (1982) has pointed out, the term is now used indiscriminately in patients' notes as if it were an end to the diagnostic process. Its use assumes that everyone — except the patient — understands what the cause of the symptoms is.

The word is doubly unfortunate because it not only suggests a unitary aetiology where none exists, but also perpetuates the 'either/or', 'organic versus psychological' dichotomy in medicine. This view does not provide an adequate framework for understanding the aetiology of many of the disorders discussed in this book. In spite of this, the term 'functional' is retained, *faute de mieux*, to describe the symptoms of patients with the more common syndromes often ascribed to a psychological aetiology.

More recently, the term 'somatization' has been introduced to describe patients with somatic complaints that do not have an organic basis. It is a generic term that subsumes a wide range of clinical phenomena. It is not a psychiatric diagnosis and it no longer means what it did to Stekel in 1908 — '... a deep-seated neurosis akin to the mental mechanism of conversion'. The term is now used to describe the variety of processes that lead patients to seek medical help for bodily symptoms which are misattributed to organic disease (Murphy, 1989). It is best seen as a process rather than a disease entity, and it can be acute, subacute or chronic (Rosen *et al.*, 1982). In general, acute and subacute forms are seen more frequently in primary care whereas chronic somatization is more likely to be found in the general hospital.

Many definitions of somatization have been proposed, but the following is both concise and should be acceptable to most:

A tendency to experience and communicate somatic distress and
symptoms unaccounted for by pathological findings, to attribute them
to physical illness, and to seek medical help for them (Lipowski, 1988).
Lipowski has made the important point that somatization does *not* imply
that the patient may not have a concurrent physical illness. On the contrary,
in some cases it can actually coexist with, mask, and be facilitated by such an
illness.

Somatic presentations of psychological illness are often considered to be
uncommon or atypical. This belief, enshrined in textbooks of psychiatry, was
not challenged until recently partly because psychiatry was taught to post-
graduates in psychiatric ward settings. But in general hospitals and general
practice settings somatic presentations of psychiatric illness are the *norm*.

## Prevalence of somatization

### Primary care

In a UK study of somatization in primary care almost 20% of patients who
presented to their doctors with new episodes of illness fulfilled research
criteria for somatization. That is to say, the patients consulted for somatic
complaints, ascribed these to physical disease, and had a treatable psychiatric
disorder (Goldberg & Bridges, 1988).

A physical disease was demonstrated in about 70% of these somatizing
patients, but did not, by itself, account for the patients' symptoms. The
authors observed that when somatization occurred only *half* of all psychiatric
disorders were detected by the family doctor, whereas 95% of those patients
who reported psychological symptoms at the initial interview were correctly
identified (Bridges & Goldberg, 1985).

### General hospitals

A substantial proportion of the patients referred to psychiatrists in general
hospitals satisfy criteria for somatization. Thomas (1983) estimated that they
are responsible for 30% of referrals to a UK liaison service, while Katon *et al.*
(1984) claimed they formed 38% of patients seen on a liaison service in the
USA.

## Factors contributing to somatization

These can be grouped together under a number of headings, which range from
biological through the psychological to social and cultural.

*Morbid states of emotion* are accompanied by bodily feelings, and Tyrer *et al.* (1980) have shown that certain anxious and hypochondriacal patients have greater awareness of bodily function than phobic patients. Increased awareness of bodily sensations can result in more intense emotion which can in turn further increase somatic symptoms.

What determines whether some individuals report somatic sensations at a relatively low level of emotional distress? Traits of anxiousness and health-consciousness (hypochondriasis) are obvious candidates, but little is known about the ways in which hypochondriacal traits become acquired in childhood.

An inability to verbalize distressing emotions is thought to predispose to somatization. Thus, *alexithymic* individuals are said to display a diminished capacity for affective and psychological expression; that is, they lack the words for feelings. But the concept of alexithymia has been difficult to define and is simplistic. Like a related concept, Type A behaviour, the explanatory power of alexithymia suffers by neglecting crucial *interactive* components between the person exhibiting the traits and the specific events and circumstances which elicit the adverse consequences of such an interaction. In a study that reported the impact of specific life events on an individual's capacity to respond using appropriate affective language, Andrews and House (1987) found an excess of events relating to conflicts over speaking out before the onset of functional dysphonia. Their methodology took account of a specific type of event, how it was appraised, and the type of complaint which this conflict led to.

In another interesting series of studies, Pennebaker and Susman (1988) have suggested that inability to disclose traumatic childhood events may lead to adverse health outcomes. They hypothesize that inhibition of thoughts, feelings and behaviours is associated with psychological work, which may be manifest in the short term by increases in autonomic nervous activity. Furthermore, if the effects of inhibition are cumulative it follows that traumas that occurred earlier in life would produce more health problems than traumas that occurred recently. The authors have produced data to support these suggestions, which demand further investigation.

Ideas borrowed from cognitive psychology have made an important contribution to the understanding of somatization. In particular, the patient's *attributional style* determines not only how symptoms are perceived but also what treatments are sought. This somatic focusing prevents any psychological understanding and obscures the need for personal change. However, it has also been suggested that somatization serves an adaptive function for the patient by avoiding the stigma of mental illness. It may also lessen the responsibility for the life predicament the patient happens to be in. Goldberg and Bridges (1988) believe that this blame avoidance function of somatization is its key feature.

Attributions have assumed central importance in the cognitive–behavioural treatments of patients with functional somatic complaints, and this issue will be discussed further in the chapters of this book (see also Hawton *et al.*, 1989).

*Cultural factors* play an important part in somatization. Somatic symptoms have been variously described as 'communicative acts' (Kirmayer, 1984) and 'coded messages' (Racy, 1980), whereby the individual, having troubles in various areas of life, conveys these in bodily terms. That is to say, physical symptoms can be seen as part of a process of making meaning out of experience.

The importance of cultural factors has been shown by Kleinman and his colleagues in their study of mental health in the Chinese. The Chinese medical care system does not recognize or deal with psychosocial issues in illness. Kleinman and Kleinman (1985) studied 100 patients in Hunan diagnosed by Chinese psychiatrists as 'neurasthenics' and found that no fewer than 87% fulfilled the criteria for major depressive disorder (using a structured psychiatric interview). However, all the patients had sought help for somatic symptoms such as headaches, dizziness and chest pains. Only 9% articulated depression as one of their main complaints. In Chinese culture a diagnosis of neurasthenia sanctions a medical sick role for patients who would otherwise bear the stigma of mental illness.

Somatization has also been viewed as a means of entry to the sick role. Patients who are viewed as legitimately sick find that their symptoms allow them to control interpersonal relationships, obtain release from obligations, receive attention and sympathy from others and, sometimes, enjoy financial gain. I have already pointed out that in Chinese society somatic illness is an effective and legitimate way to request care and help from others, while psychological problems are not. Complaints of sadness, loneliness and anxiety are regarded as trivial and not worthy of serious attention, whereas headaches, fatigue and abdominal discomfort are taken more seriously.

## Somatization and the medical model

As Eisenberg (1977) has pointed out, in Western medicine it is typically not until the explanatory power of the biological model has been thoroughly exhausted that the practitioner begins to consider the patient's subjective illness experience in more detail. The diagnosis of somatization is thus, in most cases, a diagnosis by elimination (Kirmayer, 1984). How has this state of affairs come about? One reason is that medicine has become more specialized, and the 'organ specialist' has replaced the generalist. As a consequence each specialist becomes more concerned to exclude serious organic disease in the 'organ of interest' rather than consider the psychosocial context of the illness.

Although Todd (1984) has criticized this preoccupation among physicians 'to exclude', it remains prevalent in general hospitals. Regrettably, our current clinical concepts are inescapably dualistic. The principle on which clinical assessment is based is to exclude organic pathology — often system by system. The longer this process is pursued the greater the likelihood that a spurious abnormality will be found. Such positive findings may be coincidental, and their detection may lead the physician to pursue further false clues which do not benefit the patient. The most extreme examples of 'excluding' are seen with chronic complainers, who have the potential to provoke doctors into wasting an enormous amount of resources (see Chapter 12, p. 301).

This excluding process may be taken to extremes, as this following remark made by a group of American cardiologists illustrates:

> For most patients referred for evaluation of chest pain, particularly when atypical in nature, exercise T1-201 scintigraphy (thallium scan) can provide a *degree of reassurance nearly equal to that of coronary angiogram* [my italics] (Pamelia *et al.*, 1985).

This implies that investigations are being used, not in an attempt to establish a diagnosis, but to reassure the patient about the *absence* of a disease. It also implies a misuse of high technology medicine, especially as there is now unequivocal evidence from a number of studies that half the patients with chronic chest pain and normal coronary arteries have psychiatric illness as defined by standardized criteria (Katon *et al.*, 1988; Beitman *et al.*, 1989; Chambers & Bass, 1990).

This approach to investigations, prevalent in a litigation conscious medical health care system, is not without risk. The reasons are as follows: (i) psychiatric illness (and crucial psychosocial issues) are not dealt with and therefore not adequately treated; (ii) there is evidence that some functional disorders are made *worse* by repeated reassurance (Warwick & Salkovskis, 1988, see Chapter 3, p. 57); (iii) it is possible that repeated invasive investigations, though negative, may increase a patient's conviction that he/she has an organic disease; and (iv) invasive tests can cause disease. This misuse of high technology medicine is often seen in patients with thick hospital files with multiple unexplained somatic symptoms and it has rightly been condemned by a British physician: '... if high technology rightly used is the apogee of modern medicine, this mismanagement of the chronic complainers is its nadir. We should collectively hang our heads in shame at what we have done and are still doing' (Todd, 1987).

## Somatization and the psychiatrist

Since the 1960s psychiatrists have been working more closely with colleagues in general hospitals and primary care settings, and dealing with patients that do not fit neatly into categories of either psychosis or neurosis. Patients with acute and subacute forms of somatization are not found in the ICD because hospital based psychiatrists seldom see such patients (Goldberg *et al.*, 1989). Those with chronic somatization sit uneasily in categories derived by psychiatrists and psychologists and referred to as somatoform disorders (see Chapter 2, p. 10).

Another reason for the lack of interest shown in these patients by psychiatrists is that until recently the general hospital has not been a place where psychiatrists have worked. This physical segregation of psychiatrists from other practitioners has also encouraged the view that psychiatrists are not 'proper doctors'. Although this is changing, there is a need to establish more training posts for psychiatrists in the general hospital. Both physicians and medical students would benefit from the educational opportunities consequent upon such a move, and eventually so would patients.

Furthermore, general hospital psychiatry (or liaison psychiatry) has relatively low status in the UK, and the Royal College of Psychiatrists has expressed the view that there is an insufficient body of knowledge and skills to justify the establishment of liaison psychiatry as a separate subspecialty. But if large mental hospitals are closing and the psychiatrists of the future are being trained to work in district general hospitals, then it is essential that general hospital based training schemes be established. Only in this way will a new generation of psychiatrists gain experience in the detection and management of these patients, who occupy a disproportionate amount of physicians' time but whom psychiatrists, with few exceptions, have largely ignored. One reason for this is that psychiatric training schemes tend to place more emphasis on major mental illness (the psychoses) at the expense of minor mental illness. Indeed, it is possible for junior psychiatrists to complete their training without having any experience of those disorders that are commonplace in non-psychiatric settings.

What can psychiatrists do to change the status quo in this neglected aspect of psychiatric practice? Collaborative research with physicians and surgeons represents one way in which advances can be made in this field. Such interdisciplinary research has service implications, and it is commonplace for referral rates to psychiatrists to increase once research links have become established. Fruitful links are more likely to be forged if the psychiatric department is situated in the general hospital. Another important step would be to include general hospital psychiatry attachments in all psychiatric training schemes. This would, of course, require either more consultant posts in liaison psychiatry or, at the very least, consultant posts with designated sessions in liaison psychiatry as part of the job description. Regrettably, there is little evidence that such training posts are being established or that consultant posts with a bias towards general hospital psychiatry are being created.

Psychiatrists also need to take account of the training of medical students, over half of whom become family doctors. Medical student education remains disease orientated and decontextualized. In particular, the training in psychiatry does little to prepare the GP for the range of psychiatric illnesses that are encountered in primary care.

It is time for psychiatrists to direct more of their attention to this shifting army of patients with somatoform disorders. Where psychiatrists have particularly failed these patients, as well as their physician colleagues, is in assigning inadequate resources to the study of these disorders, in particular into studies of intervention. It is hoped that this book will stimulate both more interest and more research in these common but neglected psychiatric disorders.

# References

Andrews, H. & House, A. (1987). Functional dysphonia: establishing a new dimension to life events and difficulties, in *Life Events and Illness* (Eds. Brown, G. & Harris, T.), Guilford Press, New York.

Beitman, B.D., Mukerji, V., Lamberti, J.W. *et al.* (1989). Panic disorder in patients with chest pain and angiographically normal coronary arteries, *American Journal of Cardiology*, **63**, 1399–1403.

Bridges, K.W. & Goldberg, D.P. (1985). Somatic presentations of DSM-III psychiatric disorders in primary care, *Journal of Psychosomatic Research*, **29**, 568–569.

Chambers, J.B. & Bass, C. (1990). Chest pain with normal coronary anatomy. A review of natural history and possible aetiological factors, *Progress in Cardiovascular Diseases*, (in press).

Eisenberg, L. (1977). Disease and illness. Distinctions between professional and popular ideas of sickness, *Culture, Medicine and Psychiatry*, **1**, 9–23.

Foville, A.L. (1834). Dictionnaire de medecine et de chirugie pratiques, in *Historical Origins of the Concept of Neurosis* (Ed. Lopez-Pinero, J.M.), Cambridge University Press, 1983.

Freud, S. (1894). On the grounds for detaching a particular syndrome from neurasthenia under the description 'anxiety neurosis', in *The Standard Edition of the Complete Psychological Works of Sigmund Freud*, volume III, Hogarth Press, London, 1962.

Goldberg, D.P. & Bridges, K.W. (1988). Somatic presentations of psychiatric illness in primary care settings, *Journal of Psychosomatic Research*, **32**, 137–144.

Goldberg, D.P., Gask, L. & O'Dowd, T. (1989). Treatment of somatisation: teaching technique of reattribution, *Journal of Psychosomatic Research*, **33**, 689–695.

Hawton, K., Salkovskis, P.M., Kirk, J. & Clark, D.M. (1989). *Cognitive Behaviour Therapy for*

*Psychiatric Problems*, Oxford Medical Publications.

Katon, W., Hall, M.L., Russo, J. *et al.* (1988) Chest pain: relationship of psychiatric illness to coronary angiographic results, *American Journal of Medicine*, **84**, 1–9.

Katon, W., Ries, R.K. & Kleinman, A. (1984). A prospective study of 100 consecutive somatisation patients, *Comprehensive Psychiatry*, **25**, 305–314.

Kirmayer, L. (1984). Culture, affect and somatisation, *Transcultural Psychiatry Research*, **21**, 237–262.

Kleinman, A. & Kleinman, J. (1985). Somatisation: the interconnections in Chinese society among culture, depressive experiences, and the meanings of pain, in *Culture and Depression* (Eds. Kleinman, A. & Good, B.), University of California Press.

Lopez-Pinero, J.M. (1983). *Historical Origins of the Concept of Neurosis*, Cambridge University Press.

Lipowski, Z.J. (1988). Somatization: the concept and its clinical application, *American Journal of Psychiatry*, **145**, 1358–1368.

Mayou, R.A. & Hawton, K. (1986). Psychiatric disorder in the general hospital, *British Journal of Psychiatry*, **149**, 172–190.

Murphy, M. (1989). Somatisation: embodying the problem, *British Medical Journal*, **298**, 1331–1332.

Pamelia, F.X., Gibson, R.S., Watson, D.D., Craddock, G.B., Sirowatka, J. & Beller, G.A. (1985). Prognosis with chest pain and normal thallium-201 exercise scintigrams, *American Journal of Cardiology*, **55**, 920–926.

Pennebaker, J.W. & Susman, J.R. (1988). Disclosure of traumas and psychosomatic processes, *Social Science and Medicine*, **26**, 327–332.

Racy, J. (1980). Somatization in Saudi women: A therapeutic challenge, *British Journal of Psychiatry*, **137**, 212–216.

Rosen, G., Kleinman, A. & Katon, W. (1982). Somatization in family practice: a biopsychosocial approach, *Journal of Family Practice*, **14**, 493–502.

Sicherman, B. (1977). The uses of a diagnosis: doctors, patients, and neurasthenia, *Journal of the History of Medicine*, **32**, 33–54.

Stekel, W. (1908). *Nervose angstzustande und ihre behandlung*, Urban and Schwartzenberg, Berlin and Vienna.

Thomas, C.J. (1983). Referrals to a British liaison psychiatry service, *Health Trends*, **15**, 61–64.

Todd, J.W. (1984). Wasted resources: investigations, *Lancet*, **ii**, 1146–1147.

Todd, J.W. (1987). Specialists should also be generalists: a discussion paper, *Journal of the Royal Society of Medicine*, **80**, 153–156.

Trimble, M. (1982). Functional diseases, *British Medical Journal*, **ii**, 1768–1770.

Tyrer, P., Lee, I. & Alexander, J. (1980). Awareness of cardiac function in anxious, phobic and hypochondriacal patients, *Psychological Medicine*, **10**, 171–174.

Warwick, H.M. & Salkovskis, P.M. (1988). Hypochondriasis, in *Cognitive Therapy: a clinical casebook* (Eds. Scott, J., Williams, J.M. & Beck, A.T.), Croom Helm, London.

Wessely, S. (1990). Old wine in new bottles: Neurasthenia and 'ME', *Psychological Medicine*, **20**, 35–53.

# 2
# Classification of the Somatoform Disorders

M.R. MURPHY

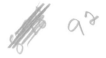

## Definition

The term 'somatoform disorders' was introduced in the third edition of the *Diagnostic and Statistical Manual of Mental Disorders* (DSM-III) (American Psychiatric Association, 1980) to describe a new class of psychiatric syndromes whose essential feature is: 'physical symptoms suggesting physical disorder for which there are no demonstrable organic findings or known physiological mechanisms and for which there is positive evidence, or a strong presumption, that the symptoms are linked to psychological factors or conflicts'.

The six conditions classified as somatoform disorders in DSM-III-R are: body dysmorphic disorder, conversion disorder, hypochondriasis, somatization disorder, somatoform pain disorder, and undifferentiated somatoform disorder. These diagnoses encompass what has previously been called hysteria (Hyler & Spitzer, 1978) or abnormal illness behaviour (Pilowsky, 1969).

Somatoform disorders are distinguished from factitious disorders: in the former patients have no voluntary control of their symptoms, while in the latter physical symptoms are produced intentionally. This distinction is sometimes difficult to make in practice because patients do not readily admit to deliberate simulation of symptoms, while doctors are understandably reluctant to suggest this. The distinction from factitious disorder is therefore usually based on impression or inference (see also section on malingering,— Chapter 8).

Another diagnostic difficulty arising from the DSM-III-R definition of somatoform disorder is deciding whether a symptom has a 'known physiological mechanism'. The DSM-III-R gives this guideline: 'Although the symptoms of somatoform disorders are "physical", the specific pathophysiological processes involved are not demonstrable or understandable by existing laboratory procedures and are conceptualized most clearly by means of psychological constructs'. This presumably means that symptoms arising from increased autonomic activity (demonstrable by laboratory procedures and not a psychological construct) are not 'somatoform'. This gives rise to difficulty with the diagnosis of somatization disorder and hypochondriasis, conditions in which autonomic overactivity is often present. Other mechanisms such as hyperventilation or hypothalamo–pituitary–gonodal disturbances can also produce physical symptoms in emotionally disturbed patients (see Chapter 7, p. 192), but tests for these mechanisms are seldom performed in routine clinical work.

The ambiguity surrounding the pathogenesis of somatoform symptoms is most obvious with the DSM-III-R description of somatization disorder (SD). Here it is acknowledged that some of the symptoms listed as criteria also occur in panic disorder, and should only be counted towards a diagnosis of SD if they also occur outside a panic attack (which has a minimum requirement of four symptoms for diagnosis). This suggests that symptoms of autonomic overactivity and other pathophysiological correlates of anxiety are, in practice, often included in the diagnosis. As a taxon, somatoform disorder does not therefore fully subsume the description of one of its members — a departure from a basic principle of classification. This is presumably done to achieve the appearance of conceptual consistency for the somatoform disorders — a goal that the task force responsible for DSM-III set itself. The result, however, makes a Procrustean bed of somatoform disorder.

The major diagnostic problem that arises from the ambiguity is in distinguishing somatoform disorders from anxiety disorders. It is common for criteria of both types of disorder to be satisfied in the same patient (Boyd *et al.*, 1984). This is particularly true of hypochondriasis or somatization disorder with concurrent panic disorder. This association and overlap is considered in more detail later in this chapter and in Chapter 12, p. 301.

### Somatoform disorders and neurosis

The need for a new category of somatoform disorder arose with the DSM-III when the concept of neurosis was abandoned. As a consequence disorders previously regarded as neuroses had to be redefined and reclassified. Thus, while anxiety neurosis, neurotic depression, hypochondriasis and hysteria (conversion and dissociative type) had been classified as members of one category, in the DSM-III-R they are found in four separate categories: anxiety disorders, mood disorders, somatoform disorders and dissociative disorders respectively.

The elimination of neurosis was part of the American Psychiatric Association's attempt to make the DSM-III descriptive and 'atheoretical with regard to (what were believed to be) unproved etiological assumptions' (Bayer & Spitzer, 1985). The concept of neurosis most prevalent in the USA before the DSM-III (and enshrined in the DSM-II) was aetiological and assumed 'an underlying process of intra-psychic conflict resulting in symptom formation that served unconsciously to control anxiety' (Bayer & Spitzer, 1985). Freeing diagnostic concepts of psychodynamic inference was seen as a step towards creating a classificatory system that was 'reliable and could provide the basis for testable hypotheses' (Bayer & Spitzer, 1985).

In the 1988 draft version of the International Classification of Diseases (ICD-10), the World Health Organization (WHO) has followed the American lead and includes a category of somatoform disorders. As in the DSM-III, this innovation is related to an attempt to eliminate the concept of neurosis as 'a major organizing principle'. There are, however, differences between the two concepts of somatoform disorder (Table 2.1). Firstly, the ICD-10 has combined somatoform disorders with 'stress-related' and 'neurotic' disorders to form a single overall group that emphasizes their historical association with earlier concepts of neurosis and their likely psychogenic aetiology. Thus, despite its demotion from 'organizing principle', the term neurosis is retained. Secondly, conversion disorders are excluded from the ICD-10 group of somatoform disorders and grouped instead with 'dissociative' disorders, thus retaining the traditional conceptual unification of hysteria that dates from the 19th century. Thirdly, the ICD-10 includes 'psychogenic autonomic dysfunction' as a form of somatoform disorder.

**Table 2.1.** Comparison of the DSM-III-R and ICD-10 (1988 Draft) classificatons of somatoform and related disorders

| DSM III-R (1987)<br>*Somatoform disorders* | ICD-10 (1988 Draft)<br>*Neurotic, stress-related and*<br>*somatoform disorders* |
|---|---|
| Conversion disorder | (F44) Dissociative and conversion disorder<br>(F45) Somatoform disorders |
| Somatization disorder | .0 Multiple somatization disorder |
| Undifferentiated somatoform disorder | .1 Undifferentiated somatoform disorder |
| Hypochondriasis | .2 Hypochondriacal syndrome |
| No specific category | .3 Psychogenic autonomic dysfunction |
| Somatoform pain disorder | .4 Psychogenic pain |
| Body dysmorphic disorder | No specific category<br>(F48) Other neurotic disorder |
| No specific category | .0 Neurasthenia (fatigue syndrome) |

Other minor differences between DSM-III-R and ICD-10 are the absence of a specific category of 'body dysmorphic disorder' from the ICD-10 (such cases are to be classified as variants of the hypochondriacal syndrome instead — 1988 draft), and the inclusion of 'neurasthenia (fatigue syndrome)' in the ICD-10 broad F4 grouping, not as a somatoform disorder, but *sui generis*.

As the DSM-III concept of somatoform disorders has been in use for a decade, the work cited in this chapter relates mainly to the DSM-III. Nevertheless, it is relevant to the ICD-10 and may already have influenced its compilers.

## Criticisms of the concept of somatoform disorder

Much of the criticism of the DSM-III category of somatoform disorder applies to the DSM-III and psychiatric diagnosis in general. The more specific criticisms have been along the following lines:

1  Division of patients on the basis of presenting symptoms is superficial. The categories thus convey little information about patients whose psychopathology is likely to be heterogeneous. Psychiatric classification should be based on something 'deeper' than physical symptoms.

2  The individual disorders are not qualitatively distinct but rather merge into each other. Moreover, the distinctions made in the DSM-III are not valid; most patients have clinical features from different diagnostic categories rather than being 'pure' cases.

3  Many of the concepts, including medical help-seeking behaviour, numbers of symptoms and hypochrondriacal attitudes are better described in dimensional rather than categorical terms.

4  The clinical descriptions of specific disorders are derived from hospital based experience and are not representative of the large population of somatizing patients in community and primary care settings. They reveal more about the referral process between community and specialist care than they do about the psychopathology of the patients (Goldberg, 1984). There is undue emphasis on chronic as opposed to the more common problems of acute and subacute somatization.

5  Making diagnoses gives the spurious impression of understanding and leads to naïve assumptions about disease entities (Kendell, 1983).

6  The diagnostic criteria for somatization disorder are too restrictive for clinical use, particularly outside the USA (Deighton & Nicol, 1985; Escobar, 1987). As a consequence most cases end up in a 'residual' category (undifferentiated somatoform disorder). By contrast, diagnoses other than somatization disorder can be criticized for being insufficiently operationalized to allow research.

The reliability, validity and effects of psychiatric diagnoses and their classification are the subject of debate by both psychiatrists and lay observers. Referring to the dispute that followed the publication of Rosenhan's influential paper suggesting that the diagnosis of mental illness is inherently unreliable, Sokal (1974) suggested that: '... many controversies could be avoided, or at least the area of disagreement narrowed and the point under contention refined, if proper principles of classification were adhered to'. Sokal was referring specifically to the 'existence and desirability of polythetic taxa' (discussed below). An outline of some recent ideas in the field of taxonomy (defined as the theoretical study of classification, its bases, principles and rules) is given below with the aim of clarifying some of these criticisms. However, it is important to appreciate that there are different schools of thought in taxonomy and that classifications must not be judged correct or incorrect, but as more or less relevant to their purpose. For example, distinctions that are important in psychiatric research may have little practical relevance to a clinician or health service administrator (Cawley, 1983).

## Classification: general considerations

Classification involves the recognition of similarities and differences between things, organisms, concepts, activities, etc., and the arrangement of these into groups on the basis of their relationships. The formation of categories and their elaboration into classificatory systems is not simply an academic matter. Without being conscious of it we allocate everything we encounter to one or other class. This cognitive activity is essential to the way we cope with life. The way we construct categories and classify things is the subject of recent empirical investigation in cognitive psychology (see Lakoff, 1987), and results of this research are beginning to influence the way psychiatric taxonomists approach their task (Jablensky, 1988). In science, the main purpose of a classification is to describe the relationship of entities or concepts to each other and to similar entities or concepts, and to simplify these relationships so that general statements can be made about classes of entities/concepts. A successful classification should allow us to summarize 'bundles' of information by describing them in simple terms. In this way we achieve a cognitive economy that facilitates memory and the manipulation of information.

A further justification for classifications is that they are heuristic and lead to the generation and testing of hypotheses. A more contentious aspect of scientific classifications is that they are often assumed to reflect natural processes. For example, in biology categories may be thought to represent evolutionary processes. This last aspect of classification is based on a complex set of currently disputed assumptions (see Sokal, 1974 for review).

Critics of psychiatric classification often focus on the lack of clear boundaries between diagnostic categories, a criticism that has often been made of the somatoform disorders. This critique is based on a set of assumptions about what psychiatric classifications *should* be like. The assumption that categories *should* have clear boundaries presupposes a 'classical' view of categorization — a doctrine implicit in the aphorism that classification is 'the art of carving nature at the joints'. Attempts to validate psychiatric diagnoses have often been attempts to demonstrate 'natural' boundaries between related psychiatric disorders. However, a British psychiatric taxonomist, having recently reviewed the spectacular failure of these endeavours, concluded that psychiatrists may have to accept the idea that 'nature has no joints' (Kendell, 1989).

It is important to appreciate that the 'classical' view of categories is not empirically derived but is part of 'a philosophical position arrived at on the basis of a priori speculation' (Lakoff, 1987). This position is often taken for granted in psychiatric nosology (as well as other academic disciplines), and rather than being seen as a theory it is accepted 'as an unquestionable, definitional truth' (Lakoff, 1987). However, as Lakoff points out, the evidence is that most useful categories in both scientific work and daily life do not fit the classical assumptions; it has been empirically demonstrated that most categories *lack specific defining characteristics; many do not have clear boundaries;* and most show considerable *heterogeneity* of features.

An alternative to the classical view of categorization called 'prototype theory' has evolved from empirical research. Proponents of this view point out that some members of a category are better examples of that category than others. This would not be so if categories were defined *only* by properties that *all* members shared. It has been shown that subjects overwhelmingly agree in their judgements of how good an example of a category a member is, even when they disagree about the boundary of a category (Rosch, 1975). For example, an orange is a good example of a fruit and few would disagree about its classification; the classification of a tomato by contrast leads to disagreement with some saying that it is a vegetable and not a fruit (botanists class it as a fruit). Best examples are called prototypes: 'the more prototypical of a category a member is rated, the more attributes it has in common with other members of the category and the fewer attributes in common with members of contrasting categories' (Rosch, 1978). In the case of somatoform disorders, somatization disorder is obviously more prototypical than body dysmorphic disorder. Empirical analysis has demonstrated that members of a category are not grouped together because they share a fixed set of common properties but rather because they are united by 'family resemblances' (Wittgenstein, 1953).

Prototype theory has made more sense of existing classifications (including those of mental illness) than approaches that adopt the classical view (Cantor *et al.*, 1980; Mezzich, 1989). But it is a branch of cognitive psychology rather than taxonomy, i.e. it asks 'how do we classify?' rather than 'what is the best way to classify?'. However, there have been independent developments in the field of taxonomy that show a parallel with the principles of prototype theory:

> Of the various principles applied in recent classificatory theory, the distinction between monothetic and polythetic classification is probably of greatest importance. Monothetic classifications are those in which the classes established differ by at least one property which is uniform among the members of each class. Such classifications are especially useful in setting up taxonomic keys and certain types of reference and filing systems . . . In polythetic classifications, taxa are groups of individuals or objects that share a large proportion of their properties but do not necessarily agree in any one property. Adoption of polythetic principles of classification negates the concept of an essence or type of any taxon. No single uniform property is required for the definition of a given group nor will any combination of characteristics necessarily define it. This somewhat disturbing concept is readily apparent when almost any class of objects is examined (Sokal, 1974).

One of the consequences of polythetic classification is that categories defy precise definition, and overlap in respect of some of their properties. This idea may be unpalatable to psychiatric taxonomists who have attempted to achieve greater reliability for diagnosis by defining boundaries more clearly and reducing overlap. Rosch (1978) has pointed out that it is also in the interests of cognitive economy for categories to be viewed as separate from each other and as clear cut as possible: 'One way to achieve this is by means of formal, necessary and sufficient criteria for category membership. The attempt to impose such criteria on categories marks virtually all definitions in the tradition of Western reason'. The DSM-III attempts to create clear boundaries between what are assumed to be a priori separate disorders.

But researchers in physical and natural sciences report that polythetic categories are more useful than these traditional approaches to classification. Psychiatrists have also started to accept these principles. Swartz *et al.* (1987) have used a multivariate technique called 'grade of membership analysis' to examine somatic symptom data from the National Institute of Mental Health Epidemiological Catchment Area (NIMH-ECA) project. This technique makes no a priori assumptions about threshold levels or clustering of physical symptoms, and scores are generated that allow individuals to be partial members of two or more groups. The 'fuzzy set' classification that emerges from this analysis describes 'mixed' syndromes and is more representative of somatization syndromes in the community (see Zadeh, 1965 for the logic of fuzzy sets).

In a study of 'medically unexplained somatic distress' in a family medicine sample, Robbins *et al.* (1989) compared patterns (covariation) of 'functional' symptoms with definitions of five 'functional somatic syndromes' described in the medical literature. These were: fibromyalgia, chronic fatigue syndrome, somatic depression, somatic anxiety and irritable bowel syndrome. They considered it possible that these were not discrete syndromes at all, 'but are perceived as such only when claimed by a particular medical speciality that focusses attention on limited aspects of distress'.

The definitions of the discrete functional syndromes were examined by estimating 'latent variable models' of distress and testing them for 'goodness of fit'. They found that one latent construct of 'functional somatic distress' did poorly in accounting for the covariation among symptoms. A two-factor model in which the latent constructs were labelled 'somatic anxiety' and 'somatic depression' did better but still failed to provide a good fit to the covariation among symptoms. The final model that hypothesized five latent constructs, corresponding to the five syndromes, fitted best and provided evidence for the convergent validity of the functional somatic syndromes. In other words, the symptoms alleged to occur with each of the syndromes were found to covary more within syndromes than between syndromes. However, it does not follow that the syndromes occur in isolation from each other. Indeed, when co-occurrence of syndromes was examined it was found that most patients who satisfied criteria for one syndrome generally did so for one or two of the others. This study demonstrated that a syndrome may have validity but still show considerable overlap with other syndromes.

## Reliability and validity of diagnosis

The unreliability of psychiatric diagnosis was demonstrated in the 1960s and 70s. The method most frequently used to study reliability was for two psychiatrists to examine the same patient independently, after which their diagnoses were compared (inter-rater reliability). The largest source of disagreement that occurred in early studies was 'criterion variance', i.e. use of different diagnostic criteria by different psychiatrists (Spitzer *et al.*, 1978). In addition, when a classificatory system was used (DSM-I, 1952), raters often had to make a choice between two categories whose criteria had both been fulfilled, but with no adequate criteria for differentiating related syndromes (Ward *et al.*, 1962).

Such lack of reliability has been a serious impediment to communication in clinical practice and research. To an extent this has been remedied by simple methods like structured interviews and the use of operational defini- tions (the DSM-III being the first psychiatric classification intended for routine clinical use to specify formal criteria). Thus, by specifying exactly what criteria must be satisfied before a diagnosis can be made, diagnoses are made more reliable. These definitions may also specify exclusion criteria that enable a decision to be made if the criteria for two diagnoses have been met, for example if a case satisfies DSM-III criteria for somatoform pain disorder and somatization disorder, only the second diagnosis should be made. The reliability of a diagnosis is thus concerned with the defining characteristics of a class and the ease with which class membership can be established.

Reliability is easily measured and has been shown to be 'acceptable' for many DSM-III-R diagnoses. For the somatoform disorders, however, only somatization disorder has been adequately operationalized to allow its reliability to be demonstrated.

Validity is concerned with the correlates of class membership and is more difficult to define. It is essentially concerned with prediction and hence practical utility. In the case of psychiatric classification a valid category is one that helps decide treatment and predict outcome. The validity of a diagnosis or a diagnostic distinction is not therefore an absolute quality, but varies with context. Various strategies have been used to establish the validity of clinical syndromes. These include: cluster analysis to identify clusters of correlated symptoms; discriminant function analysis to demon- strate a boundary between related syndromes; demonstration of different outcomes for different syndromes; responses to different treatments; family studies and the discovery of biological correlates (see Kendell, 1989 for review).

Reliability does not guarantee validity and it has been argued that the DSM-III has sacrificed validity in the pursuit of reliability. Vaillant (1984) points out that operational criteria are used simply because it is possible to get greater inter-rater reliability with them. Yet important 'hallmarks' of psychiatric disorders are abandoned because it is not possible to get such reliability, and these 'hallmarks' are what may be more valid. He uses the analogy of selecting a basketball team to illustrate this point — measuring the height of a basketball player is a far more reliable procedure than judging his/her ball-handling skill, but is unlikely to predict a player's performance and has far less relevance in establishing a winning team (see Faust & Milner, 1986 for a critique of the methodological doctrine underlying DSM-III).

The specific somatoform disorders will now be discussed with the above taxonomic considerations in mind. Comparisons between DSM-III-R and ICD-10 are made where possible.

# Body dysmorphic disorder

This diagnosis was introduced as a separate category in the 1987 revised edition of the DSM-III (DSM-III-R). It is defined as a 'preoccupation with some imagined defect in appearance in a normal-appearing person. The most common complaints involve facial flaws, such as wrinkles, spots on the skin, excessive facial hair, shape of nose, mouth, jaw, or eyebrows ...'. The description continues ... 'In some cases a slight physical anomaly is present, but the person's concern is grossly excessive'. The criteria exclude cases in which the complaint is delusional and when it arises in the course of anorexia nervosa or transsexualism.

While the term is new the concept is not; Morselli described 'dysmorphophobia' a century ago as 'a subjective feeling of ugliness or physical defect which the patient feels is noticeable to others, although the appearance is within normal limits' (Birtchnell, 1988). This older term was replaced because the disturbance is not a true phobia in that avoidance behaviour is not typical.

There are no data on the reliability or validity of this diagnosis. There are, however, some obvious problems with its definition. For example, it is assumed that a 'normal-appearing person' with an 'imagined' defect can be distinguished. But it has been demonstrated that a person's appearance, judged normal by some, will be judged abnormal by others (Harris, 1982). Such judgements are not medical but aesthetic and are likely to vary between doctors. General practitioners demonstrate this divergence in aesthetic values in their referral practices. A UK study found no significant difference in the degree of disfigurement (or psychopathology) between patients referred to surgeons and those referred to psychiatrists (Hay, 1970a). Similarly, assessment of concern as 'grossly excessive' is also a difficult value judgement. A physical anomaly may appear 'slight' in the clinic but put the patient at a social disadvantage in other situations (Lacey & Birtchnell, 1986; Dion *et al.*, 1972).

In the modern context of aesthetic surgery the DSM-III-R criteria are irrelevant, if not meaningless. A substantial number of patients seeking aesthetic facial surgery can be regarded as 'normal-appearing'. Indeed, aesthetic surgery has been defined as 'surgery which is designed to correct defects which the average prudent observer would consider to be within the range of normal' (Goin & Goin, 1986). And the evidence is that (in the eyes of its clients) aesthetic surgery frequently improves a normal appearance (Hay & Heather, 1973; Goin & Goin, 1986).

In general, the evidence from follow-up studies of cosmetic surgery patients suggests that most have a good psychosocial outcome regardless of the objective degree of anomaly (Edgerton *et al.*, 1960; Hay & Heather, 1973).

On the other hand, there is also evidence that the cosmetic complaints of a minority of patients seeking surgery may reflect significant psychopathology, the full extent of which may only later become apparent (Hay, 1970b; Connolly & Gipson, 1978). Distinguishing these patients from the larger group of cosmetic surgery candidates is the diagnostic task for which criteria are needed. The DSM-III-R definition of body dysmorphic disorder is too overinclusive to be of any value to a psychiatrist attempting to predict the outcome of surgery.

Although there is little sound research on the validity or reliability of dysmorphophobia, descriptive clinical reports suggest a prototype. In addition to the morbid preoccupation, its characteristics include: marked self-reference; an unrealistic attribution of all other problems to the cosmetic 'defect' and an unrealistic expectation of surgery; vagueness or bizarreness in the patient's description of the defect; and an association with 'sensitivity' of personality. To use Vaillant's term (1984), these are the 'hallmarks' that give the psychological entity some validity and may be useful in predicting course and outcome of treatment. It may not be easy, however, to define reliably each individual characteristic.

The ICD-10 draft (1988) has retained the term 'dysmorphophobia' to refer to 'fears relating to the presence of . . . disfigurement' and includes it as a form of the hypochondriacal syndrome. There are obvious similarities to hypochondriacal patients but the essential feature of dysmorphophobia is a preoccupation with ugliness and not a fear of disease. Most psychiatrists would have little trouble distinguishing the two and there is no empirical or heuristic reason for grouping them together. Uncertainty about the noso-logical status of dysmorphophobia in the ICD-10 is reflected in its shift from 'delusional disorder' in the 1987 draft to 'hypochondriasis' in the 1988 version.

## Somatization disorder (SD)

The criteria for this disorder are 'a history of many physical complaints or a belief that one is sickly, beginning before the age of 30 and persisting for several years'. In addition the patient must have at least 13 physical symptoms from a list of 35 specified in the manual. These are listed in 6 groups: pain, gastrointestinal, cardiopulmonary, conversion (pseudoneuro-logical), sexual and female reproductive symptoms. For a symptom to count towards the diagnosis it must satisfy three criteria: there is no pathophys-iological mechanism to account for the symptom; it has not occurred only during a panic attack; and it has caused the person to take medicine (other than over-the-counter pain medication), see a doctor, or alter lifestyle.

These criteria may appear arbitrary to anyone unfamiliar with the recent history of the concept of hysteria in the USA — summarized briefly this is as follows. In 1951 Purtell *et al.*, from the Department of Psychiatry at Washington University, St Louis, reported a study of 50 patients who had been investigated for numerous unexplained physical complaints. The authors found a consistent pattern of symptoms that generally only occurred in women and began early in life. They also noted a greater number of hospital admissions and major surgical operations when they compared these patients with controls. They concluded that this was a distinct syndrome and that the picture they described was similar to the descriptions of hysteria offered by Briquet in 1859 and Saville in 1909 (see Mai & Merskey, 1980 for discussion of Briquet's 1859 treatise).

Since the early 1960s numerous research reports on hysteria from the St Louis department have been published in UK and USA journals and the name Briquet's syndrome was introduced to avoid the pejorative connotations of the term hysteria. The main claims made in this work are that the diagnosis has a high level of reliability (Spitzer *et al.*, 1978); that it has good validity (Guze, 1975) and is stable over time (Perley & Guze, 1962); that it is common, with a prevalence of 1–2% in women (Woodruff *et al.*, 1971); that it is familial and affects 10–20% of first degree female relatives (Cloninger *et al.*, 1975).

On the basis of their family studies the St Louis group have claimed that there is a spectrum of related disorders, and that:

> Hysteria and sociopathy have a common familial origin, whether genetic, social, or both. The earliest manifestations of the adult disorders may take the form of the hyperactive child syndrome. As the child matures, various forms of delinquency and antisocial behaviour may become evident. The clinical picture in adolescence and adulthood will depend in part on the sex of the individual. Briquet's syndrome will predominate in females and the sociopathic constellation will predominate in males (Guze, 1975).

For the operational definition of Briquet's syndrome, Perley and Guze (1962) listed 59 symptoms divided into 10 groups (see Chapter 12, p. 301). The diagnosis requires a minimum of 20 symptoms which must come from at least nine of the groups. Unlike the DSM-III criteria for SD they include 'anxiety attacks', 'depressed feelings' and other complaints that are not unexplained physical symptoms. But this set of criteria was judged too long and complex for routine clinical work, and an abridged set of 35 symptoms is currently used to establish a DSM-III-R diagnosis of somatization disorder.

Inevitably, this redefinition has created discordance between the two diagnoses: it is possible to satisfy criteria for Briquet's syndrome without satisfying those for somatization disorder and vice versa. In a study of 90 female psychiatric outpatients who received *either* diagnosis, only 71% received *both* diagnoses (Cloninger *et al.*, 1986). The implication of this finding is that claims made for the validity of Briquet's syndrome cannot be assumed to hold good for SD. For instance, there is evidence that the familial associations of Briquet's syndrome may not be true for SD (Cloninger *et al.*, 1986). It has also been argued that the rationale for reducing the number of symptoms is misguided since the symptoms which have been dropped are elicited routinely in psychiatric assessments (Cloninger, 1986). Both the DSM-III-R criteria for SD and the Perley–Guze criteria for Briquet's syndrome are given in Chapter 12, p. 303.

The exclusion of psychological symptoms such as anxiety attacks also represents an attempt to make the criteria 'conceptually consistent'. Yet it is common for patients satisfying these criteria to show also the features of panic disorder/agoraphobia and mood disorder. A community survey found that subjects with SD were 96 times more likely to have panic disorder, 27 times more likely to have agoraphobia and 25 times more likely to have major depression than people without somatization disorder, suggesting a shared diathesis for these three syndromes (Boyd *et al.*, 1984). This has led to the suggestion that SD, 'rather than being categorically distinct from affective and anxiety disorder ... actually may be a collection of these and other syndromes aggregating in a complex form' (Orenstein, 1989). To embody such a view of SD, a classificatory system has to take more account of pathogenesis than does the DSM-III-R.

## Undifferentiated somatoform disorder

This DSM-III-R category is defined as a 'residual to somatization disorder': it is diagnosed in cases that 'do not meet the full symptom picture of somatization disorder'. Its diagnostic criteria are: one or more physical complaints that either cannot be explained by organic pathology or pathophysiological mechanisms, or are grossly in excess of what would be expected from organic findings; duration of more than 6 months; and occurrence not exclusively during the course of another disorder (including a sleep disorder and sexual dysfunction).

It is stated that (i) although the diagnosis can be made in cases of a single symptom, more commonly multiple symptoms are present; and (ii) there is no evidence that the disorder is more common in females and there is no age requirement for its diagnosis. The ICD-10 (1988 draft) includes an equivalent category.

Research carried out in the community has shown that more patients with functional somatic symptoms can be classified in this category than in any of the other somatoform categories. In practice, clinicians and researchers seem understandably reluctant to use a 'residual' category to classify an extremely common type of clinical problem. But this residual category has been introduced because most patients with chronic somatization fail to satisfy criteria for SD. In other words, the vagueness and lack of definition that makes this category unattractive is a consequence of the restrictive criteria for SD.

Deighton and Nicol (1985) surveyed all young women in a large group family practice in North East England and identified 49 patients with the highest rate of functional complaints whom they regarded as 'eligible for Briquet's syndrome'. Only two satisfied the criteria. Those who did not shared many of the features associated with Briquet's, suggesting that this syndrome does not represent a sharp qualitative departure from lesser degrees of morbidity. It is not surprising that patients with multiple somatic symptoms that fail to satisfy criteria for Briquet's should resemble cases that do. If followed up many of these subthreshold cases would develop further symptom episodes and become cases. These findings challenge the usefulness of the syndrome.

By abandoning the qualitative features of Briquet's syndrome (vagueness, dramatism) in the description of SD the diagnosis is reduced even further to a symptom count. The requisite number of symptoms is less for SD but they are more uniformly somatic symptoms. This suggests that the distinction between SD and a subgroup of undifferentiated somatoform disorder may simply be one of severity or chronicity, or both.

This has led Escobar and Canino (1989) to suggest that DSM-III-R somatization disorder could technically be described as 'Somatic Symptom Index-13' (SSI-13). It follows that undifferentiated somatoform disorder could be described as SSI-1 to SSI-12. Escobar *et al.* (1987) have explored the use of subsyndromal symptom counts in an effort to investigate the validity of a broader category. Using large data sets from epidemiological studies they found that an index of four symptoms for men and six for women (SSI-4 and SSI-6) predicted similar correlates and outcomes to SSI-13 (somatization disorder). Furthermore, the prevalence of this subthreshold syndrome was *100 times* higher than for SD. This supports the argument put forward by Deighton and Nicol (1985) and other authors (Bhattacharya & Bharadwaj, 1977) that a less restrictive definition is more useful both clinically and as a basis for research. The St Louis group, on the other hand, have justified their definition of Briquet's syndrome by presenting data to show that the familial associations (a criterion of validity) demonstrated for this disorder are not found when abridged criteria (DSM-III-R) are used (Cloninger *et al.*, 1986).

This raises the possibility that, although discontinuity at the clinical descriptive level cannot be easily demonstrated, mild and severe cases of the disorder may have different aetiologies. The choice of symptom threshold for inclusion as a case should therefore depend on the question that is addressed when making the diagnosis.

In a discriminant function analysis of data on female adoptees with somatization, Cloninger *et al.* (1984) identified 'two discrete groups of somatizers who differ in their frequency and severity of disability'. The first, 'high frequency somatizers', had more frequent psychiatric complaints, abdominal pain and back pain; while the second group, 'diversiform somatizers', had less frequent disability but a greater diversity of complaints when they were ill. The data used in the study were derived from registers of the Swedish National Insurance Board and not by interview or self-report, so that it is not clear how these two groups compare with clinical categories. However, in a cross-fostering analysis of data on the same subjects, the 'high frequency somatizers' often had biological fathers who had a history of criminality — an association found in patients with Briquet's syndrome (Bohman *et al.*, 1984).

# Multiple somatization disorder (ICD-10)

The ICD-10 definition of multiple somatization disorder (MSD) is less restrictive than the DSM-III-R category in three respects: (i) it does not specify how many symptoms a patient should have; (ii) there are no specified criteria (other than the absence of an organic explanation) that have to be satisfied before a symptom can be counted towards the diagnosis; and (iii) there is no specified age of onset. The essential requirement is 'at least 2 years of multiple and variable physical symptoms for which no adequate physical explanation has been found'. Additional requirements for a 'definite diagnosis' are refusal to accept the reassurance of several different doctors that there is no physical explanation for the symptoms, and impairment of social functioning attributable to the disorder.

This broader definition will thus allow the diagnosis of multiple somatization disorder in cases failing to meet DSM-III-R criteria. The category is thus likely to be considerably more heterogeneous, to show less inter-rater relibility, and cannot be assumed to have the same clinical or sociodemographic characteristics as Briquet's, for example the association with sociopathy in first degree male relatives. The ICD-10 category of undifferentiated somatoform disorder is for cases of less than 2 years' duration and 'less striking symptom patterns'.

# Conversion disorder

An essential difference between this and other somatoform disorders is that 'an alteration or loss of physical functioning' is required for the diagnosis, i.e. it is not diagnosed on the basis of symptom complaints alone. Pain is therefore not classified as a conversion symptom even if the examiner believes that conversion is the mechanism of symptom production. The diagnosis of somatoform pain disorder should be considered instead (see below).

Most typical examples of conversion suggest neurological disease, e.g. paralysis, seizures, or anaesthesia. The DSM-III-R, however, also gives pseudocyesis and vomiting as examples of conversion (see Chapter 8, p. 207 for further discussion).

Unlike other somatoform disorders an episode of conversion is usually of short duration with sudden onset and resolution, although it can be recurrent. Such episodes are also a feature of SD and can occur in the course of other psychiatric illness such as depression and schizophrenia. When conversion symptoms occur in these contexts, conversion disorder should not be diagnosed.

In view of the DSM-III's espousal of a descriptive atheoretical approach to classification, conversion disorder is a unique concession to psychodynamic theory. Not only is the term 'conversion' (which implies an unconscious mental mechanism) retained, but the text that accompanies the diagnostic criteria endorses Freud's explanation of hysterical conversion in terms of primary and secondary gain.

Several studies have demonstrated the unreliability of an initial diagnosis of conversion; these are discussed in Chapter 8, p. 209. The sources of error in the medical assessment of a patient with undiagnosed neurological disease that give rise to the mistaken diagnosis of conversion include: natural variation in disease processes; limitations in medical knowledge and methods of assessment; and a tendency for distressed patients to exaggerate their complaints. In addition, positive evidence of psychiatric disturbance is also unreliable. On the basis of eight clinical studies of putative conversion symptoms, Cloninger (1986) concluded that the only 'psychiatric inclusion criteria' that reliably predicted absence of physical disease were: (i) a previous history of conversion; (ii) a previous history of unexplained somatic complaints; and (iii) a previous model for symptoms. Features which failed to predict the absence of physical disorder were (i) current anxiety or dysphoria; (ii) emotional stress before onset; (iii) secondary gain; (iv) improvement with suggestion or sedation; (v) histrionic personality in the absence of a previous history of conversion; and (vi) *la belle indifférence*. In other words, it is unwise to attach much significance to any of these last six features when considering a diagnosis of conversion — they occur too frequently in patients with neurological disorders to be of diagnostic value.

## Somatoform pain disorder

Pain is the most common complaint in medicine (Merskey & Spear, 1967); it is also a common way for psychiatric disorder to present, particularly depression (von Knorring *et al.*, 1983). In the case of somatoform disorders it is usually present in SD and common in hypochondriasis. It is not, however, a sufficient symptom for the diagnosis of conversion disorder. In the 1980 edition of the DSM-III, criteria for psychogenic pain disorder were identical to those for conversion disorder, with the difference that in the former the symptom was limited to pain. It was thus a requirement of the diagnosis for psychological factors to be 'etiologically involved in the symptom', as it was for conversion disorder. The reason given for separating pain from conversion symptoms was that psychogenic pain tended to be chronic while other conversion symptoms are usually transient.

The term 'psychogenic pain disorder' was replaced by the current term 'somatoform pain disorder' in response to the criticism that the former term was 'stigmatising' (Williams & Spitzer, 1982). The description of the disorder and the criteria for its diagnosis were also modified. This was, in part, to take account of the findings from a study of patients with chronic pain published in 1982 (Blumer & Heilbronn, 1982). The revised criteria include:

1  Preoccupation with pain for at least 6 months.
2  Either (a) or (b):
    (a)  appropriate evaluation uncovers no organic pathology or pathophysiological mechanisms (for example a physical disorder or effects of injury) to account for the pain;
    (b)  when there is related organic pathology, the complaint of pain or resulting social or occupational impairment is grossly in excess of what would be expected from the physical findings.

These revised criteria no longer require any judgement about the aetiological role of psychological factors. The ICD-10 has also included a caveat in its description of somatoform pain that allows the diagnosis to be made without evidence of psychological aetiology.

Somatoform pain disorder is therefore a diagnosis of exclusion and is based on the presence of a single symptom. The term thus describes a diagnostic problem rather than a discrete syndrome. Indeed, it might be asked why a diagnosis based on these criteria should be regarded as a mental disorder at all.

Problems also arise with the classification of regional pain syndromes for which there are competing physical and psychological aetiological theories. Atypical facial pain is a good example. Claims have been made for temporomandibular joint disease, cervical spine disease and vasomotor dysfunction, whereas others regard it as a conversion symptom or as a 'symptom of an underlying depressive state' (Lascelles, 1966).

Other chronic regional pain syndromes, such as low back pain, headache, and chronic pain whose site is not specified, have also frequently been described as variants of depression (Roy *et al.*, 1984). The evidence for these claims is, on the whole, unsatisfactory. Many studies have demonstrated that chronic pain sufferers frequently report depressive symptoms and depressed subjects frequently report pain. But failure to specify diagnostic criteria for depression, poor sampling methods, varying selection criteria, lack of suitable controls and the use of unreliable techniques for measuring pain and depression have all undermined this research effort (see Gupta, 1986, for critical review).

The most recent and influential case for regarding chronic pain as a 'variant of depressive disorder' has been argued by Blumer and Heilbronn (1982). They have described a syndrome called 'the pain prone disorder' which they claim is 'a well defined psychobiological disorder with characteristic clinical, psychodynamic, biographic, and genetic features'. They conceive this as 'a form of masked depression, ... associated with a number of characteristic traits'. To explain why this essentially depressive disorder is dominated by pain, they combine clinical observations with psychodynamic inference in a narrative replete with meaningful connections. They also present empirical data from a clinical study comparing 'pain patients' with rheumatoid arthritis sufferers to support their claims. However, the methodology (the choice of controls, in particular) in this study and the authors' interpretation of their findings have been challenged (Turk & Salovey, 1984).

Nevertheless, the American Psychiatric Association (APA) have included several features of 'pain-prone disorder' in the DSM-III-R description of somatoform pain disorder under the heading of predisposing factors, for example, a history of 'workaholism'. But it is clear from Blumer and Heilbronn's own data that the clinical features they describe are neither sensitive nor specific enough to be diagnostic criteria in the DSM-III sense. They have not delineated a syndrome with clear boundaries, rather they have described a prototype based on their clinical experience. Nor have they made a convincing case for chronic pain as 'masked depression'. In Popperian terms this is a scientifically spurious hypothesis as it cannot be refuted by failing to demonstrate depression (Popper, 1963).

The relationship between chronic pain syndromes and depression (like that for anxiety disorders and SD) is a good example of why psychiatric taxonomists need to consider polythetic principles of classification more seriously. As Sokal (1974) has pointed out '... classifications need not be hierarchic and the clusters may overlap (intersect). The whole idea of hierarchic, non-overlapping (mutually exclusive) classifications which is so attractive to the human mind is currently undergoing re-examination. *For studies in a variety of fields the presentation of taxonomic structure as overlapping clusters or as ordinations appears far preferable'* (my italics).

Like body dysmorphic disorder, the concept of somatoform pain disorder is virtually meaningless to a psychiatrist working in the consultation–liaison field. The fact that the patient has been referred to a psychiatrist usually indicates that the criteria for its diagnosis have already been satisfied, i.e. the referring physician cannot account for the pain in organic terms. To make a 'diagnosis' that denotes little more than this is hardly making a diagnosis.

## Hypochondriasis

The DSM-III-R and the ICD-10 concepts of hypochondriasis differ little from Gillespie's 1928 definition of hypochondria. This emphasized the patient's preoccupation with having a physical disorder 'far in excess of what is justified', as well as disease conviction that showed an 'indifference to the opinion of the environment, including irresponsiveness to persuasion' (Gillespie, 1928). The DSM-III-R (1987) diagnostic criteria for hypochondriasis are shown in Table 2.2.

As with hysteria there has been doubt about the existence of hypochondriasis as a separate entity. Much of this arose after a case note study by Kenyon (1964) of 512 patients with hypochondriacal complaints. Kenyon con-

**Table 2.2.**   DSM-III-R criteria for hypochondriasis

| | |
|---|---|
| A | Preoccupation with the fear of having, or the belief that one has, a serious disease, based on the person's interpretation of physical signs or sensations as evidence of physical illness |
| B | Appropriate physical evaluation does not support the diagnosis of any physical disorder that can account for the physical signs or sensations or the person's unwarranted interpretation of them, *and* the symptoms in A *are not* just *symptoms of panic attacks* |
| C | The fear of having, or belief that one has, a disease persists despite medical reassurance |
| D | Duration of the disturbance is at least 6 months |
| E | The belief in A is *not of delusional* intensity, as in Delusional Disorder, Somatic Type (i.e. the person can acknowledge the possibility that his or her fear of having, or belief that he or she has, a serious disease is unfounded) |

cluded that there was no evidence to support the view that hypochondriasis was a primary neurotic syndrome as described by Gillespie, but rather that, '... on the available evidence, hypochondriasis is always part of another syndrome, most commonly an affective one'. He recommended that the word hypochondriacal be retained only as an adjective to describe either symptoms present in other disorders or personality traits.

While widely quoted and influential, Kenyon's study is methodologically flawed and does not justify his conclusion. Apart from the limitation of being a retrospective case note study, it was conducted in a psychiatric hospital population, introducing a selection bias towards the coexistence of other psychiatric disorders. No operational definitions of hypochondriasis or other disorders were used, and there is no statistical analysis of the data to support his interpretation of them. It has even been suggested that Kenyon's own data could be used to *support* the argument for the existence of primary hypochondriasis (Appleby, 1987).

Subsequent studies have supported the notion of a hypochondriacal syndrome. Pilowsky (1967) devised a questionnaire called the 'Whiteley Index' to investigate the concept of hypochondriasis. After establishing items which reliably distinguished hypochondriacal from non-hypochondriacal patients, the responses were used in a factor analysis. Principal component analysis identified three factors, each reflecting a different dimension of hypochondriasis. The factors were described as: 'bodily preoccupation', 'disease phobia' and 'conviction of the presence of disease with non-response to reassurance' (disease conviction). Subsequent similar work by Pilowsky and others has supported the validity of primary hypochondriasis (Pilowsky, 1970; Bianchi, 1973).

Barsky *et al.* (1986) devised a set of operational criteria derived from the DSM-III criteria for hypochondriasis and assessed them in a random sample of 92 consecutive medical outpatients. The patients were assessed with the Whiteley Index, a somatic symptom self-report scale (derived from the sub-scales of a number of different inventories), a structured interview and a review of medical records. They found that disease conviction, disease fear, bodily preoccupation, and somatic symptoms were significantly intercorrelated. In other words, they showed that these characteristics tend to occur together in the same individuals. They concluded that, in accord with previous work, there was considerable 'internal validity' and consistency in the syndrome.

When Barsky *et al.* (1986) examined the distribution of hypochondriacal attitudes and somatic symptoms they found that there was no evidence of bimodality, nor any discontinuity in measured variables between the most highly hypochondriacal individuals and the group as a whole. They therefore concluded that hypochondriasis was best viewed as a dimension of illness behaviour rather than as a discrete category.

In this study the strongest psychiatric correlate of hypochondriacal attitudes (Whiteley Index score) was the Beck Depression Inventory Score, which accounted for 33% of the variance. The degree of depression also emerged as a powerful predictor of somatic symptoms, accounting for 26% of the variance. Although these are strong correlations, it is also clear that a fairly high proportion of hypochondriasis could not be accounted for by depression. Thus the two conditions showed partial overlap. Overlap with anxiety disorders was not assessed in this study but the somatic symptoms commonly reported by most hypochondriacal patients were those of autonomic arousal.

### The distinction between hypochondriasis and anxiety disorders

It is suggested in the DSM-III-R that while hypochondriacal 'concerns' occur in a wide range of psychiatric disorders 'rarely will there be longstanding preoccupation with hypochondriacal symptoms'. However, when criteria for both hypochondriasis and another disorder are met, both diagnoses can be made, provided that the symptoms are 'not just symptoms of panic attacks'. Hypochondriacal interpretations of panic attack symptoms are extremely common (Noyes *et al.*, 1986) and cognitive models of panic give them a causal role in the pathogenesis of some panic attacks (Clark, 1988). It has been suggested that an important difference in the development of panic attacks as opposed to hypochondriasis is the nature of the patient's illness beliefs. For example, if hypochondriacal beliefs concern an immediately catastrophic event such as a heart attack, the patient will selectively attend to sensations consistent with this belief. When the patient detects an innocuous change in heart rate, symptoms may rapidly increase as fear leads to autonomic arousal. Further symptoms are then taken as evidence of medical catastrophe and a panic attack ensues. However, a patient who believes he/she has cancer does not anticipate immediate catastrophe and does not therefore develop the same level of arousal or need to seek immediate medical attention (Warwick & Salkovskis, 1990).

### The distinction between hypochondriasis and somatization disorder

While hypochondriasis is defined by a set of beliefs, attitudes and fears, somatization disorder (SD) is defined by past medical history, i.e. two different variables are used to classify cases (Table 2.3). There is therefore no reason to expect the categories to be mutually exclusive, nor any taxonomic principle that prevents a particular patient from being classified as a case of both hypochondriasis and SD.

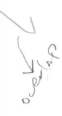

**Table 2.3.** Differences in diagnostic criteria and associated features between somatization disorder and hypochondriasis in DSM-III-R

| Somatization disorder | Hypochondriasis |
|---|---|
| Emphasis is on multiple physical symptoms | Preoccupation, fear and/or belief concerns serious disease |
| At least 13 symptoms | Number of symptoms unspecified |
| Symptoms not due to pathophysiologic mechanisms | Symptoms from normal sensations or minor abnormalities |
| Chronic, onset before 30, usually in teens | Duration of at least 6 months and can begin at any age |
| Much more common in females | Sex ratio equal |
| Associated with antisocial personality and interpersonal difficulties | Associated with obsessive compulsive personality traits |
| Familial associations have been reported | No information on familial associations |

Nor is there any empirical evidence of a boundary between these two clinical syndromes. The DSM-III-R thus specifies that both diagnoses can be made. Nevertheless, there is widespread resistance to the idea of making more than one diagnosis, and in practice psychiatrists have used a diagnostic hierarchy or exclusion criteria to differentiate between two diagnoses when criteria for both are satisfied. This taxonomic procedure was used extensively in the DSM-III (1989). For example, if a patient satisfied criteria for panic disorder and SD, only the diagnosis of SD was made and panic disorder was considered to be 'due to' SD. It seems logically suspect to say that one disorder (somatization disorder), defined solely by a set of operational criteria, can 'cause' another disorder. In the DSM-III-R however this exclusion criterion has been dropped and both diagnoses can be made concurrently.

The assumptions underlying exclusion criteria are not explicit in the DSM-III (Boyd *et al.*, 1984). They are presumably similar to those governing diagnostic hierarchies in the European tradition (Foulds & Bedford, 1975) and operationalized in the PSE/CATEGO system (Wing *et al.*, 1974). Such assumptions are of course *theoretical* with regard to aetiology and contradict the stated goals of the APA for their classificatory system. The trend from DSM-III (1980) to DSM-III-R (1987) has thus been to abandon them and allow more than one diagnosis. This is also a step away from 'essentialist' assumptions (Lakoff, 1987) and a step towards polythetic classification. It has been suggested that the DSM-IV will be hierarchy-free and include fewer exclusion criteria (P. Salkovskis, personal communication).

In the ICD-10 it is suggested that the distinction between hypochondriasis and multiple somatization disorder is that in the former the patient is preoccupied by 'the presence of the disorder itself and its future consequences' whereas in the latter the emphasis is on individual symptoms. It is also stated that in hypochondriasis there is 'likely to be a preoccupation with only one or two possible physical disorders which will be named consistently, rather than the more numerous and often changing possibilities in multiple somatization disorder' (WHO, 1987).

There are no data on the co-occurrence of hypochondriasis and SD. It is difficult to obtain such data using the DSM-III-R definition because the criteria for hypochondriasis are not adequately operationalized. We have, however, examined a small sample of patients satisfying DSM-III-R criteria for somatization disorder using the Whiteley Index (see previously) and found, not surprisingly, that patients with somatization disorder often score in the hypochondriacal range on this scale (Bass & Murphy, in preparation). *But many do not.*

The distinction berween hypochondriasis and SD has been attacked as trivial (Vaillant, 1984). But while there is overlap, the accurate identification and analysis of hypochondriacal preoccupations and behaviours may have important treatment implications. Cognitive–behavioural formulations of hypochondriasis, compatible with the DSM-III-R definition, have been proposed and form the basis of cognitive–behavioural treatments (Warwick & Salkovskis, 1989). The outcome of this treatment still needs further evaluation but early reports suggest that it may be effective. It is therefore important to identify different cognitive sets in patients with chronic somatization. Many of our own cases of SD, while showing disease conviction, have ideas and attitudes concerning illness that are distinct from hypochondriasis. For example, patients with SD are often not seeking reassurance that they are free of serious disease (as in hypochondriasis) but rather want their illness behaviour and sick role to be sanctioned by a diagnosis of physical disorder. Thus, hypochondriacal patients may be anxious that they have multiple sclerosis and seek reassurance that they have not. By contrast, patients with SD may become angry at the suggestion that they do not have serious physical disease to legitimize their invalid status. These differences are shown as prototypical cognitive–behavioural sets in Table 2.4. Many cases will of course not be typical but show features from both sets.

## Hypochondriasis as a personality disorder

It has been argued by Tyrer *et al.* (1990) that some hypochondriacal patients have a personality disorder rather than a mental state disorder (in DSM-III terms they have an Axis II as opposed to an Axis I disorder). They have identified cases in a psychiatric patient population using the Personality Assessment Schedule (PAS) (Tyrer *et al.*, 1979) and point out how hypochondriacal

**Table 2.4.** Differences in cognitive–behavioural set between hypochondriasis and somatization disorder

| Hypochondriasis | Somatization disorder |
|---|---|
| Disease conviction focused on specific condition | Disease conviction vague |
| Preoccupation with bodily sensations and future medical catastrophe | Preoccupation with past neglect and mistreatment by doctors |
| Seeks reassurance | Seeks proof that disease is 'real' |
| Fears disease | Fears implications of health |

**Table 2.5.** Criteria for diagnosing hypochondriacal personality disorder

Excessive preoccupation with maintenance of health with associated behaviour (e.g. will only take a limited range of food and water, regular consumption of 'health-promoting' medicines in order to remain well)
The perception of minor ailments and physical symptoms is distorted and magnified in to major and life-threatening disorder
Repeated recourse to consultation with medical and associated disciplines for reassurance, investigation and treatment
Rigidity of beliefs about health and lifestyle ensures their persistence

From Tyrer *et al* (1990).

attitudes and behaviours are chronic maladaptive patterns which begin early and continue throughout life (Table 2.5).

In contrast to the association between antisocial and histrionic traits described for Briquet's syndrome, patients diagnosed with hypochondriacal personality disorder scored highly on scales measuring anxiousness and dependence. In their classification of personality disorders using the PAS, hypochondriacal personality disorder most closely resembles anankastic personality disorder (Tyrer & Alexander, 1987).

While some DSM-III-R cases may match Tyrer's description of personality disorder, there are also some which begin later in life which do not. For example, some patients first develop marked hypochondriacal features following a serious acute illness.

## Psychogenic autonomic dysfunction

Unlike the DSM-III-R, the ICD-10 has a subcategory of disorder whose essential feature is symptoms arising from autonomic overactivity. This group is further subdivided according to the organ or system regarded by the patient as the origin of the symptoms (Table 2.6).

For a definite diagnosis the following four features should be present: (i) persistent troublesome symptoms of autonomic arousal, e.g. palpitations, tremor, etc.; (ii) additional symptoms referred to a specific organ or system; (iii) preoccupation and distress about the possibility of a serious disorder of the stated organ or system that does not respond to reassurance; (iv) no evidence of a significant disturbance of structure or function of that organ/ system.

**Table 2.6.** Psychogenic autonomic dysfunction (ICD-10)

| Subcategory (organ or system) | Examples |
| --- | --- |
| Heart and cardiovascular | Cardiac neurosis<br>Neurocirculatory asthenia |
| Oesophagus and stomach | Psychogenic aerophagy<br>Gastric neurosis |
| Lower gastrointestinal | Irritable bowel syndrome |
| Respiratory | Hyperventilation |
| Urogenital | Psychogenic frequency of<br>micturition and dysuria |

Based on WHO (1987).

It is stated that psychogenic autonomic dysfunction can be differentiated from generalized anxiety disorder by the predominance of 'the psychological components of autonomic arousal and the lack of a consistent physical focus for symptoms'. This sharp dichotomy between somatic and psychological components of anxiety is difficult to sustain in clinical practice and many cases could be classified either way. As with hypochondriasis and somatization disorder the overlap of this category with hypochondriasis is inevitable because different variables are used to define different taxa in the same classificatory system. For example, 'cardiac neurosis' is given as an example of psychogenic autonomic dysfunction in the ICD-10 and as an example of hypochondriasis in DSM-III-R. In the former case it is classified by *origin of symptoms* while in the latter it is classified by *psychological characteristics*. It is not a case of one or the other being the correct classification.

## Neurasthenia

In the ICD-10 this disorder is classified under 'other neurotic disorders' rather than as a somatoform disorder, and two main types are described. The main features of the first type are mental fatigability with difficulty concentrating and inefficient thinking, while in the second it is 'feelings of bodily or physical weakness and exhaustion after only minimal effort accompanied by a feeling of muscular aches and pains'. A variety of other physical and mental symptoms are also described. The overlap of this syndrome with mood and anxiety disorders is discussed in Chapter 5, p. 116. The DSM-II (1968) included 'neurasthenic neurosis' but this diagnosis was abandoned in the DSM-III because it was rarely used in the USA.

## Prospects and conclusions

Both nosological and taxonomic properties of somatoform disorders have been criticized for their lack of clinical and research utility. The introduction of the concept has nevertheless helped to highlight the current limits of medical knowledge in this neglected area of common morbidity.

Developments in general taxonomy, cognitive science, multivariate statistics and the use of the computer offer concepts and empirical methods for creating better classifications. A few recent research and theoretical papers indicate that these techniques are being applied to the study of somatization. We also recognize that the type of classificatory system adopted should depend on the purpose or aims of those using it. To date psychiatrists have assumed the 'classical' approach to categorization and can be accused of oversimplifying and reifying complex processes. Many have been frustrated by the limitations of this position and have rejected the role of formal classification.

The WHO has recognized the importance of adapting diagnostic categories to the differing needs of psychiatrists working in clinical and research contexts by providing different versions of the ICD-10. One version will consist of a 'comprehensive description of the clinical concept' underlying each disorder (prototypical) with points on the differential diagnosis and rough diagnostic guidelines. This is intended for clinical and educational use. A second version, derived from the first, specifies precisely defined criteria for use in research (Cooper, 1988).

Finally, a multiaxial system, able to represent the complexity of cases seen in the consultation–liaison field, has also been proposed (Table 2.7; Mezzich, 1988; Lobo, 1989). (This is discussed in more detail in Chapter 3). This conceptual scheme is familiar to most psychiatrists. However, few clinicians or researchers have made full use of it in the field of somatoform disorders. We also need to develop measurement instruments for each axis if we are to make the best use of the tools of modern taxonomy. For the somato-

**Table 2.7.** Proposed multiaxial schema for ICD-10

| Facets | Axes | |
|---|---|---|
| Psychopathological | I | General psychiatric syndromes |
| | II | Developmental conditions including personality disorders and traits |
| Physical | III | Concomitant physical conditions |
| Social | IV | Abnormal psychosocial situations |
| | V | Disabilities (self-care, occupational, family, relations, social in general) |

Based on Mezzich (1988).

form disorders such as endeavour might bring clarity and aetiological understanding. Alternatively, it may simply help us to define more precisely the 'fuzziness' of our categories.

# References

American Psychiatric Association (1968). *Diagnostic and Statistical Manual of Mental Disorders*, 2nd edn, (DSM-II) Washington DC.

American Psychiatric Association (1980). *Diagnostic and Statistical Manual of Mental Disorders*, 3rd edn, (DSM-III) Washington DC.

American Psychiatric Association (1987). *Diagnostic and Statistical Manual of Mental Disorders*, 3rd edn, revised, (DSM-III-R) Washington DC.

Appleby, L. (1987). Hypochondriasis: an acceptable diagnosis? *British Medical Journal*, **294**, 857.

Barsky, A., Wyshak, G. & Klerman, G. (1986). Hypochondriasis: an evaluation of the DSM-III criteria in medical out-patients, *Archives of General Psychiatry*, **43**, 493–500.

Bayer, R. & Spitzer, R. (1985). Neurosis, psychodynamics, and DSM-III: a history of the controversy, *Archives of General Psychiatry*, **42**, 187–196.

Bhattacharya, D. & Bharadwaj, P. (1977). Reassessment of Perley–Guze criteria for the diagnosis of hysteria — a study based on 304 Indian patients, *Indian Journal of Psychiatry*, **19**, 38–42.

Bianchi, G. (1973). Patterns of hypochondriasis: a principal components analysis, *British Journal of Psychiatry*, **122**, 541–548.

Birtchnell, S.A. (1988). Dysmorphophobia — a centenary discussion, *British Journal of Psychiatry*, **153** (Suppl 2), 41–43.

Blumer, D. & Heilbronn, M. (1982). Chronic pain as a variant of depressive disease: the pain prone disorder, *Journal of Nervous and Mental Diseases*, **170**, 381–409.

Bohman, M., Cloninger, C., von Knorring, A. *et al.* (1984). An adoption study of somatoform disorders: III. Cross-fostering analysis and genetic relationship to alcoholism and criminality, *Archives of General Psychiatry*, **41**, 872–878.

Boyd, J., Burke, J., Gruenberg, E. *et al.* (1984). Exclusion criteria of DSM-III, *Archives of General Psychiatry*, **41**, 983–989.

Cantor, N., Smith, E.E., French, R.D. *et al.* (1980). Psychiatric diagnosis as prototype classification, *Journal of Abnormal Psychology*, **89**, 181–193.

Cawley, R. (1983). Psychiatric diagnosis: what we need, *Psychiatric Annals*, **13**, 772–782.

Clark, D. (1988). A cognitive model of panic attacks, in *Panic: Psychological Perspectives* (Eds. Rachman, S.J. & Maser, J.), Lawrence Erlbaum Associates, Hillsdale, New Jersey.

Cloninger, C. (1986). Diagnosis of somatoform disorders: a critique of DSM-III, in *Diagnosis and Classification in Psychiatry* (Ed. Tischler, G. ), Cambridge University Press, New York.

Cloninger, C., Martin, R., Guze, S. *et al.* (1986). Somatisation disorder in men and women: a prospective follow-up and family study, *American Journal of Psychiatry*, **143**, 873–878.

Cloninger, C., Reich, T. & Guze, S. (1975). The multifactorial model of disease transmission: III. Familial relationship between sociopathy and hysteria (Briquet's Syndrome), *British Journal of Psychiatry*, **127**, 11–22.

Cloninger, C., Sigvardsson, S., von Knorring, A. *et al.* (1984). An adoption study of somatoform disorders: II. Identification of two discrete somatoform disorders, *Archives of General Psychiatry*, **41**, 863–871.

Connolly, F. & Gipson, M. (1978). Dysmorphophobia — a long-term study, *British Journal of Psychiatry*, **132**, 568–570.

Cooper, J. (1988). The structure and presentation of contemporary psychiatric classifications with special reference to the ICD-9 and 10, *British Journal of Psychiatry*, **152** (Suppl 1), 21–28.

Deighton, C. & Nicol, A. (1985). Abnormal illness behaviour in young women in primary care setting: is Briquet's syndrome a useful category? *Psychological Medicine*, **15**, 515–520.

Dion, K., Berscheid, E. & Walster, E. (1972). What is beautiful is good, *Journal of Personal and Social Psychology*, **24**, 285.

Edgerton, M., Jacobsen, W. & Meyer, E. (1960). Surgical psychiatric study of patients seeking plastic (cosmetic) surgery: 98 consecutive patients with minimal deformity, *British Journal of Plastic Surgery*, **13**, 136–145.

Escobar, J.I., Burnam, M., Karno, M. *et al.* (1987). Somatisation in the community, *Archives of General Psychiatry*, **44**, 713–718.

Escobar, J.I. & Canino, G. (1989). Unexplained physical complaints: psychopathology and epidemiological correlates, *British Journal of Psychiatry*, **154** (Suppl 4), 24–27.

Faust, D. & Milner, R. (1986). The empiricist and his new clothes: DSM-III in perspective, *American Journal of Psychiatry*, **143**, 962–967.

Foulds, G. & Bedford, A. (1975). Hierarchy of classes of personal illness, *Psychological Medicine*, **5**, 181–192.

Gillespie, R. (1928). Hypochondria: its definition, nosology, and psychopathology, *Guy's Hospital Report*, **78**, 408–460.

Goin, M.K. & Goin, J.M. (1986). Psychological effects of aesthetic facial surgery, *Advances in Psychosomatic Medicine*, **15**, 84–108.

Goldberg, D. (1984). The recognition of psychiatric illness by non-psychiatrists, *Australian and New Zealand Journal of Psychiatry*, **18**, 128–133.

Gupta, M. (1986). Is chronic pain a variant of depressive illness? A critical review, *Canadian Journal of Psychiatry*, **31**, 241–248.

Guze, S. (1975). The validity and significance of hysteria (Briquet's Syndrome), *American Journal of Psychiatry*, **132**, 138–141.

Harris, D. (1982). Cosmetic surgery — where does it begin? *British Journal of Plastic Surgery*, **35**, 281–286.

Hay, G. (1970a). Psychiatric aspect of cosmetic nasal operation, *British Journal of Psychiatry*, **116**, 85–97.

Hay, G. (1970b). Dysmorphophobia, *British Journal of Psychiatry*, **116**, 399–406.

Hay, G. & Heather, B. (1973). Changes in psychometric test results following cosmetic nasal operations, *British Journal of Psychiatry*, **122**, 89–90.

Hyler, S. & Spitzer, R. (1978). Hysteria split asunder, *American Journal of Psychiatry*, **135**, 1550–1554.

Jablensky, A. (1988). Methodological issues in psychiatric classification, *British Journal of Psychiatry*, **152**, 15–20.

Kendell, R. (1983). Diagnosis and classification, in *Companion to Psychiatric Studies* 3rd edn. (Eds. Kendell, R. & Zeally, A.), Churchill Livingstone, Edinburgh and London.

Kendell, R. (1989). Clinical validity, *Psychological Medicine*, **19**, 45–55.

Kenyon, F. (1964). Hypochondriasis: a clinical study, *British Journal of Psychiatry*, **110**, 478–488.

Lacey, J.H. & Birtchnell, S. (1986). Body image and its disturbances, *Journal of Psychosomatic Research*, **30** (6), 623–631.

Lakoff, G. (1987). *Women, Fire, and Dangerous Things: What Categories Reveal about the Mind*, University of Chicago Press, Chicago and London.

Lascelles, R. (1966). Atypical facial pain and depression, *British Journal of Psychiatry*, **112**, 651–659.

Lobo, A. (1989). On multiaxial psychiatric diagnosis for general medical patients, *British Journal of Psychiatry*, **154** (Suppl 4), 38–41.

Mai, F. & Merskey, H. (1980). Briquet's treatise on hysteria: a synopsis and commentary, *Archives of General Psychiatry*, **37**, 1401–1405.

Merskey, H. & Spear, F. (1967). *Pain: Psychological and Psychiatric Aspects*, Ballière, Tindall and Cassell, London.

Mezzich, J.E. (1988). On developing a psychiatric multiaxial scheme for ICD-10, *British Journal of Psychiatry*, **152** (Suppl 1), 38–44.

Mezzich, J.E. (1989). An empirical prototypical approach to the definition of psychiatric illness, *British Journal of Psychiatry*, **154** (Suppl 4), 42–46.

Noyes, R., Reich, J., Clancey, J. *et al.* (1986). Reduction in hypochondriasis with treatment of panic disorder, *British Journal of Psychiatry*, **149**, 631–635.

Orenstein, H. (1989). Briquet's syndrome in association with depression and panic: a reconceptualization of Briquet's syndrome, *American Journal of Psychiatry*, **146**, 334–338.

Perley, M.G. & Guze, S.B. (1962). Hysteria: the stability and usefulness of clinical criteria, *New England Journal of Medicine*, **266**, 421–426.

Pilowsky, I. (1967). Dimensions of hypochondriasis, *British Journal of Psychiatry*, **131**, 89–93.

Pilowsky, I. (1969). A general classification of abnormal illness behaviour, *British Journal of Medical Psychology*, **51**, 131–137.

Pilowsky, I. (1970). Primary and secondary hypochondriasis, *Acta Psychiatrica Scandinavica*, **46**, 273–285.

Popper, K. (1963). *Conjectures and Refutations: the growth of scientific knowledge*, Routledge & Kegan Paul, London.

Purtell, J., Robins, E. & Cohen, M. (1951). Observations on clinical aspects of hysteria: a quantitative study of 50 hysteria patients and 156 control subjects, *Journal of the American Medical Association*, **146**, 902–909.

Robbins, J., Kirmayer, L. & Tepper, S. (1989). *Latent Variable Models of Functional Somatic Distress*. Paper prepared for the symposium 'Current concepts of somatisation'. American Psychiatric Association meetings, San Francisco.

Rosch, E. (1975). Cognitive representations of semantic categories, *Journal of Experimental Psychology*, **104**, 192–233.

Rosch, E. (1978). Principles of categorisation, in *Cognition and Categorization* (Eds. Rosch, E. & Lloyd, B.), Lawrence Erlbaum Associates, Hillsdale, New Jersey.

Roy, R., Thomas, M. & Mattas, M. (1984). Chronic pain and depression: a review, *Comprehensive Psychiatry*, **25**, 96–105.

Sokal, R. (1974). Classification: purposes, principles, progress, prospects, *Science*, **185**, 1115–1123.

Spitzer, R., Endicott, J. & Robins, E. (1978). Research diagnostic criteria: rationale and reliability, *Archives of General Psychiatry*, **35**, 773–782.

Swartz, M., Blazer, D., Woodbury, M. *et al.* (1987). A study of somatisation disorder in a community population utilizing grade of membership analysis, *Psychiatric Developments*, **3**, 219–237.

Turk, D. & Salovey, P. (1984). 'Chronic pain as a variant of depressive disease': a critical re-appraisal, *Journal of Nervous and Mental Disease*, **172**, 398–404.

Tyrer, P. & Alexander, M. (1987). Personality Assessment Schedule, in *Personality Disorders: diagnosis, management and course* (Ed. Tyrer, P.), Wright, Bristol.

Tyrer, P., Alexander, M., Ciccehetti, D. *et al.* (1979). Reliability of a schedule for rating personality disorders, *British Journal of Psychiatry*, **135**, 168–174.

Tyrer, P., Fowler-Dixon, R. & Ferguson, B. (1990). The justification for the diagnosis of hypo-chondriacal personality disorder, *Journal of Psychosomatic Research*, (in press).

Vaillant, G. (1984). The disadvantages of the DSM-III outweigh its advantages, *American Journal of Psychiatry*, **141**, 542–545.

von Knorring, L., Perris, C. & Eisemann, M. (1983). Pain as a symptom in depressive disorders. I. Relationship to diagnostic subgroup and depressive symptomatology, *Pain*, **15**, 19–26.

Ward, C., Beck, A., Mendelson, M. *et al.* (1962). The psychiatric nomenclature, *Archives of General Psychiatry*, **7**, 198–205.

Warwick, H. & Salkovskis, P.M. (1989). Cognitive therapy of hypochondriasis, in *Cognitive Therapy in Clinical Practice* (Eds. Scott, J., Williams, J. & Beck, A.), Croom Helm, London.

Warwick, H. & Salkovskis, P.M. (1990). Hypochondriasis, *Behaviour Research and Therapy*, **28**, 105–117.

Williams, J. & Spitzer, R. (1982). Ideopathic pain disorder: a critique of pain prone disorder and a proposal for a revision of the DSM-III category, psychogenic pain disorder, *Journal of Nervous and Mental Diseases*, **170**, 415–419.

Wing, J., Cooper, J. & Sartorius, N. (1974). *Description and Classification of Psychiatric Symptoms*, Cambridge University Press, Cambridge.

Wittgenstein, L. (1953). *Philosophical Investigations*. E. Hanscombe (transl). Basil Blackwell, Oxford.

Woodruff, R., Clayton, P. & Guze, S. (1971). Hysteria: studies of diagnosis, outcome, and pre-valence, *Journal of the American Medical Association*, **215**, 415–428.

World Health Organization (1987). Mental, behavioural and developmental disorders, in *International Classification of Diseases* (10th revision) Draft chapter V(F). Division of Mental Health, World Health Organization, Geneva.

Zadeh, L. (1965). Fuzzy sets, *Information and Control*, **8**, 338–358.

# 3
# Assessment and Management of Patients with Functional Somatic Symptoms

C.M. BASS

## Introduction

It is important to recall that it is often the referring physician and not the psychiatrist who first defines a clinical problem as 'psychiatric' or 'functional'. In the general hospital the decision to refer a patient to a psychiatrist commonly rests with the senior doctor under whose care the patient is admitted (or assessed in the outpatient clinic). This decision is in turn influenced by many factors, among which are the physician's attitude to psychiatry and the extent of the relationship established between psychiatrists and particular medical units (Crisp, 1968; Sensky, 1986). Another determining factor is, of course, the physician's capacity to perceive psychological factors as aetiologically relevant. The complex process whereby patients in a general hospital are recognized as psychiatrically ill, are referred to psychiatrists and subsequently treated is illustrated in Figure 3.1. A similarly complex process occurs in primary care settings (Goldberg & Huxley, 1980).

### The referral process

Many patients with functional disorders do not believe that they have a psychological problem. They may be reluctant to accept a psychological approach to treatment and may construe the referral to a psychiatrist as a sign that the physicians are not taking their symptoms seriously. 'Preparing' the patient for referral is therefore an important practical step, and needs to be dealt with tactfully by the clinician.

Referral is more likely to be successfully accomplished when close service links are established between the Department of Psychological Medicine and medical or surgical units. The most satisfactory arrangement is for a designated consultant psychiatrist (and his/her team or 'firm') to have links with a specific medical or surgical specialty, e.g. cardiology, neurology or obstetrics. At King's College Hospital there are both service and collaborative

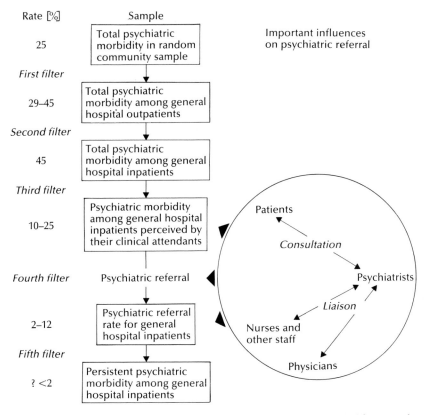

**Fig. 3.1.** The pathway to psychiatric attention in the general hospital (modified from Sensky & Greer, 1985, after Goldberg & Huxley, 1980). Each prevalence figure relates to psychiatric morbidity or referral rates in the sample adjacent to it (below the second filter in the figure, the rates refer to total general hospital inpatients).

research links between psychiatric teams and specified medical units. Collaboration is more likely to occur if the Department of Psychiatry is located within the district general hospital and not separate from it.

It is likely that close links between physicians and psychiatrists will also improve treatment compliance. An example of such an arrangement is often seen in the Pain Clinic, where the psychiatrist or psychologist works alongside the medical staff and is involved in the patient's initial medical assessment.

**The patient's attitude to psychiatric referral**

This will partly depend on how the referring physician explains the need for referral. 'I can't find anything wrong with you, I think you need to see a psychiatrist' is likely to be equated with 'you are imagining your symptoms, I think you are mad'. The patient will feel understandably angry about such a referral and this may become apparent at the initial psychiatric assessment.

An advantage of close liaison with medical colleagues is that the psychiatrist and physician can discuss the way in which the referral should be made. A better way of preparing a patient for referral to a psychiatrist might be as follows:

> I'm happy say that we have ruled out serious disease as a cause of your symptoms. But I can see that the pain (or other complaint) remains a major problem for you. I am concerned about the difficulties that you've been having at home and how tense they make you — that certainly won't help you get well. I have a colleague who is a psychiatrist with an interest in persistent pain (or other symptom) who often advises me in cases like your own. I would like to get his/her opinion about how best to proceed . . . .

It is important at this stage of the referral to avoid giving the message that the patient is not genuine, not ill, bothers doctors unnecessarily, or is 'mad'. The patient should also perceive that the physician and psychiatrist are collaborating in his/her management and that the patient is not being simply 'packed off'. An effective way of communicating this is for the physician to see the patient again after the initial psychiatric assessment. Physician and psychiatrist can then jointly plan their respective management strategies in the intervening period.

If anger or resentment at the referral become apparent during an interview, then these negative emotions should be dealt with. For example, in response to a surly and abusive patient who balks at the imputation of psychological illness implicit in the referral, the psychiatrist might say: 'You seem to be very upset/angry about being here; can you say why that is?' As well as allowing the psychiatrist to clarify his/her role, such questions encourage honesty about feelings and put them on the agenda for discussion. Responses to such open questions may also provide some insight into the patient's attitudes and explanatory models of illness (see below).

## The history

Certain aspects of the clinical history are of particular importance, in particular an *illness history*. Regrettably, a doctor eliciting a medical history is usually interested only in recording details of previous episodes of physical illness and/or operations. But an illness history is more than this; the emphasis is directed towards *somatic complaints* which may have occurred during periods of adversity or life change (although the patient may not make such a link). Some patients have a tendency to react to life stressors with a characteristic symptom or array of complaints, for example a habitual tendency to experience nausea or vomiting in response to adverse life experiences. It is important to elicit this information because it has <u>predictive</u> <u>utility</u>, i.e. it makes a current diagnosis of a 'functional' disorder more likely.

data ?

It is useful to begin this part of the history by enquiring about *parental illness*, specially during the patient's formative years (0–16 years). For example, was one or both parents chronically sick or handicapped and what impact did this have on the patient's life? How did this illness affect the parent's ability to care for the child, i.e. did it lead to a change in the *quality of care*?

Physical illness in childhood can have an enduring psychological effect, specially if it is accompanied by parental overconcern and injudicious advice from doctors. For this reason it is always important to ask about *illnesses and hospitalizations in childhood*. For example, in what circumstances did this occur? Did it lead to separation from parents or prolonged absence from school? What impact did it have on developmental issues? What was the child told about the illness; was he/she advised to avoid physical exercise or given special dietary advice?

The patient's perception of his/her early experiences of rearing by both parents can be assessed by using the Parental Bonding Instrument or PBI (Parker *et al.*, 1979). Although this scale assumes parental consistency throughout infancy, childhood and early adolescence, it has acceptable reliability and validity. It provides measures of parental care and overprotection, and norms for a general population have been described (Parker *et al.*, 1979).

In a subgroup of patients with a particular somatic symptom or group of symptoms, there may be a past history of unexplained physical complaints involving *different* organ systems. It is essential to obtain as much information as possible about these past illnesses, and to record the details of previous hospital admissions, results of any investigations, trials of treatment and/or operations for each hospital or illness episode. This should include what the patient was told about his/her physical complaints by previous physicians and surgeons. To obtain this data may require extensive correspondence with the medical records departments of many different hospitals, but these efforts may yield crucial information about the patient.

The medical histories of patients who persistently somatize are more likely to contain details of 'complaint behaviour' than evidence of ascertainable organic disease. For example, the non-inflamed appendix, normal gastrointestinal series, normal coronary angiogram, etc. The presenting somatic complaints may be the most recent of a number of unexplained physical symptoms which have occurred at intervals throughout the patient's life. It is important to identify these chronic complainers, who may satisfy DSM-III-R criteria for somatization disorder or ICD-10 criteria for multiple somatization disorder. Such patients require a specific treatment approach (see below).

Another group of patients whose complaints require detailed attention and documentation are those with chronic idiopathic pain. Again, it is necessary to record the duration of the pain and its response, if any, to previous treatment. Does the pain bear any relation to environmental or psychological factors? A relative or spouse should be able to describe the pain behaviours and avoidance behaviour exhibited by the patient (Philips, 1987). Is there any inconsistency in complaint behaviour or disability? i.e. is the patient relatively mobile about the house but unable to walk to the local shops?

## Psychiatric assessment

Ideally the initial psychiatric interview should take place in a psychiatric outpatient clinic within the general hospital. At this initial interview it may be necessary to allow the patient to discuss his/her previous medical experiences and to discover what he/she has been told by other doctors. It is not uncommon for patients with functional somatic symptoms (FSSs) to have visited many doctors and to have had disagreements or other difficulties with medical staff. It is important for the psychiatrist not to become involved in criticizing medical colleagues.

No attempt will be made in the present chapter to outline a comprehensive scheme for psychiatric history taking or examination. This is covered in textbooks of general psychiatry and summarized in a recent publication by the Institute of Psychiatry (Notes on Eliciting and Recording Clinical Information, 1983). The purpose here will be to focus on those aspects of clinical enquiry which assume particular importance in patients with functional somatic symptoms. A proposed multiaxial approach to assessment based on ICD-10 will be used throughout (Mezzich, 1988). This is particularly relevant to patients with FSSs, in whom the aetiological contribution of psychosocial stressors, personality, and physical illness needs to be fully assessed. All these factors have a bearing on the course and outcome.

### Axis I: general psychiatric syndromes

Mental state assessment should be as comprehensive as for all psychiatric patients, but certain aspects should be given particular emphasis. In particular, enquiring about features of affective or phobic disorder should be as thorough as possible, and it is essential to ascertain the patient's attitude to the symptoms.

## Affective disorder

Of patients with functional somatic symptoms attending the general hospital, about <u>half</u> have been shown to have affective disorders (notably depressive and anxiety/panic disorders; Katon *et al.*, 1984; Lloyd, 1986; Table 3.1). For this reason it is important for the psychiatrist to have a detailed knowledge of the ways in which these disorders present somatically.

Depression is often experienced in a very physical fashion (Paykel & Norton, 1982; Fig. 3.2). These patients may be so preoccupied with the physical symptoms that the depression may remain hidden or, or if it is evident, be seen as a reaction to the physical suffering. Delay in accurate diagnosis and treatment can be very serious, as the following case illustrates:

> This 67-year-old retired motor mechanic was admitted to the accident and emergency department after a serious suicide attempt. He had lacerated his neck, both arms and ankles and was found by his wife exsanguinating in his bath. He required surgery to severed nerves and tendons in his left arm. Interview after this emergency surgery revealed that he had complained of unremitting lower abdominal pain for 18 months which had failed to respond to multiple interventions. After retirement 2 years previously he began to experience pain in the left groin associated with nocturia and frequency. A prostatectomy failed to alleviate his pain and further investigations including a

**Table 3.1.** DSM-III diagnoses (%) in patients referred for psychiatric evaluation of unexplained somatic symptoms

| | Katon *et al.* (1984) (*n* = 100) | Slavney & Teitelbaum (1985) (*n* = 100) | Lloyd (1986) (*n* = 85) |
|---|---|---|---|
| Affective disorders | 48 | 9 | 33 |
| Somatoform disorders | 29 | 34 | 11 |
| Psychological factors affecting physical disorder | 9 | 14 | — |
| Substance use/alcoholism | 8 | 1 | — |
| Adjustment disorder | 7 | 8 | — |
| Factitious disorder | 4 | 1 | — |
| Eating disorder | — | 1 | 4 |
| Generalized anxiety | — | — | 14 |
| Panic disorder | 4 | — | 4 |
| Anxiety disorders, unspecified | — | 7 | — |
| Schizophrenia | — | — | 2 |
| Other diagnosis | 4 | 10 | 12 |
| No psychiatric diagnosis | — | 15 | 18 |

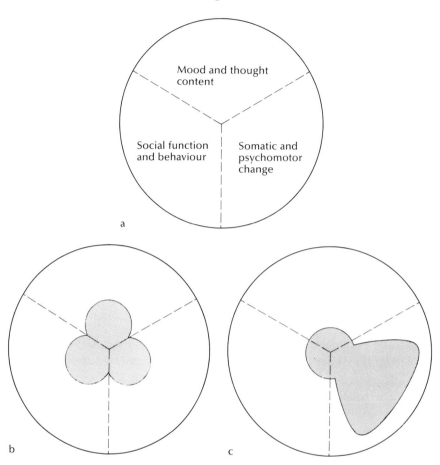

**Fig. 3.2.** (a) and (b) Typical presentations of depression. (c) Predominantly somatic manifestations of depression (reproduced with permission from Paykel & Norton, 1982).

gastroscopy and barium enema revealed minimal diverticular disease. He was informed that this was probably not the cause of his pain. After 6 months of further symptoms he requested a private opinion but after further blood tests and X-rays was told that no cause of his pain could be detected. Although reassured by these negative tests his symptoms continued to bother him, but to a lesser extent. Two subsequent episodes of haematuria led to another prostatectomy. A pain specialist told him that he would have to live with his symptoms. In desperation he tried to contact the private doctor for a further consultation, only to find that he had retired. He then attempted suicide. Psychiatric enquiry revealed a premorbidly obsessional and conscientious man and habitual worrier. His wife said that he became distressed by changes in routine and always had difficulty articulating emotional problems. The only relevant past history had occurred at the age of 42, when he had abdominal pain following stress at work and required anti-depressants. His wife said that the symptoms were similar in nature to those of his current illness. In his recent history he complained of loss of appetite, weight loss of half a stone in the last year, an inability to enjoy food, initial and late insomnia, social withdrawal, anergia, loss of interest in hobbies, and low mood. In addition he reported episodes of sweating, chest tightness, globus sensation, tinnitus and trembling that often occurred on waking but were *not* accompanied by subjective anxiety. A diagnosis of severe depression following retirement in an obsessional personality was made and he responded over the next 6 weeks to a course of dothiepin. After 9 months the dothiepin was gradually withdrawn, and 2 years after his suicide attempt he remains well with no recurrence of pain.

Because depression is so common in general hospital psychiatric practice, it is good practice to screen for its presence routinely. The Hospital Anxiety and Depression Scale (HADS) (Zigmond & Snaith, 1983) is a useful instrument which takes only 2 minutes to complete and yields composite scores of both anxiety and depression.

The physiological basis of the symptoms in anxiety is a result (in part) of an increase in activity of the autonomic nervous system, both sympathetic and parasympathetic (Bass, 1985). Increase in muscle tension may also contribute to symptoms. This may be localized, as in the globus sensation and the temporomandibular joint syndrome, or generalized, as in fatigue or anergia (see Chapter 5, p. 104).

### A phobic diathesis

Somatization is very common in patients with phobic disorders and panic attacks (Katon *et al.*, 1984). Hyperventilation occurs in approximately two-thirds of patients with panic anxiety (Magarian, 1982; Gardner & Bass, 1989) and it is important to know about its diverse somatic manifestations. These are shown in Table 3.2, together with suggested pathophysiological mechanisms.

The diagnosis of agoraphobia is surprisingly easy to miss in a patient with somatic complaints who does not make the link between physical symptoms, fear, and situations which bring on the symptoms. The patient may not attribute being housebound to a psychiatric illness, and often does not spontaneously report avoidance. Agoraphobia may only be identified by direct enquiry into the physical symptoms experienced in specific situations.

**Table 3.2.** Hyperventilation: common modes of presentation and suggested pathophysiological mechanisms. (Reproduced with permission from Gardner & Bass, 1989).

| System | Symptom(s) | Suggested mechanism and evidence |
|---|---|---|
| Cardiac | Chest pain (pseudoangina) <br> Chest pain (angina) <br> Palpitations | Spasm and/or fatigue of intercostal muscles[1] <br> Coronary vasoconstriction and spasm[2] <br> Paroxysmal dysrhythmia[3] |
| Neurological | Dizziness, syncope <br> Unilateral somatic symptoms e.g. paraesthesiae, clumsiness | Cerebral vasoconstriction[4] <br> Alkalosis affecting peripheral nerves[5] |
| Respiratory | Air hunger, sighing | ?Enhanced proprioception from overexpanded intercostal muscles and/or lungs |
| Gastrointestinal | Dry mouth <br> Flatulence, abdominal distension <br> Retrosternal pain (pseudoangina) | Mouth-breathing <br> Aerophagy[6] <br> ?Increase in oesophageal contractility[7] |
| Psychiatric | Poor concentration, forgetfulness. Wide variety of psycho-sensory experiences, e.g. hallucinations, euphoria, depersonalization <br> Anxiety, panic | Cerebral vasoconstriction[8,9] <br><br><br><br> Any hyperventilation-induced symptom can induce fear/panic if interpreted in a catastrophic fashion[10] |
| General | Weakness, listlessness | Increase in sympathetic nervous system activity[11] and or hypokalaemia[12] |

*References*
1 Friedman, M. (1945). *American Heart Journal*, **30**, 557.
2 Crea, F., Davies, G. & Chiercha, S. (1985). *American Journal of Cardiology*, **58**, 18.
3 Wildenthal, K., Fuller, D.S. & Shapiro, W. (1968). *American Journal of Cardiology*, **21**, 436.
4 Wyke, B. (1963). *Brain Function and Metabolic Disorders*, Butterworths, London.
5 Blau, J.N., Wiles, C.M. & Solomon, F.S. (1983). *British Medical Journal*, **286**, 1108.
6 McKell, T.E. & Sullivan, A.J. (1947). *Gastroenterology*, **9**, 6.
7 Herrington, J.P., Burns, T.W. & Balart, L.A. (1984). *Digestive Diseases and Sciences*, **29**, 134.
8 Okel, B.B. & Hurst, J.W. (1961). *Archives of Internal Medicine*, **108**, 157.
9 Allen, T.E. & Agus, B. (1968). *American Journal of Psychiatry*, **125**, 632.
10 Clark, D. (1986). *Behaviour Research and Therapy*, **24**, 461.
11 Breggin, P.R. (1964). *Journal of Nervous and Mental Disease*, **139**, 558.
12 Pearson, M.G., Quadiri, M.R. & Finn, R. (1986). *British Journal of Clinical Practice*, **40**, 28.

For example, are the symptoms of dizziness, breathlessness and paraesthesiae worse in crowds, shops, public transport? Does the sweating, shaking, and hand tremor only occur when the person is aware of being scrutinized or observed? Does the patient report any *avoidance behaviour*? For example, are crowds, public transport, enclosed spaces, restaurants, etc. avoided because of a fear of experiencing distressing physical symptoms? It is always important to elicit an avoidance profile in such patients, and in the clinic this can be quantified by the Fear Questionnaire (Marks & Mathews, 1979). The following case illustrates the *situational* component of somatic symptoms, which had (incorrectly) been ascribed to thyroid disease:

> A 34-year-old married woman was referred from the Endocrine Clinic with a provisional diagnosis of hyperventilation. She gave a 6 year history of palpitations, hot flushes, breathlessness and trembling of her limbs. Investigations for thyrotoxicosis performed in another hospital 2 years previously had revealed 'borderline' thyroid function tests. Further blood tests at our hospital had revealed normal full blood count and ESR, electrolytes, thyroid function and thyroid autoantibodies and ECG. Close enquiry revealed that she had left her job as a supermarket check-out operator because of anxiety and trembling whenever observed by her superiors. In her current job as a shop assistant her hands would tremble and legs go weak whenever she was observed writing by customers. Holding drinks and eating in front of others also brought on her symptoms, but travel on public transport and standing in queues were negotiated without discomfort. This woman had classical social anxiety, and experienced somatic symptoms of anxiety *only* in social situations. That is to say, her awareness of rapid heartbeat, flushing sensations, sweating, shaking, trembling of the extremities and short shallow breathing were particularly marked when she was aware of being *scrutinized*, e.g. when writing, speaking, eating or drinking in front others. She dealt with her social anxiety by avoiding parties and social functions. She responded well to an exposure programme.

If apprehension and/or panic accompany the physical symptoms, it is important to determine whether any fears are entertained during an attack. Rachman *et al.* (1987) recently demonstrated that in claustrophobic subjects certain *cognitions* are almost invariably associated with specific *somatic symptoms*, in particular breathlessness. Many patients fear heart disease, multiple sclerosis or strokes, and these fears should be enquired after using carefully chosen open questions. The interviewer should also ask about recent illness in the patient's family, and whether the patient has witnessed the death of a close friend or relative. The emotional response to that experience should be elicited.

*Attitudes to illness and illness beliefs*

The patient's attitude to his/her illness should always be ascertained. He/she may harbour the belief that the symptoms are due to serious underlying physical disease or, alternatively, make light of the symptoms and deny their significance despite the presence of moderate or severe handicap. The most florid discrepancies or 'mismatches' between physical disability and emotional concern are often seen in patients with pseudoneurological syndromes characterized by loss of function of one or more limbs or parts of limbs (Lader & Sartorious, 1968, and see Chapter 8, p. 222), but they are also evident in pain patients and patients with chronic symptomatic hyperventilation (Bass & Gardner, 1985).

Patients with illness fears, morbid preoccupation with disease and disease conviction are commonplace in general hospital settings and these illness attitudes must be explored before embarking on any treatment procedure. If the patient holds very firm views about the cause of his/her symptoms, it is important to determine the conviction with which they are held (McKenna, 1984). Patients with hypochondriacal delusions may require treatment with neuroleptic drugs.

Because illness attitudes have such an important bearing on treatment adherence and outcome, it is helpful to use standardized questionnaires and inventories to compliment the clinical impression. The best known of these is the illness behaviour questionnaire or IBQ (Pilowsky *et al.*, 1984) — a 62-item questionnaire that yields seven factors. But elevated IBQ scores should not be used as indicators of abnormal illness behaviour without corroborating medical information; this may be more misleading than accepting a patient's symptom reports at face value (Zonderman *et al.*, 1985). Furthermore, major psychometric weaknesses have been demonstrated in the IBQ, and an alternative scoring system using a shortened 37-item version has been developed that includes three factors: affective and hypochondriacal disturbance, life disruption and social inhibition (Main & Waddell, 1987). A shortened 14-item version of the IBQ (the Whiteley Index) has been shown to discriminate between hypochondriacal and nonhypochondriacal patients and is useful for routine clinical use (Pilowsky, 1967). Another self-report scale which offers promise is the Illness Attitude Scale (IAS) developed by Kellner *et al.* (1987).

**Axis II: personality disorders**

Certain personality traits may predispose an individual to develop a functional disorder in the face of adverse life circumstances (see later), and so it is essential to build up a picture of a patient's personality before the onset of the current illness episode. This may prove to be difficult. A patient's judgement about his/her own premorbid personality is often retrospectively altered by chronic illness, and it is not uncommon for a patient (and often spouse or partner as well) to present an idealized picture of how things were before the onset of the current illness. Nevertheless, an attempt at assessment of personality should be made, preferably by using a structured interview schedule. These have good inter-rater reliability, good temporal reliability, and avoid significant contamination of personality assessment by current mental disorder (Tyrer, 1987). The most promising are the Personality Assessment Schedule or PAS (Tyrer *et al.*, 1979) and the Structured Assessment of Personality (SAP) (Mann *et al.*, 1981). Both require prior training and informant interviews are essential in the SAP and advisable in the PAS.

The criteria used for the diagnosis of DSM-III personality disorders are based, with the exception of antisocial personality disorder, on inadequate evidence (Tyrer, 1988). Too much reliance is placed on questions to the subject and not enough on interviews with an informant. Furthermore, the reliance on a categorical rather than a dimensional classification minimizes the chances of detecting a number of traits that might be associated with somatization, e.g. dependent, obsessional, hypochondriacal characteristics.

Using the PAS, Tyrer and his colleagues (Tyrer *et al.*, 1990) have asserted that patients with hypochondriacal personality disorder have common characteristics that justify a separate diagnosis. They assessed 1000 psychiatric outpatients using a standardized psychiatric interview as well as the PAS and found that hypochondriacal personality disorder occurred in 2.5% of the total sample and 8.6% of a group with affective psychoses. The criteria for diagnosing hypochondriacal personality disorder are given in Chapter 2. Tyrer's findings are important because they suggest that a subgroup of patients with FSSs may have an associated personality disturbance which may prove intractable. This issue is discussed in more detail by Bass and Murphy in Chapter 12, p. 301.

Although not strictly a personality disorder, *alexithymia* has attracted considerable interest from clinicians. It refers to an enduring characteristic (more a 'cognitive style' than a personality disorder) which is thought to predispose individuals to somatization. Alexithymic individuals characteristically show a striking difficulty in recognizing and describing their own feelings, and they have difficulty distinguishing between emotional states and bodily sensations (Taylor, 1984). Alexithymia is a difficult concept to operationalize, and until recently no sufficiently reliable and valid instrument for measuring it has been developed. Although Taylor and his colleagues (1988) recently demonstrated the criterion validity of the Toronto Alexithymia Scale (or TAS), they also found that alexithymic patients did not report more somatic complaints than those rated non-alexithymic. This challenges the view that alexithymic individuals are prone to somatize.

## Axis III: concomitant physical conditions

The relationship between physical disorders and psychiatric illness is variable and complex. It is essential to recognize this in our classification (Goldberg, 1984). First, psychiatric illness may be a relatively direct consequence of disease, as in the example of the patient who becomes depressed following a myocardial infarction. Second, physical disease and psychiatric disorder may coexist, but the emotional distress may serve not only to aggravate physical complaints but also to delay recovery from the physical illness. Third, the patient may have a psychiatric illness which presents to the physician as a physical symptom. This is interpreted as a sign of disease and may be treated as such.

It has been established in both primary care and general hospital settings that physical illness and psychiatric disorder often coexist (Mayou & Hawton, 1986; Goldberg & Bridges, 1988). For this reason the contribution of physical illness must be assessed. Unfortunately it is often far from clear whether the physical problem is contributing to psychopathology or whether it is merely coincidental. It is helpful to divide physical problems into those that are currently active and those which are of historical interest. A disease in the latter group, for example tuberculosis in childhood, may contribute to current understanding of the patient because it led to profound disturbances in childhood adjustment and family life.

Some patients with numerous complaints have a trivial coexisting physical disorder which is considered to be aetiologically significant, for example an anxious patient with non-cardiac chest pain but trivial valvular heart disease may undergo an unnecessary valvotomy. Such a patient will be doubly disadvantaged. That is to say, he/she will have insignificant physical disease which is treated, and psychiatric illness which is not.

## Axis IV: abnormal psychosocial situations or stressors

This axis includes problems which are often of aetiological significance. One potential form of psychosocial stressor is a life event, which is more likely to lead to morbidity if it is appraised in a certain way, for example death of a spouse leading to profound grief. There is now impressive empirical data to support the relation between the experience of distressing life events and the onset of functional symptoms (Creed, 1981; Craig & Brown, 1984; Scaloubaca *et al.,* 1988). Moreover, certain types of life event are likely to be aetiologically relevant, in particular those which carry the threat of loss (Creed, 1985). In a fascinating study House and Andrews (1988) found that women with functional dysphonia had experienced significantly more events linked to conflicts over speaking out in the year before the onset of the complaint than a community comparison group.

It is essential to include carefully chosen open questions about recent life events, and the patient's reply should be corroborated by those of a reliable informant. Cohen (1982) drew attention to the importance of precipitating (and predisposing) factors when he urged that the following questions be asked in all patients with 'functional' complaints: (i) *why* is the patient ill?; (ii) why is the patient ill *now?*; (iii) why is this particular person ill in this particular way?

The Social Interview Schedule (SIS) is a semistructured interview designed to obtain information on social conditions, attitudes and functioning (Clare & Cairns, 1978). It is ideal for use in patients with FSSs. The schedule examines each subject's life from three main standpoints: first, material conditions, i.e. what the person has in terms of living conditions, money, etc; second, social functioning, e.g. management of social activities and relationships; and third, social satisfaction, i.e. the subject's satisfaction with various aspects of his/her life situation such as housing and parental role.

### Axis V: disabilities

It is important to establish the impact of the symptoms on the patient's life. For example, the patient may have restricted his/her social and recreational life, may be absenting him/herself from work and unable to function with his/her family, or, in rare circumstances, be in receipt of invalidity or disability benefits *despite the absence of ascertainable disease.* The various disabilities experienced by the patient should be assessed. Suitable rating scales include the Psychosocial Adjustment to Illness Scale or PAIS (Derogatis, 1986) and the Sickness Impact Profile (Bergner *et al.,* 1981).

It is always difficult to assess whether the symptom(s) result in gains for the patient. But an attempt should be made to determine whether the complaints avert or diminish conflict or provide a solution to an apparently insoluble life problem. Regrettably, information of this nature, because it is based on inference, is difficult to support or refute.

Time should also be spent in attempting to get as complete a picture as possible of any benefits the patient receives, i.e. invalidity, mobility, or attendance allowances. These disability payments should be summated and compared with the salary the patient last received when in gainful employment. Tact should be exercised when collecting this information, because the patient may balk at the implication that his/her illness is financially remunerative.

*The family doctor*

The general practitioner is likely to have information about not only the patient's complaint behaviour but also his/her domestic and family circumstances. A telephone conversation with the family doctor may yield essential information which the patient may not have disclosed. If the family doctor can be persuaded to part with the patient's complete medical file, so much the better. Collection of 'objective' data is of the utmost importance in patients with functional somatic symptoms, especially in those with chronic symptoms or multiple unexplained somatic complaints. For example, past records might reveal a pattern of persistent and repetitive complaint behaviour that has driven more than one family practitioner to distraction. These patients may be consulting numerous doctors at different practices, and as a consequence may be in receipt of a number of medications and (often contradictory) advice about their symptoms.

*The patient's family*

There may be advantages in conducting the interview with the patient in the presence of one or more family members. This may be particularly apposite in those patients with chronic pain or persistent unexplained complaints, when family members may have been exposed to months or years of complaint behaviour. Because the patient is more likely to have a psychosocial problem than a biomedical disease, an interview which takes account of the patient's role in the family 'system' may provide information which is unlikely to become apparent if the patient is interviewed alone (Watson, 1985). An essential component of this interview involves an assessment of the attitudes of each family member. Evidence that they share the patient's hypochondriacal or morbid beliefs about the complaints is likely to have an adverse influence on the prognosis, and suggests that family therapy may be an appropriate treatment (see later).

# Management

Patients with functional complaints take up a considerable amount of time in medical outpatient clinics, yet the space given to the management of these disorders in medical textbooks is nugatory. This is regrettable, especially as early detection and management is essential; delay in diagnosis and treatment may lead to subtle but unalterable changes in the nature of the disorder and the patient's attitude towards it.

In this chapter a range of treatment approaches will be described. I will be concerned with the management of those patients who have experienced symptoms for at least 3 months, and who have often undergone investigations or tests that have failed to demonstrate objective pathology. An exhaustive account of all available treatments will not be attempted, and, wherever possible, only those treatments that have been subjected to (or are susceptible to) controlled evaluation will be described.

Before describing specific treatments, some general principles need to be outlined.

*Engaging the patient*

Some patients will have had numerous examinations and investigations before referral. If the physician has not explained the results of these before referral, the patient should be told that these have not provided the answer to what was wrong, but that if there had been serious disease present the tests would have revealed it. These remarks should be accompanied by an explanation that the patient does have a genuine disorder to account for the symptoms, that it is not going to lead to harm, and that it has a good prognosis.

This involves listening to the patient — taking a full history of the complaint and exploring the patient's health beliefs. Goldberg *et al.* (1989) have stressed the importance of the preliminary stage of the interview, which they have termed 'feeling understood'. It is essential to prepare the ground in this way, otherwise the patient will not engage in any meaningful way with the treatment plan. Goldberg and his colleagues have proposed a three-stage model to encourage somatizing patients to *reattribute* their bodily symptoms, and relate them to psychological problems. These stages are *feeling understood*, *changing the agenda*, and *making the link* between bodily symptoms and emotional disorder, and they are described in more detail by Craig and Boardman (Chapter 4, p. 93). Practical examples of 'making the link' in patients with functional bowel disorders are described by Creed in Chapter 6, p. 157.

Although reattribution is the aim when working with patients with morbid health beliefs and disease conviction, one should guard against moving the patient from a belief in an organic aetiology to belief in a psychological one. This would not only be an unrealistic aim, it would usually replace one distortion of reality with another. As Watts (1982) has pointed out, the aim should be 'to encourage patients to see the full range of aetiological factors that apply. Patients will initially have a crude dichotomy of aetiologies, believing they must either have genuine symptoms with an organic aetiology or that they have psychological symptoms that are simply "all in the mind"'. Regrettably, it is not only the patient who is likely to adopt this 'either/or' dichotomy; the idea is widespread in our culture.

*Adverse responses to negative investigations*

It is useful to assess the patient's response to being informed that investigations are normal. A range of responses are possible, but in general an attitude of disbelief or dismay, anger or resentment following these disclosures carries a poor prognosis (see also Chapter 8, p. 226). The reasons for these attitudes should be explored, but in some cases the patient's disease conviction remains unshakeable. Some of these patients may ultimately find their way to alternative practitioners or allergy clinics (Stewart & Raskin, 1985). Conversely, some patients react to the information about the absence of disease with a sense of relief and gratitude. Responses of this nature are more likely to be associated with a favourable outcome. Another group of patients may express relief at the absence of organic disease, but nevertheless relentlessly pursue a physical explanation for their symptoms as the following case illustrates:

> A 49-year-old previously fit lorry driver was referred from the cardiology service in 1987 with a 3 year history of episodic palpitations. During the first episode of symptoms he was admitted to an intensive care unit and told that he had had 'some form of heart attack'. He continued to experience symptoms whilst driving and visited two accident and emergency departments; at one he was told that he had Wolf–Parkinson–White syndrome whereas at another he was reassured that his heart was entirely normal. Although an exercise test, 24-hour tape, echocardiogram and catecholamine screen were within normal limits, an initial diagnosis of paroxysmal atrial tachycardia was made and he was treated with digoxin and verapamil and advised not to drive. For the next 2 years he remained relatively well apart from occasional palpitations, but then his symptoms changed in quality and included pressure on the chest, breathlessness, flatulence and audible belching. These episodes, some of which were thought to be attributable to overbreathing, lasted about an hour and were associated with sweating, choking sensations, and restlessness. Barium meal, gastroscopy and respiratory function tests were all normal. Ranitidine and maxolon provided no relief. At the initial psychiatric interview he was angry and frustrated because the doctors

could not agree about the diagnosis, but there was a marked lack of conspicuous anxiety or depression. He had been off work for 11 months. Following 2 minutes of voluntary overbreathing he began belching frequently and experienced most of his usual somatic symptoms. The results of this test were discussed with him and he was encouraged to reattribute his somatic symptoms to 'overbreathing attacks' rather than to serious heart disease.

Because aerophagy was considered to contribute to his symptoms he was also treated with a course of physiotherapy directed at breathing retraining. But he requested more physical investigations, and for the next 6 months he continued to visit medical outpatient clinics. Eventually his exasperated GP made a 'final' referral to a gastroenterologist, who made a diagnosis of hyperventilation and referred him back to the psychiatric department. Predictably, he declined this referral.

In a subgroup of patients, especially those with chronic persistent fatigue who have visited numerous specialists without having received an 'acceptable' diagnosis, one of the main functions of treatment is to allow the patient to call a halt without loss of face. It is necessary to share with the patient the uncertainty concerning the topic, to admit that there are some disorders for which medicine does not possess all the answers, and to help the patient accept that there will never be the 'ultimate opinion' or the 'final specialist' (Wessely *et al.*, 1989). In essence the doctor is inviting the patient to collaborate in a process of rehabilitation, with the assistance of the doctor and other professionals, who might include a nurse therapist, occupational therapist, physiotherapist and others. Regrettably some patients, like the one just described, are unwilling to undertake such a venture.

## Reassurance

Reassurance is probably the most widely used but poorly understood psychotherapeutic manoeuvre in medical practice. It is frequently given to patients with FSSs after tests have proved negative, and often results in alleviation of anxiety and concerns about physical symptoms. Patients who *respond* to reassurance usually have somatic concerns in the context of an anxiety or depressive illness. These illness concerns may recede with the treatment of the primary disorder (Noyes *et al.*, 1986). However, a plausible explanation for somatic complaints should always be attempted. For example, common symptoms such as globus or stabbing chest pain may be ascribed to 'overstretching or tension in the muscles'. This explanation should be congruent with the patient's sociocultural background. This approach offers information that is relevant to the patient's clinical condition (Warwick & Salkovskis, 1985), and is more likely to be effective than bland reassurance 'that the tests are all normal so there is nothing to worry about'. The timing of reassurance is also important, as Kessel (1979) has stressed. It is less likely to be useful if given prematurely, before the results of the investigations are known, or before the patient has been allowed to air his/her concerns. Conversely, reassurance is more likely to be effective when it is accompanied by information that the therapist has been successful in managing patients with similar complaints.

Information intended to reassure must be accurate. For example, if a doctor provides a patient with information about the duration of symptoms that turns out to be false, this may aggravate the patient's illness (Philips, 1988). The patient may also lose faith in what doctors say and interpret further reassurance as an attempt to 'fob off' the complaints.

In many cases reassurance may be all that is required. But patients with hypochondriasis are important to identify because in this group repeated reassurance may be counterproductive. Indeed, the diagnosis of this disorder is contingent upon the patient's illness beliefs persisting *despite medical reassurance* (DSM-III-R, 1987). Hypochondriacal patients have illness fears that have usually persisted for at least 6 months (and often many years) and they commonly ascribe their physical complaints to serious organic disease, prompting repeated presentation with trivial symptoms and disproportionate anxiety. It is this fear and preoccupation with disease that leads to the need for reassurance.

Physicians often deal with this reassurance-seeking by repeated reassurance, ordering further tests, or regular clinical appointments — with detrimental consequences. Warwick and Salkovskis (1985) have drawn attention to the fact that this kind of reassurance can exacerbate the patient's problems. It seems that this occurs because such reassurance serves the same function as rituals in obsessive–compulsive disorder — that is a short term reduction in anxiety and a longer term return of and increase in fear and the urge to seek further reassurance. Salkovskis and Warwick (1986) have devised a cognitive–behavioural treatment strategy for patients with hypochondriacal symptoms which is based on this premise that the illness is sustained by the seeking of reassurance from physicians and repeated checking of bodily state (see below).

*Withdrawing unnecessary medication*

This issue provides another opportunity to assess the patient's attitudes to his/her symptoms and motivation for change. Both patient and clinician may be faced with a dilemma when, after months or years of symptoms and/or disability, a critical examination fails to reveal evidence of relevant organic disease. Referral to a psychiatrist may follow, when it will be important to discuss with the patient the possibility of gradual withdrawal of unnecessary medication. This phase of management requires skilful handling, for in effect the psychiatrist is inviting the patient to negotiate the transition from a 'sick' to a 'healthy' mode of living. Each patient's response to this suggestion should be carefully noted, as it usually has an important bearing on prognosis. It is essential that the doctor has not only gained the patient's trust, but also satisfied him/herself that there is an alternative explanation for the genesis of the complaint *before* this topic is broached. Prolonged unemployment and being in receipt of disability payments increase the likelihood of the patient remaining in the sick role. The following case illustrates the dilemma for the patient when a psychological disorder is incorrectly ascribed to an organic aetiology:

> This 29-year-old single unemployed woman was referred from the gastroenterology service with an 8 year history of faecal incontinence. A diagnosis of ulcerative colitis had been made at another hospital 8 years previously and she had been prescribed sulphasalizine. However, her GP was unimpressed by this diagnosis and requested a psychiatric opinion because her main complaints were a fear of faecal incontinence when travelling from home. Further investigations failed to establish the presence of inflammatory bowel disease, and the gastroenterologist diagnosed a neurotic disorder. Close enquiry revealed that she had complained of intermittent constipation and diarrhoea since early childhood. She had visited her family doctor on a regular basis between the ages of 11 and 20 with abdominal pains and gastrointestinal symptoms, for which laxatives and analgesics had been prescribed. For the previous 8 years she had reported fear of incontinence, worse in public places, and as a consequence avoided going out or travelling on public transport. Journeys away from home were infrequent and she always carried toilet paper and perfume with her in case she was incontinent. Before leaving the house there would be considerable anticipatory anxiety with frequent visits to the toilet and loose bowel motions. Abdominal cramps and diarrhoea would occur whenever she became excited, anxious or angry. She had been unemployed since the diagnosis of ulcerative colitis 8 years previously. She was informed that the symptoms were the consequence of an emotional rather than physical disorder and expressed an interest in attempting to overcome her difficulties. Drug treatment was withdrawn and she read a lay book on fears and phobias. She

participated in an exposure programme, purchasing a bicycle and travelling gradually further distances away from home. At the time of writing there is much less avoidance behaviour and she is actively seeking employment.

## Physical treatments

*Drug treatment*

In many patients with FSSs evidence of a mood disorder can be obtained. Drug treatment of this disorder, especially when it is associated with acute or subacute somatization, may lead to resolution of the physical complaints. However, a problem with compliance may arise with a patient who is convinced that his/her symptoms have an organic basis. The patient may protest that psychotropic drugs are inappropriate, because the problem is not 'mental'. It is not uncommon for patients with FSSs to have been prescribed a psychotropic drug by a GP or hospital doctor before referral to a psychiatrist. However, the patient may not have been told what benefits and possible side-effects to expect, especially when tricyclic antidepressants are used. Dosage may not have approached therapeutic levels before treatment is abandoned. To achieve acceptable compliance, the patient has to be told what symptoms can be expected to improve, when this is likely to happen, what side-effects to expect, and how long to persist with the drug if benefits do not become apparent. Furthermore, each patient should be seen at regular intervals to assess the drug's efficacy.

The choice of drug treatment depends on the underlying psychiatric disturbance. Medication may be used either in conjunction with other nonpharmacological methods or as the main form of treatment. The most important drugs are tricyclic antidepressants, monoamine oxidase inhibitors and betablockers.

*Tricyclic antidepressants*   These drugs have been shown to be of benefit to patients whose hypochondriacal complaints are associated with depression (Kellner *et al.*, 1986). They should be considered only after detailed assessment of the nature of the mood disturbance and its causes. In some depressed patients the somatic complaints may show a diurnal variation, and symptoms may be reported more often in the morning when the mood is at its lowest. It may be difficult to decide whether the depressive symptoms are primary or secondary to the persisting pains or worry. In these cases it may be best to give the depression the benefit of the doubt and treat it. In some patients hypochondriacal concern may be completely relieved by antidepressants.

Dothiepin is an effective antidepressant, has some sedative action, and fewer anticholinergic side-effects than amitriptyline. Treatment should begin with small dosage, e.g. 25 mg at night, increasing in 25 mg increments to a therapeutic dosage of 150 mg per day (less in older patients).

There is a considerable body of research evidence to support the efficacy of TCAs, in particular imipramine, in the treatment of patients with panic attacks. Some investigators, for example Mavissakalian (1986) have even suggested that imipramine reduces the frequency of panic attacks and associated hypochondriacal symptoms independently of any antidepressant effect, although high doses in excess of 200 mg daily may be required.

At present there is no consensus about the most appropriate treatment for patients with panic attacks, and the topic continues to generate lively and acrimonious debate (Klein, 1988; Lelliott & Marks, 1988). These issues will become clearer with the publication of the results of controlled studies comparing imipramine, behavioural and cognitive therapy in patients with panic. At present the treatment adopted for these patients depends, to a large extent, on the orientation of the clinician and the acceptability of the treatment to the patient.

This latter point is important in panic patients, who are often exquisitely sensitive to somatic sensations and may not be able to tolerate the common side-effects of the TCAs such as drowsiness, dry mouth and blurred vision. For this reason it is important to commence treatment with relatively small doses, e.g. 25 mg on and gradually increase the dose during the subsequent 2–3 weeks to the therapeutic range of 150 mg. Of the classical tricyclics anticholinergic activity is strongest with amitriptyline and imipramine and least with desipramine (Pinder, 1988).

*Monoamine oxidase inhibitors*   These drugs are particularly useful for patients with FSSs associated with anxiety. The type of patient most likely to respond has panic attacks accompanied by multiple autonomic symptoms such as palpitations, trembling and chest tightness (Bass & Kerwin, 1988). Mood may be depressed but usually retains its *reactivity* (complete, albeit transient, remission from depressed mood due to positive environmental factors). Somatic features of anxiety may be accompanied by loss of interest, irritability with anergia and there may be initial rather than late insomnia (Liebowitz et al., 1988). Phobias, panic attacks and depersonalization may complete the clinical picture (Tyrer & Shawcross, 1988). Evidence of a stable and moderately well adjusted premorbid personality predicts good response, but MAOIs are contraindicated in those patients with alcohol problems and/or a previous history of impulsive self-poisoning.

Phenelzine is usually begun at 15 mg daily in the morning for three days, followed by 30 mg in the morning for four days, followed by 45 mg in divided dosage (9 am and midday) for one week. If at the end of a week on 45 mg the patient continues to have panic attacks, the dose should be raised to 60 mg and held there for 2 weeks. Again, if the patient is not panic free, one can progress to 75 mg daily and, 1 week later, if necessary, to 90 mg per day. Once a patient is panic free, the patient requires support and encouragement to re-enter phobic situations that have been avoided.

These drugs are quite safe if used carefully, in selected patients who understand the dietary restrictions and drug interactions. Common side-effects include anticholinergic symptoms, orthostatic hypotension, anorgasmia (reversible), daytime drowsiness (overcome by prescribing drug at night), and hyperalertness. Treatment should be continued for 6–9 months and the drug tapered at a rate of 15 mg per week. Rapid withdrawal is more likely to result in an unpleasant withdrawal syndrome. There is a risk of relapse in 30–60% of patients.

Some patients with severe, recurrent panics and multiple somatic symptoms are unable to tolerate small doses of MAOIs as outpatients, and for these a brief hospital admission may be required. In this setting the dose of phenelzine (or tranylcypromine) can be gradually increased over 7–14 days, when side-effects may be closely monitored and compliance encouraged. Apparently intractible patients may benefit from this procedure, as the following case report demonstrates:

> This 38-year-old married woman was referred for assessment of her panics and cardiorespiratory symptoms. She had a 12 year history of multiple somatic complaints, and had been investigated in many different hospital departments. Her complaints included back pain, gastrointestinal symptoms (normal barium series and gall bladder ultrasounds), persistent headaches and cardiorespiratory symptoms (normal exercise test and echocardiogram). An admission to a psychiatric hospital and 4 years of outpatient treatment of her panics with imipramine — 50 mg on, valium — 10 mg tds and propranolol — 20 mg tds, had not proved helpful. She had two teenage children, was premorbidly stable, and worked as a shop assistant. By the time of referral she was addicted to lorazepan — 1 mg tds.
>
> A diagnosis of anxiety disorder with predominantly cardiorespiratory symptoms was made. She had 2 to 3 uncued (unprovoked) panics daily and avoided crowds, public transport and travelling far from home unaccompanied. Symptoms of palpitations, stabbing chest pain and breathlessness were accompanied by characteristic catastrophic thoughts. She also reported chronic fatigue, and was mildly depressed but with mood reactivity.

During the next 3 years she failed to respond to a course of relaxation and breathing exercises, outpatient group treatment for chronic somatizers, as well as a course of betablockers. Very small doses of imipramine (10 mg) and phenelzine (15 mg) led to intolerable side-effects which acted as a focus for further catastrophic thoughts. During this 3 year period her symptoms continued and she admitted herself to the A&E department on 6 separate occasions.

Admission to hospital was precipitated by an ativan overdose. Because of her chronic symptomatology she was assessed for somatization disorder using the Diagnostic Interview Schedule (Robins *et al.*, 1981), but attained only 11 of the 13 symptoms required to establish this diagnosis. Because of her symptom profile inpatient treatment was commenced with phenelzine — 15 mg daily, increasing by 15 mg increments every 3 days until a dose of 60 mg was reached. After initial deterioration (she became more depressed and tearful) there was dramatic improvement in the third week. During her month in hospital lorazepan was tapered from 3 mg to 1 mg per day. She was discharged symptom free after four weeks. Improvement was maintained one year later on 45 mg of phenelzine daily. She was panic free, there was no avoidance behaviour or irritability and she had more energy. Her depression had lifted and family members were astonished at her change. Her confidence was such that she had discontinued lorazepan. She was reluctant to withdraw from phenelzine, despite a weight gain of 2 stones and a craving for carbohydrates.

This patient illustrates two important points. First, a patient who almost satisfied diagnostic criteria for somatization disorder improved dramatically on treatment with MAOI. Second, inability to tolerate the side-effects of phenelzine as an outpatient should not discourage the use of MAOIs in appropriate patients. We have found that a brief (3–4 weeks) inpatient admission to stabilize patients on these drugs can prove very cost-effective.

*Benzodiazepines*  Because of the risks of dependence and severe withdrawal symptoms, special care has to be taken when prescribing these drugs. Because they are best used for periods of no more than 2 weeks in regular dosage, or in intermittent flexible dosage, the author considers them to be inappropriate for patients with functional complaints or hypochondriacal symptoms. Nevertheless, Noyes *et al.* (1986) found that hypochondriacal preoccupation in patients with panic disorder and multiple somatic symptoms was reduced after 6 weeks of treatment with the triazolodiazepine alprazolam. But these patients were recruited by newspaper advertisement, and no information was provided about long term follow-up or withdrawal symptoms after stopping alprazolam, a known complication of this drug (Pecknold *et al.*, 1988).

*Beta-adrenergic blockers*   The case for betablockers in the treatment of somatic symptoms of anxiety has probably been overstated. That they reduce sympathetically mediated symptoms such as palpitations, tremor and sweating is undisputed (Hallstrom, 1984). But this is the sum total of their anxiogenic action. They do not affect any other somatic symptoms or have a direct affect on psychic symptoms (Tyrer *et al.*, 1980). By minimizing the cardiovascular symptoms the drugs may reduce the apprehension or panic that such symptoms are capable of inducing. They therefore reduce psychic anxiety indirectly. Nevertheless, they are useful in patients complaining of palpitations and who have a tachycardia in excess of 90 beats per minute, when the dose should be titrated against the pulse rate. If hyperventilation complicates the disorder it is safer to use a more cardioselective betablocker such as metoprolol (50–100 mg bd) to reduce the possibility of inducing bronchospasm.

## Psychological treatments

### Introduction

There has been a resurgence of interest in the psychological treatment of functional disorders in the last decade. Cognitive–behavioural treatments have been the most widely studied, and some of these will be described. Patients with unexplained somatic symptoms may also be amenable to a 'systems' approach, when members of the patient's immediate social network may be invited to attend treatment sessions. This is particularly applicable when the symptom(s) are considered to serve a particular function for the family, e.g. to prevent a spouse from leaving home, or when the family's illness model is maintaining a member in the sick role.

### Cognitive–behavioural treatment (CBT)

Of all the neurotic illnesses, those characterized by anxiety and hypochondriacal symptoms have usually been associated with a poor long term prognosis (Greer & Cawley, 1966). However, recent work by Warwick and Salkovskis (1988) has suggested that even this potentially intractible disorder may respond to CBT (Fig. 3.3). These authors suggest that three main mechanisms operate to increase anxiety, preoccupation with illness and the misinterpretation of bodily variations that characterize this disorder. These

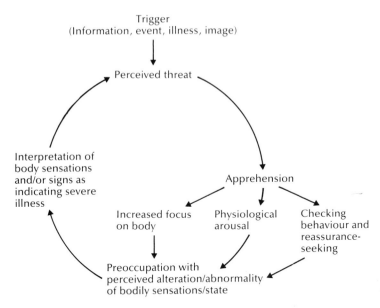

**Fig. 3.3.** Cognitive model of hypochondriacal problems. (Reproduced with permission from Warwick & Salkovskis, 1988).

are (i) *increased physiological arousal* (which leads to increased occurrence of autonomically mediated sensations); (ii) *selective attention* (normal variations in bodily function or previously unnoticed aspects of appearance or bodily function may be noticed more readily than had previously been the case); and (iii) *avoidant behaviours*; the hypochondriacal patient has become conditioned to stimuli associated with illness that causes anxiety, i.e. bodily sensations such as palpitations, chest pain, and signs such as a skin blemish. The patient attempts to neutralize the anxiety associated with these interoceptive cues by behaviour (reassurance-seeking) which is more typical of the obsessional patient. Although this avoidance behaviour serves to terminate exposure to the feared stimuli, it prevents habituation from taking place. These avoidant behaviours are considered important because they prevent the patient from learning that the things which are feared do not actually happen.

Warwick and Salkovskis believe that reassurance-seeking and its provision is of fundamental importance in maintaining hypochondriasis, and that inappropriate reassurance ('all the tests are normal so there can't be anything wrong') can exacerbate the problem. They have also suggested that it is helpful to devise a behavioural experiment demonstrating the effects of reassurance (Salkovskis, 1989). This experiment is also a useful engagement strategy in patients who demand a 'final test' before treatment. In such patients a final physical examination is arranged on the strict understanding that it is unnecessary for the patient's physical health, but may be helpful in the psychological assessment. The patient is asked to rate beliefs in specific health related thoughts and need for reassurance before and after the test. If, as is usual, anxiety is reduced only briefly, this is used as a basis for discussion about the way in which reassurance maintains health anxiety. It also helps to engage the patient in treatment and establishes a collaborative relationship.

In a recent study they demonstrated the efficacy of a novel treatment, based on their cognitive–behavioural model, in two patients with hypochondriacal illnesses (Salkovskis & Warwick, 1986). Both patients were incapacitated by anxious preoccupation with physical disease, and their importunate behaviour had led to severe deterioration in relationships at work and at home. After inpatient treatment with a combination of behavioural techniques that involved withholding reassurance both patients showed reduction in health anxiety, illness conviction and need for reassurance.

Improvement in health anxiety and social functioning was reported in a further 17 patients with illness phobia who were treated with a combination of exposure to illness cues and response prevention (Warwick & Marks, 1988). This included live exposure to feared stimuli (e.g. visiting hospital, reading literature relating to the feared illness), satiation (e.g. repeatedly writing the fears down on paper), paradox (e.g. exercising to try to 'bring on a heart attack'), and the banning of reassurance-seeking (banning visits to hospital for examination and tests, teaching relatives how to withhold reassurance when asked for it). Although these studies are uncontrolled, they highlight the need for controlled, prospective study with follow-up in such patients.

### Cognitive–behavioural treatment in chronic pain

Although there have been many behaviourally oriented treatment programmes for patients with chronic pain (Linton, 1986), the process whereby the patients improve in these programmes remains to be determined. One of the most comprehensive recent studies included measures of behaviour, cognitions and subjective report in a chronic pain sample (Philips, 1987). In this 9-week outpatient study of 40 patients with chronic pain, 25 were allocated to treatment (in groups of 5–7 individuals) and 15 were placed on a waiting list. All patients had pain of at least 6 months' duration and were assessed comprehensively with a variety of standardized instruments which measured not only mood, pain intensity and self-efficacy, but also reports of avoidance and complaint behaviour, two of the most important aspects of pain behaviour. The findings were impressive; there was significant clinical improvement in 83% of the treated cases. Philips found that changes in self-efficacy ratings and in the expressed control over the pain problem were highly correlated with the rating of the pain problem. That is to say, one of the most important effects of treatment was the development of a sense of control and mastery over pain. The author concluded that the reduction in avoidance behaviour may be a crucial and preliminary step which results in important and enduring changes in attitude as well as subjective experience. Thus pain behaviours have to change first before experiential or attitudinal changes occur (cognitive lag) (Rachman & Hodgson, 1974). Details of the treatment programme are available in a manual (Philips, 1988).

*Psychotherapy*

Kellner (1983) has described a psychotherapeutic technique which he claims to be effective in hypochondriacal patients. Unlike Warwick and Salkovskis, Kellner advocates physical examination and reassurance as cornerstones of treatment. For example, he remarks: 'when a patient telephones in a state of panic and afraid that he is dying, an immediate appointment for a physical examination and reassurance lead often to rapid (albeit temporary) relief of symptoms; this procedure appears to save a great deal of time and verbal psychotherapy'. Like Warwick and Salkovskis (1988), Kellner admits that such reassurance produces only *brief* respite, but asserts that 'with repetition, reassurances that were initially ineffective, or effective only for a short time, tended to have longer effects, were more frequently recalled, and when recalled carried more conviction. This confidence in the therapeutic benefit of reassurance is not in accordance with the views of Warwick and Salkovskis (1988).'

Kellner's treatment strategy includes accurate information and explanation about the psychophysiological processes involved, emphasis on the innocuousness of the symptoms, making the patient aware of his/her selective perception of bodily sensations, and use of deliberate suggestion when this is in accord with the prognosis. When the patient has recurrences of symptoms and fears, physical examinations are repeated and the patient is reassured. Using this approach, Kellner claims that 64% of 34 patients with hypochondriacal neurosis were improved after a follow-up period of 2 years. But these results must be interpreted with caution, because the study was uncontrolled, many patients received additional psychotropic drugs, and the number of treatment sessions was not standardized.

*Group psychotherapy*

There are very few published controlled studies of the efficacy of group psychotherapy in patients with circumscribed functional syndromes. Of those studies that have been published, most are uncontrolled and have not used standardized measures to define patient groups or outcome criteria. Chronic somatizers or 'untreatable' patients have attracted most interest, but the studies leave much to be desired (e.g. Mally & Ogston, 1964; Roskin *et al.*, 1980).

*Family therapy*

It has already been emphasized that family members in frequent contact with a patient may serve to reinforce hypochondriacal attitudes and act as 'maintaining factors' in somatization. Members of the same family are likely to learn shared attitudes and beliefs, including those concerning disease. Intuitively, family therapy should be potentially helpful in somatizing patients (Watson, 1985), but there is no objective evidence at present to suggest that family therapy intervention can lead to symptomatic improvement in somatizing patients.

*Management of the chronic somatizer*

Patients who persistently somatize psychological distress may present the physician with formidable management problems. They usually have long histories of multiple unexplained physical symptoms and may have undergone an excessive number of surgical operations. The hospital notes may run to many volumes. Typically, these patients have a history of marital discord and occupational difficulties and, although they may have received treatment for psychiatric problems in the past, often do not disclose this information. These patients have been described by American psychiatrists as suffering from somatization disorder (American Psychiatric Association, 1987), a perplexing disorder which is described in greater detail in Chapter 12, p. 301).

A psychiatrist may be asked to assess one of these patients, but regrettably this is usually late in the course of the illness. Not surprisingly, the referral is often resented by the patient. Careful history taking may reveal evidence of numerous previous admissions to other hospitals, an excessive number of surgical procedures, and possibly a history of suicide threats. Current emotional problems and/or life stresses are usually minimized or denied.

Despite these discouraging signs, many patients with chronic somatization can be engaged in psychological treatment of a supportive nature. Indeed, Smith *et al.* (1986) carried out a controlled trial that demonstrated the value of a single psychiatric assessment followed by advice to primary care physicians on management. This important study and guidelines on the management of these patients are described in more detail in Chapter 12.

## Conclusions

Assessment of patients with functional somatic symptoms demands considerable skill. Judicious use of open and closed questions and exploration of illness beliefs are of paramount importance. The assessment may be made doubly difficult when the patient brings to the consultation views about his/her illness that are discrepant with those of the psychiatrist. The assessment may require more than one interview and should lead to a multiaxial formulation of the patient's problem.

Treatment of these patients requires flexibility and ingenuity on the part of the therapist, who has a wide range of physical and psychological treatments at his/her disposal. Management depends on many factors, in particular the duration and severity of the disorder. Patients with acute (weeks) and subacute (up to 6 months) somatization may require different treatment from those with more intractable chronic somatization, who may have reported symptoms for many years.

## References

*References with an asterisk contain information about rating scales and questionnaires that have been referred to in the text. All are useful in patients with FSSs.

American Psychiatric Association (1987). *Diagnostic and Statistical Manual of Mental Disorders (DSM-III-R)* 3rd edn, revised, Washington DC.
Apley, J. & Hale, B. (1973). Children with recurrent abdominal pain: how do they grow up? *British Medical Journal*, **i**, 7–9.
Bass, C. (1985). Physical symptoms of anxiety, *British Journal of Clinical Practice*, **39** (Suppl 38), 34–38.
Bass, C. (1990). The frequent attender in general practice, *Update*, **40**, 494–501.
Bass, C. & Gardner, W.N. (1985). Respiratory and psychiatric abnormalities in chronic symptomatic hyperventilation, *British Medical Journal*, **i**, 1387–1390.
Bass, C. & Kerwin, R. (1988). MAOIs in psychiatry: underprescribed or obsolete? *British Medical Journal*, **298**, 345–346.
*Bergner, M., Bobbitt, R.A., Carter, W.B. & Gilson, B.S. (1981). The sickness impact profile: development and final revision of a health status measure, *Medical Care*, **19**, 787–805.
*Clare, A.W. & Cairns, V.E. (1978). Design, development and use of a standardised interview to assess social maladjustment and dysfunction in community studies, *Psychological Medicine*, **8**, 589–605.
Cohen, S.I. (1982). The evaluation of patients with somatic symptoms — the 'difficult' diagnostic

problem, in *Medicine and Psychiatry: A Practical Approach* (Eds. Creed, F. & Pfeffer, J.), Pitman, London.

Corney, R.H., Strathdee, G., Higgs, R., King, M., Williams, P., Sharp, D. & Pelosi, A.J. (1988). Managing the difficult patient: practical suggestions from a study day, *Journal of the Royal College of General Practice*, **38**, 349–352.

Craig, T.K. & Brown, G.W. (1984). Goal frustration and life events in the aetiology of painful gastrointestinal disorder, *Journal of Psychosomatic Research*, **28**, 411–421.

Creed, F.H. (1981). Life events and appendicectomy, *Lancet*, **i**, 1381–1385.

Creed, F. (1985). Life events and physical illness, *Journal of Psychosomatic Research*, **29**, 113–123.

Crisp, A.H. (1968). The role of the psychiatrist in the general hospital, *Postgraduate Medical Journal*, **44**, 267–276.

Derogatis, L.R. (1986). The psychological adjustment to illness scale (PAIS), *Journal of Psychosomatic Research*, **30**, 77–91.

Gardner, W.N. & Bass, C. (1989). Hyperventilation in clinical practice, *British Journal of Hospital Medicine*, **41**, 73–81.

Goldberg, D. (1984). The recognition of psychiatric illness by non-psychiatrists, *Australian and New Zealand Journal of Psychiatry*, **1B**, 128–133.

Goldberg, D. & Bridges, K. (1988). Somatic presentations of psychiatric illness in primary care setting, *Journal of Psychosomatic Research*, **32**, 137–144.

Goldberg, D., Gask, L. & O'Dowd, T. (1989). The treatment of somatisation: teaching techniques of reattribution, *Journal of Psychosomatic Research*, **33**, 689–695.

Goldberg, G. & Huxley, P. (1980). *Mental Illness in the Community*, Tavistock, London.

Greer, S. & Cawley, R.H. (1966). Some observations on the natural history of neurotic illness, *Archdale Medical Monograph, No. 3*, Australian Publishing Company, Sydney.

Hallstrom, C. (1984). Practical aspects of the use of beta-blockers in anxiety states: morbid anxiety, *Postgraduate Medical Journal*, **60** (52), 26–28.

House, A.O. & Andrews, H.B. (1988). Life events and difficulties preceding the onset of functional dysphonia, *Journal of Psychosomatic Research*, **32**, 311–319.

Katon, W., Ries, R.K., Kleinman, A. (1984). A prospective study of 100 consecutive somatisation patients, *Comprehensive Psychiatry*, **25**, 305–314.

Kellner, R. (1983). Prognosis in treated hypochondriasis, *Acta Psychiatrica Scandinavica*, **67**, 69–79.

*Kellner, R., Abbott, P., Winslow, W.W. & Pathak, D. (1987). Fears, beliefs, and attitudes in DSM-III hypochondriasis, *Journal of Nervous and Mental Diseases*, **175**, 20–24.

Kellner, R., Fava, G.A., Lisansky, J., Pavine, G.I. & Zielezny, M. (1986). Hypochondriacal fears and beliefs in DSM-III melancholia: changes with amitriptyline, *Journal of Affective Disorders*, **10**, 21–26.

Kessel, N. (1979). Reassurance, *Lancet*, **i**, 1128–1133.

Klein, D.F. (1988). The cause and treatment of agoraphobia, *Archives of General Psychiatry*, **45**, 389–392.

Lader, M. & Sartorius, N. (1968). Anxiety in patients with hysterical conversion symptoms, *Journal of Neurology, Neurosurgery and Psychiatry*, **31**, 490–495.

Lelliot, P. & Marks, I.M. (1988). The cause and treatment of agoraphobia, *Archives of General Psychiatry*, **45**, 388–389.

Liebowitz, M.R., Quitkin, F.M., Stewart, J.W. *et al.* (1988). Antidepressant specificity in atypical depression, *Archives of General Psychiatry*, **45**, 29–37.

Linton, S.J. (1986). Behavioural remediation of chronic pain: a status report, *Pain*, **24**, 125–143.

Lloyd, G.G. (1986). Psychiatric syndromes with a somatic presentation, *Journal of Psychosomatic Research*, **30**, 113–120.

McKenna, P.J. (1984). Disorders with overvalued ideas, *British Journal of Psychiatry*, **145**, 579–585.

Magarian, G.J. (1982). Hyperventilation syndromes; infrequently recognised common expressions of anxiety and stress, *Medicine*, **61**, 219–236.

Main, C.J. & Waddell, G. (1987). Psychometric construction and validity of the illness behaviour questionnaire in British patients with chronic low back pain, *Pain*, **28**, 13–25.

Mally, M.A. & Ogston, W.D. (1964). Treatment of the 'untreatables', *International Journal of Group Psychotherapy*, **14**, 369–374.

*Mann, A.H., Jenkins, R., Cutting, J.C. & Cowen, P.J. (1981). The development and use of a standardised assessment of abnormal personality, *Psychological Medicine*, **11**, 839–847.

Marks, I.M. (1985). Syndromes of anxiety, *British Journal of Clinical Practice*, **39** (Suppl 38), 23–26.

Marks, I.M. (1987). *Fears, Phobias, and Rituals*, Oxford University Press, London.

*Marks, I.M. & Mathews, A.M. (1979). Brief standard self-rating for phobic patients, *Behaviour Research and Therapy*, **17**, 263–267.

Mavissakalian, M. (1986). Imipramine in agoraphobia, *Comprehensive Psychiatry*, **27**, 401–406.

Mayou, R.A. & Hawton, K. (1986). Psychiatric disorder in the general hospital, *British Journal of Psychiatry*, **149**, 172–190.

Mezzich, J.E. (1988). On developing a psychiatric multiaxial schema for ICD-10, *British Journal of Psychiatry*, **152** (Suppl 1), 38–43.

*Notes on Eliciting and Recording Clinical Information* (1983). The Department of Psychiatry Teaching Committee, The Institute of Psychiatry, London; Oxford University Press, London.

Noyes, R., Reich, J., Clancy, J. & O'Gorman, T.W. (1986). Reduction in hypochondriasis with treatment of panic disorder, *British Journal of Psychiatry*, **149**, 631–635.

Orenstein, H. (1989). Briquet's syndrome in association with depression and panic: a reconceptualisation of Briquet's syndrome, *American Journal of Psychiatry*, **146**, 334–338.

*Parker, G., Tupling, H. & Brown, L.B. (1979). A parental bonding instrument, *British Journal of Medical Psychology*, **52**, 1–10.

Paykel, E.S. & Norton, K.R. (1982). Masked depression, *British Journal of Hospital Medicine*, **28**, 151–157.

Pecknold, J.C., Swinson, R.P., Kuch, K. & Lewis, C.P. (1988). Alprazolam in panic disorder and agoraphobia: results from a multicenter trial. Discontinuation effects, *Archives of General Psychiatry*, **45**, 429–436.

Philips, H.C. (1987). The effects of behavioural treatment on chronic pain, *Behaviour Research and Therapy*, **25**, 365–377.

Philips, H.C. (1988). *The Psychological Management of Chronic Pain: A treatment manual*, Springer, New York.

*Pilowsky, I. (1967). Dimensions of hypochondriasis (The Whitely Index), *British Journal of Psychiatry*, **113**, 89–93.

*Pilowsky, I., Spence, N., Cobb, J. & Katsikitis, M. (1984). The illness behaviour questionnaire as an aid to clinical assessment, *General Hospital Psychiatry*, **6**, 123–130.

Pinder, R.M. (1988). The benefits and risks of antidepressant drugs, *Human Psychopharmacology*, **3**, 73–86.

Rachman, S., Levitt, K. & Lopatka, C. (1987). Panics — I The links between cognitions and bodily symptoms, *Behaviour Research and Therapy*, **25**, 411–423.

Rachman, S. & Hodgson, R. (1974). Synchrony and desynchrony in fear and avoidance, *Behaviour Research and Therapy*, **12**, 311–318.

Robins, L.N., Helzer, J.E., Croughan, J. et al. (1981). National Institute of Mental Health Diagnostic Interview Schedule, *Archives of General Psychiatry*, **38**, 381–389.

Roskin, G., Mehr, A., Rabiner, C.J. & Rosenberg, C. (1980). Psychiatric treatment of chronic somatising patients: a pilot study, *International Journal of Psychiatry in Medicine*, **10**, 181–188.

Salkovskis, P.M. (1989). Somatic problems, in *Cognitive Behaviour Therapy for Psychiatric*

*Problems* (Eds. Hawton, K., Salkovskis, P.M., Kirk, J. & Clark, D.M.), Oxford Medical Publications.

Salkovskis, P.M. & Warwick, H.M. (1986). Morbid preoccupations, health anxiety and reassurance: a cognitive behavioural approach to hypochondriasis, *Behaviour Research and Therapy*, **24**, 597–602.

Scaloubaca, D., Slade, P. & Creed, F. (1988). Life events and somatisation among Students, *Journal of Psychosomatic Research*, **32**, 221–229.

Sensky, T. (1986). The general hospital psychiatrist: Too many tasks and too few roles? *British Journal of Psychiatry*, **148**, 151–158.

Slavney, P.R. & Teitelbaum, M.L. (1985). Patients with medically unexplained symptoms: DSM-III diagnoses and demographic characteristics, *General Hospital Psychiatry*, **7**, 25–35.

Smith, G.R., Monson, R.A. & Ray, D.C. (1986). Psychiatric consultation in somatization disorder: a randomised control study, *New England Journal of Medicine*, **314**, 1407–1413.

Stewart, D.E. & Raskin, J. (1985). Psychiatric assessment of patients with '20th-century disease' ('total allergy syndrome'), *Canadian Medical Association Journal*, **133**, 1001–1006.

Taylor, G.J. (1984). Alexithymia: concept, management, and implications for treatment, *American Journal of Psychiatry*, **141**, 725–732.

*Taylor, G.J., Bagby, M., Ryan, D.P. *et al.* (1988). Criterion validity of the Toronto Alexithymia Scale, *Psychosomatic Medicine*, **50**, 500–509.

*Tyrer, P. (1987). *Personality Disorders. Diagnosis, Management and Course*, Wright, Bristol.

Tyrer, P. (1988). What's wrong with DSM-II personality disorders? *Journal of Personality Disorders*, **7**, 281–291.

*Tyrer, P., Alexander, M.S., Cicchetti, D.V., Cohen, M.S. & Remington, M. (1979). Reliability of a schedule for rating personality disorders, *British Journal of Psychiatry*, **135**, 168–174.

Tyrer, P. Fowler-Dixon, R. & Ferguson, B. (1990). The justification for the diagnosis of hypochondriacal personality disorder, *Journal of Psychosomatic Research* (in press).

Tyrer, P., Lee, I. & Alexander, J. (1980). Awareness of cardiac function in anxious, phobic and hypochondriacal patients, *Psychological Medicine*, **10**, 171–174.

Tyrer, P. & Shawcross, C. (1988). Monoamine oxidase inhibitors in anxiety disorders, *Journal of Psychiatric Research*, **22**, 87–98.

Warwick, H.M. & Marks, I.M. (1988). Behavioural treatment of illness phobia and hypochondriasis, *British Journal of Psychiatry*, **152**, 239–241.

Warwick, H.M. & Salkovskis, P.M. (1985). Reassurance, *British Medical Journal*, **290**, 1028.

Warwick, H.M. & Salkovskis, P.M. (1988). Hypochondriasis, in *Cognitive Therapy: a clinical casebook* (Eds. Scott, J., Williams, J.M. & Beck, A.T.), Croom Helm, London.

Watson, J.P. (1985). Frame of reference and the detection of individual and systemic problems, *Journal of Psychosomatic Research*, **29**, 571–577.

Watts, E. (1982). Attributional aspects of medicine in *Attributions and Psychological Change* (Eds. Antari, C. & Brewin, C.), Academic Press, London.

Wessely, S., David, A., Butler, S. & Chalder, T. (1989). The management of the post-viral fatigue syndrome, *Journal of the Royal College of General Practitioners*, **39**, 26–29.

*Zigmond, A.S. & Snaith, R.R. (1983). The hospital anxiety and depression scale, *Acta Psychiatrica Scandinavica*, **67**, 361–370.

Zonderman, A.B., Heft, M.W. & Costa, P.T. (1985). Does the illness behaviour questionnaire measure abnormal illness behaviour? *Health Psychology*, **4** (5), 425–436.

# 4
# Somatization in Primary Care Settings

T.K.J. CRAIG AND A.P. BOARDMAN

## Illness behaviour: symptom perception and consultation

A significant proportion of consultations in primary care settings are for complaints which cannot be adequately accounted for by any known organic pathology. In many instances, the only abnormality seems to lie in the intensity of the complaining itself and the resistance that the patients show to reassurance or explanations which fail to confirm their belief that physical illness is present. To understand how such misunderstandings and resistances arise, we need to look at how humans evaluate their own health status and what factors lead them to consult physicians.

### The perception and evaluation of symptoms

What people know about illness affects what sensations they regard as serious and what actions should be taken when these arise. But even if differences in past experience and knowledge about disease are taken into account there is a wide variation in the tolerance of discomfort and in the interpretation placed on bodily sensations. The main factors which lead people to interpret a bodily sensation as a sign of illness fall into two broad groups. First, there are characteristics of the sensations themselves; their frequency, intensity and susceptibility to non-illness interpretations. Symptoms which are frequent or highly visible (fever, chest pain, a broken leg) are more likely to be identified as abnormal and symptoms which interfere with routine social activity are more likely to be regarded as serious than more medically dangerous symptoms which have only minimal social impact. Second are characteristics of the person and their evaluative process. Mechanic (1983) reviews extensive evidence to suggest that *introspection* is a critical personal orientation in the illness perception process. He points out that results from studies investigating such varied issues as impaired self-esteem, objective self-awareness, pain response, self-consciousness and ego defense mechanisms all support the hypothesis that preoccupation with the self increases the prevalence of reported physical and psychological symptoms. Introspective individuals complain, for example, that keeping health diaries makes them feel worse and have more symptoms (Mechanic, 1986); they report more physical illnesses, are more upset by stressful life events and are heavier users of medical care (Mechanic, 1979, 1980; Greenley & Mechanic, 1976). He suggests that the price of sensitivity (associated with many valued attributes including creativity, empathy, and artistic expression), may well be an exaggeration of the experience of distress and illness.

**Determinants of consultation**

In the UK, if symptoms are reported, then the general practitioner (GP) is likely to be the first official port of call. Factors which promote consultation include the severity of symptoms, stressors in the social environment, family attitudes to illness and the coexistence of a mood disorder.

*Symptom severity*

Although most people suffer some abnormal sensations much of the time, only a few will take these sensations to doctors for advice (Banks *et al.*, 1975; Demers *et al.*, 1980; Hannay, 1980; Last, 1963; Roughman & Haggerty, 1972; Scambler *et al.*, 1981; White *et al.*, 1967). In a health diary study of women aged 20–44 years, Banks *et al.* (1975) found that, on average, women reported symptoms 10 days out of 28. These symptoms occurred in episodes of more than one day's duration and there was one consultation for 37 symptom episodes. But with one exception the symptoms recorded most frequently were not those which were most commonly reported. For example, of 184 episodes of headache only one was taken to the doctor compared with 1 in 14 episodes of chest pain. The exception concerned emotional symptoms, which accounted for an estimated 1160 episodes in the year, ranking third behind 'headache' and 'changes of energy', and led to consultation at a rate of 1 consultation per 46 episodes. Similar findings have been reported in other studies (Dunnell & Cartwright, 1972; Morell & Wale, 1976; Scambler *et al.*, 1981). This suggests that many symptoms are perceived as mild and unobtrusive, a conclusion given some support by the work of Ingham and Miller (1982). In a study comparing recent GP attenders with controls who had not seen their GP for at least 3 months, these authors found that the symptoms reported by the controls were, on average, less severe than those reported by the consulters.

*Sociodemographic factors*

Although symptom severity plays an important part in the decision to consult it is rarely the major reason for visiting the doctor (Mechanic, 1969). In general practice high consultation rates are characteristic of the elderly, the very young, and women in the age group 15–44 years (Banks *et al.*, 1975; Hannay, 1980; Marsh & McNay, 1974; Morrell *et al.*, 1970).

The near universal observation that women report more acute illnesses and are greater users of health care services than men of similar age may be due to several factors. For example, in the USA, consultations connected with pregnancy, gynaecological disorders and breast disease account for 79% of the reported female excess in utilization between the ages of 15 and 24 and 31% of the excess between the ages of 45 and 64 (e.g. Waldron, 1983). But even after taking account of these disorders women report higher symptom rates, reflecting a greater concern with health, a tendency towards 'introspection' and increased risk of emotional disorders (Mechanic, 1976; Waldron, 1983). There may also be sex differences in tolerance of discomfort, as significant differences between the sexes in responses to pain are said to be apparent from early childhood and increase with age (Mechanic, 1964). Finally, some studies have attempted to link broader sociocultural factors to this differential sex ratio — for example the fact that women are less likely to be employed and therefore have more time to attend consultations — though the evidence is patchy and inconclusive (Mechanic, 1976).

In the UK, other factors associated with high consultation rates include large family size, low social class, low educational attainment, unemployment and poor quality housing. But most of this sociodemographic data suffers from the fundamental weakness of cross-sectional and crude approximations of the social processes that shape consultation.

*Life stress and social support*

Both the stress of moving house and that of living with aircraft noise are associated with increased consultation (Bain & Philip, 1975; Watkins *et al.*, 1981); and consultation rates seem to be correlated with many other stressful life experiences (Miller *et al.*, 1976). Ingham (1980) reported a small but significant association between life events and consultation. But, except for psychiatric disorder (anxiety and depression), stress was not found to contribute to consultation once the severity of symptoms was taken into account. This observation appears to fit much of the data linking stress and consultation, and it seems that much of the correlation can be explained by the association between stress and disorders of mood.

There is little doubt that an individual's decision to seek expert medical advice is greatly influenced by his/her social milieu. The majority of symptoms taken to GPs are discussed first with a lay person (usually a relative) and these lay consultants often initiate the referral process directly (McKinlay, 1973; Scambler *et al.*, 1981; Suchman, 1964; Zola, 1973). Friedson (1970) argues that these studies point to certain general principles concerning consultation: illness is confirmed only if the sufferer shows evidence of symptoms that others in his/her social group believe represents disease and if he/she interprets bodily sensations in a way that other people find plausible. Help-seeking is organized by a 'lay referral system' comprising a lay culture which is more or less congruent with the beliefs of the medical profession, as well as a 'network of personal influences' which provides lay consultants to whom the individual can turn for advice and ultimately for sanctioning to seek professional help (Friedson, 1970). Of course, social networks can both promote or inhibit professional consultation. The precise direction of this influence depends partly on the wider cultural context.

In a classic study of the response to pain among patients in the USA, Zborowski (1952) noted that patients of Jewish and Italian extraction tended to respond in a more emotional manner than 'Old Americans' (i.e. those with ancestral origins linked to the earlier, largely British settlers), who were more stoical in their expressions of discomfort, while patients of Irish origin tended to deny pain. Although the Jewish and Italian patients shared a similar behavioural response to pain, they also differed in a number of ways. Jewish patients were more concerned with the implications for their future health and were concerned with the broader disease which lay behind the symptom, while the Italians sought immediate relief and were happy once this was obtained, with less desire to know why the pain arose and what implications it might have for the future.

*The family*

In trying to explain these differences, Zborowski (1952) emphasized the different family atmospheres and cultures at play during the patients' formative years. Jewish and Italian patients grew up in a family atmosphere of caution in relation to illness; mothers were concerned about their children's health and participation in sports, and constantly warned their offspring to avoid chills, fights and threatening situations. In contrast, the 'Old American' family emphasized the need to take pain 'like a man', not to cry or demonstrate behaviour which in that culture might connote moral weakness. He argued that such 'training' does not discourage the use of doctors, but rather ensures that their use is based on physical rather than emotional needs.

Similar arguments relating overprotective maternal attitudes to later anxieties about illness are raised by other workers and seem to have some empirical support. For example, Tessler (1980) found that first born children were more frequent users of health services, and in a longitudinal study of health service utilization which tracked children over a 16-year period, Mechanic (1976) found that later illness behaviour was in part determined by maternal attitudes to such matters as risk-taking, time off school or reduced occupational activity.

### Emotional disorders

Mood is a potent determinant of both the perception of illness and the decision to consult. A variety of studies suggest that emotional states influence the general sense of well-being, and people reporting poor health are often depressed, alienated and less satisfied with life (Apple, 1960; Baumann, 1961; Maddox, 1962). Prospective studies of health service utilization suggest that the level of psychological distress is a significant factor in predicting the utilization of general medical services even when other key variables such as past health status and severity of symptoms are controlled (Burvill & Knuiman, 1983; Shepherd *et al.*, 1966; Tessler *et al.*, 1976). There is also a close association between physical and psychiatric disorder. This probably represents the joint contribution of several different processes — psychiatric disorder can arise as a reaction to physical discomfort; both psychiatric and physical illnesses may occur independently; neurotic illness may increase the risk of later physical illness, and finally, psychiatric disorder can be mistakenly perceived as physical illness by some patients (Craig, 1989; Murphy & Brown, 1980; Sims, 1973).

Of course, it is not only sufferers who can misperceive psychiatric disorder. Lay beliefs about illness can at times exert pressures which appear quite perverse to professionals. Myalgic encephalomyelitis (ME) is a currently popular label for a syndrome which was first described in the middle of the last century (see Chapter 5, p. 110). Self-help groups have been widely established and the ME Association is now Britain's fastest growing charity. Political interest in the disorder has even resulted in legislation to mandate official research in the USA. Although the evidence is still inconclusive, it appears likely that some cases of ME are the result of viral infection. But it is equally apparent that many patients who are labelled (by themselves, their families and the medical profession) as suffering from ME may actually have an emotional illness. The consequence of this labelling is often to deny the sufferer appropriate psychological treatment. Furthermore, to suggest that psychological assessment should be carried out as a matter of routine in ME cases is viewed with horror by some sections of society. The popular appeal of 'alternative medicine', with its emphasis on diet, viruses and allergies, may well stem from its active rejection of psychological explanations for illness, which however accurate, remain universally unpopular, stigmatizing and resisted.

**Factors that promote the chronicity of symptoms**

Psychiatric disorders, particularly those involving depression or anxiety, also contribute to the persistence of somatic symptoms. A number of studies suggest that recovery following surgery is retarded if the patient was anxious preoperatively (Johnston & Carpenter, 1980; Sime, 1976; Wolfer & Davis, 1970). These effects have been demonstrated both for levels of postoperative pain (where the mechanism is believed to be a lowering of the pain threshold in anxious patients), postoperative organ function (where the mechanism may be a reluctance to participate in the postoperative physiotherapy), and even in terms of wound healing (where some investigators suggest that the autonomic arousal and associated increase in circulating catecholamines and corticosteroids retard healing — Mathews and Ridgeway, 1981).

There is also some evidence that, in addition to psychiatric disorder, more permanent personality attributes may affect recovery. For example, Parbrook *et al.* (1973) found that peptic ulcer patients who had high scores on the neuroticism subscale of the Eysenck Personality Inventory reported greater pain, had more postoperative infections and experienced more chest complications. Similarly, chest complications and reduced vital capacity following cholecystectomy are reported to be more prevalent in patients with high neuroticism scores (Dalrymple *et al.*, 1973). Perhaps the most intriguing observations, from a somatization point of view, are reported in studies of coping styles of surgical patients. For example, Cohen and Lazarus (1973) assessed patients' coping style by analyzing responses to a semistructured interview. They classified patients as exhibiting an 'avoidant' style on the basis of ratings of denial of the threat of the forthcoming surgical procedure and on their unwillingness to discuss thoughts about the operation. The postoperative outcome of these patients was contrasted with those who exhibited a 'vigilant' coping style characterized by being overtly alert to threatening aspects of the operation, seeking out knowledge about the medical condition and by the readiness to discuss thoughts about the operation. Remaining subjects were classified in an intermediate group. The avoidant group experienced fewer complications and were discharged much earlier than the vigilant group.

Similar observations have been made in non-surgical medical conditions. For example, Querido (1959) reported data on 1630 hospital inpatients who

were examined in terms of an index of current psychosocial stress, psychological state and the outcome of their illness 6–18 months later. The rating of psychological distress while the patient was in hospital was a better predictor of outcome than the clinician's assessment of prognosis. High levels of distress made an important contribution to recovery, independently of the nature of the physical disorder involved. In a follow-up study of patients with peptic ulceration, Rutter (1963) found that anxiety and depression scores at a first hospital visit were better indicators of prognosis than any available measure of physical state. Similarly, the amount of time off work for symptoms of chronic obstructive bronchitis was not predicted by standard measures of illness severity (e.g. FEV and $PCO_2$), but was highly correlated with a combination of psychological variables (Rutter, 1979). Finally, Cay *et al.* (1973) found that while physical factors were related to outcome 4 months after a myocardial infarction, after 1 year follow-up only psychosocial factors distinguished between those who had returned to work and those who continued to be disabled.

To summarize, both the perception of illness and the tendency to seek help are influenced by factors in the individual's domestic and social life. Psychiatric disorders, particularly those involving mood, exert a powerful influence on the onset and course of physical illness. In some instances these processes may outweigh the extent and influence of any coexisting physical disorder, and it is to this that we now turn.

## Somatization disorders

### Classification and definitions

The term somatization was first introduced by psychoanalytic writers to refer to a hypothetical process, closely allied to the concept of conversion, in which unconscious defense mechanisms suppressed the experience of anxious affect and permitted only the visceral expression of this neurosis to gain conscious awareness (e.g. Menninger, 1947). As with many classifications from this school of thought, it was an attempt at an aetiological taxonomy that dealt with a presumed reason for symptom formation. Later researchers have moved away from resorting to explanations that require unconscious mechanisms, but typically retain the link with emotion. Most authors would agree that the root of the disorder is a tendency to experience and communicate somatic symptoms which are unaccounted for by pathological findings, to attribute these to physical illness and to seek medical help for them (Lipowski, 1988).

The diagnostic categories included in the overall group of somatoform

disorders described in DSM-III-R (APA, 1987) have been widely adopted and have provided the basis for much research effort (see p. 10). But they are unsatisfactory starting points for understanding the process of somatization. The patients who form the basis of the classification are a highly skewed sample of the larger population of somatization in the community and many of the descriptive features say more about the factors that govern referral to hospital than they do about the phenomenon of somatization itself. Such definitions are also unlikely to provide the basis for sound aetiological research, as the factors which contribute to chronicity may well differ from those which brought about the disorder in the first place.

   A more useful classification is provided by Rosen *et al.* (1982). These authors distinguish *acute somatization* which lasts days or weeks, and develops out of stressful conditions, from *subacute somatization* which lasts for several months and originates in a prolonged stress response or actual psychiatric disorder (commonly depression and anxiety). Finally, these are both distinguished from *chronic somatization*, which lasts for years and results from either psychiatric or physical illness in which psychosocial stressors in local contexts of power (e.g. family conflicts, insufficient resources and employment difficulties) are the chief sources of symptom amplification and disability.

### Somatization in primary care and the community

Not surprisingly, when defined in terms of chronicity and resistance to treatment, these disorders are uncommon in primary care settings. For example, in a study of women aged 16–25 on the list of one group practice in Newcastle, Deighton and Nicol (1985) found a prevalence rate for Briquet's syndrome (somatization disorder q.v.) of no more than 2.04 per 1000. Similarly, studies in the USA suggest population prevalence rates of around 4 per 1000 for the same disorder (Swartz *et al.*, 1986). Although these extreme forms of the disorder are rare in primary care, acute and subacute conditions may be much more common. The process of somatization, in the sense described by Lipowski (1988), subsumes many diverse manifestations of emotional disorder. Of the 10–15% of the general population who experience symptoms of anxiety and depression in any single year (Brown & Harris, 1978; Surtees *et al.*, 1986) the vast majority will see their family doctor at least once for complaints related to their mood. Many of these people are not recognized as suffering from any form of emotional disorder largely because they do not complain directly of misery. Rather, they present a variety of physical aches and pains which sidetrack the unwary physician into a fruitless search for somatic pathology.

In the last two decades there have been numerous surveys of the psycho-logical health of patients in medical and surgical wards of general hospitals and of attenders at primary care settings. Most of these studies suggest that between one-quarter and one-third of patients have diagnosable psychiatric illnesses (Goldberg, 1970; Goldberg *et al.*, 1976; Hoeper *et al.*, 1979; Skuse & Williams, 1984). Rates of this magnitude turn up time and again and this suggests that depression, with or without anxiety, is one of the most common disorders in primary care (Katon *et al.*, 1982). As many as three-quarters of these patients visit their family doctor complaining of physical symptoms for which no organic cause can be found (Kellner, 1966). Similarly, as many as half of all patients who are referred on to secondary care medical services have no organic basis for their complaints (e.g. Mayou, 1973; MacDonald & Bouchier, 1980). These patients also account for a disproportionately high number of laboratory investigations, drug prescriptions and surgical opera-tions (Anderson *et al.*, 1977; McFarland *et al.*, 1985).

This data suggests that the problem of somatization in primary care is largely that of somatic presentations of emotional disorders. In an important study, Bridges and Goldberg (1985) examined new onsets of disorders in general practice, and defined somatization as comprising four essential criteria:

1   The patient must seek medical help for somatic manifestations of a psychiatric illness;
2   He/she must attribute these somatic complaints to physical rather than emotional disease;
3   Psychiatric disorder must be present and detectable by standardized research criteria;
4   Treatment of the psychiatric disorder should cause the somatic manifesta-tions to disappear or revert to the level that they were before the episode of psychiatric disorder.

This definition has the distinct advantage of emphasizing that somatiza-tion is a *process* rather than a discrete disorder and therefore it can occur even when there is coincidental organic illness. Bridges and Goldberg (1985) con-ducted detailed interviews with a stratified sample of 497 people presenting at general practices in Manchester with a new inception of illness. Approxi-mately one-third of the total number fulfilled DSM-III criteria for psychiatric diagnoses. The majority of these psychiatric disorders were accompanied by physical symptoms. The most common explanation for this association was the somatic presentation of an emotional disorder (approximately 19% of inceptions), but independent physical and emotional illness accounted for approximately 10% of all presentations.

Similar findings were reported in a recent study of members of a health maintenance organization in the USA. MacFarland *et al.* (1985) found that 13% of enrolees were consistently high users of medical services, and that these patients had a particularly high prevalence of depression, complained of more physical symptoms and more often described anxiety as a presenting symptom than low frequency users. But they also had more episodes of demonstrable organic illness and died earlier than low users.

## Aetiology: the perception of bodily discomfort

Somatization is essentially a disorder of appraisal. Bodily symptoms are ubiquitous, yet some individuals seem more ready than others to ascribe illness explanations to these. Recent research in this field can be divided into (i) studies which demonstrate that somatizing patients are more aware of bodily functioning than either healthy persons or, more importantly, people with purely physical disease; and (ii) evidence which implicates a disorder of learning, personality or mood to account for this heightened awareness.

### *Somatizing patients are more aware of body functioning*

Individuals differ widely in their reactions to pain (Barsky, 1979; Melzack, 1973). Disease conviction is associated with low pain thresholds and tolerance to experimentally induced pain (Merskey & Evans, 1975). Chronic somatizers seem to be more sensitive to a wide range of internal bodily cues, even when these are not part of the symptoms which currently concern them. For example, hypochondriacal and anxious patients estimated their heart rate more accurately than other patients (Tyrer *et al.*, 1980), and hypochondriacal students were more sensitive than nonhypochondriacal students in a two flash fusion task (Hanback & Revelle, 1978). This heightened perception of bodily function may reflect a wider tendency to overestimate sensation. In one study, subjects were classified as 'augmenters' or 'reducers' according to the accuracy with which they could recall the dimensions of a shape which was presented to them briefly. Augmenters (who overestimated the size of the object) showed a markedly reduced tolerance to induced pain and scored higher on the Minnesota Multiphasic Personality Inventory hypochondriasis scale (Petrie, 1967). A more recent study (Tyrer *et al.*, 1990) suggests that this tendency to heightened awareness of bodily function may occasionally be sufficiently intense to justify a psychiatric diagnosis of hypochondriacal personality disorder. Using a structured interview for assessing personality disorders, these authors identified a small group of patients (2.5% of 1000 psychiatric consultations) in whom there was a lifelong preoccupation with the maintenance of health, a distorted perception of minor ailments and the excessive use of both medical and lay health agencies (see Chapter 2, p. 32).

## Somatizing patients may have 'learned' deviant patterns of interpretation of bodily sensations

Although the research evidence is relatively weak, there are a few studies which suggest that this process begins early in life under the influence of the family environment. A growing child often spends more time in the company of the mother, who may be unduly preoccupied with health and illness. Such a mother is likely, in turn, to influence the extent to which the child attends to bodily complaints (Mechanic, 1980). It has also been suggested that a child may learn that complaining of physical symptoms can result in increased parental attention or a means of avoiding undesirable obligations (e.g. Mechanic, 1980; Apley & Hale, 1973). The evidence that adult somatization might develop from a family environment which encourages the somatic expression of distress comes from two sources. First, there are studies which suggest that children exposed to serious physical illness in their close family are at greater risk of somatization when they grow up (Hartvig & Sterner, 1985; Mechanic, 1980; Kriechman, 1987; Shapiro & Rosenfeld, 1986). Second, there is evidence that functional somatic symptoms in children bear close resemblance to concurrent symptoms in other adult family members (Apley, 1958; Apley & Hale, 1973; Christensen & Mortensen, 1975; Oster, 1972; Davidson & Wasserman, 1966).

## Episodes of acute somatization seem to arise in the presence of disordered mood

The factors reviewed so far, such as a heightened awareness of bodily function, are not sufficient on their own to explain onset. We can afford to make this statement since the somatizing patients will, like their non-somatizing counterparts, have experienced many symptomatic episodes in the past which neither led to disease labelling nor to consultation. Some additional process must be present at key points in time which, coupled with this 'constitutional' susceptibility, triggers the episode. Given present understanding, a disorder of mood is the most likely candidate.

There is extensive evidence linking somatization phenomena with mood disorder. More patients with functional symptoms are depressed or anxious than are patients with physical disease and they are also more likely to have experienced the sort of severe life events which are common precipitants of affective disorder (Bass & Wade, 1984; Craig & Brown, 1985; Creed, 1981; Craig, 1989). Depressed patients have more functional somatic symptoms, including non-specific aches and pains, than other general medical and surgical patients (Katon *et al.*, 1982; von Knorring, 1975; Sternbach, 1974; Bradley, 1963; Lindsay & Wyckoff, 1981). Furthermore, hypochondriacal complaints tend to be correlated with anxiety and depression (Sheehan *et al.*, 1980; Bianchi, 1973). Indeed, anxiety and depression are so commonly associated with hypochondriasis that some authors doubt whether the latter is an independent syndrome at all (e.g. Kenyon, 1964; Ladee, 1966). Others have suggested that it is the manifestation of a personality tendency to perceive bodily sensations as abnormal which is triggered or amplified by a disorder of mood (e.g. Kellner, 1982; Pilowsky, 1970).

A pattern to much of this data is now emerging. Mood disorder is associated with physical symptoms in two ways. First, the mood disorder serves to draw attention to a physical sensation that otherwise might have been ignored. This may be the mechanism behind the clinical presentation of the irritable bowel syndrome, where a disorder of gut motility is probably present but not symptomatic until the patient's attention is brought to focus on his/her bodily function by the occurrence of severe stressors or the onset of emotional disorder (Craig, 1989; Creed, 1981; see also Chapter 6, p. 146). Second, the symptoms which the patient perceives and which are presented to the doctor are actually symptoms of the mood disorder itself. For example, it is proposed that the headache associated with feeling tense is the result of increased tension in voluntary muscles (Malmo & Shagass, 1949; Sainsbury & Gibson, 1954); preoccupation with cardiac symptoms typify many anxiety neuroses and these symptoms tend to resolve as the levels of fearfulness abate (Lader & Marks, 1971). Other symptoms are associated with changes in the body's biochemistry, as may occur when hyperventilation results from acute anxiety (Bass & Gardner, 1985). In general, the evidence for links between somatic presentation and these physiological states is fairly good (Grings & Dawson, 1978) and is supported by experimental manipulation (e.g. Tyrer *et al.*, 1980). It is not that the somatic symptoms replace the experience of affect; usually they coexist and can be easily identified if the right questions are asked. Subjects tend to have a consistent pattern of physiological responses to stress across different situations and across time (Lacey *et al.*, 1953; 1958). That is to say, similar somatic symptoms recur in future episodes of stress (Cloniger *et al.*, 1984).

In the general practice setting, the second of these two mechanisms is the most likely explanation for non-organic bodily complaints, i.e. patients suffering from depression and anxiety complain of bodily sensations that are part of a mood disorder. In fact, it may be that this is more typical of first presentations of depression than are complaints of psychological distress. Hence, most cross-cultural studies suggest that although the core vegetative symptoms such as insomnia, weight loss and muscle pains occur in all cultures, the cognitive changes such as sadness, guilt and self-depreciation are less common presentations in non-Western societies (Marsella, 1979; 1980). For example, in studies of traditional Arab cultures where stoicism is highly valued, complaints of sadness, guilt and self-depreciation are uncommon while complaints of gastrointestinal symptoms and other somatic complaints are usual. However, as the culture becomes more Westernized, the form of depression approaches that seen in the West (Racy, 1980).

The conclusions of studies of individual societies are reinforced by a few impressive multinational research programmes. In a study sponsored by the World Health Organization, the general health questionnaire was administered to 1624 patients in primary health care clinics in Colombia, India, Sudan and the Philippines. The most common presenting symptoms in the total sample were headaches, abdominal pains, cough, genitourinary complaints and dizziness. Fourteen per cent of the subjects were thought to have a psychiatric disorder detectable by Western semistructured psychiatric interview schedules (the Present State Examination — Wing *et al.*, 1974). Primary diagnoses were depression, anxiety, schizophrenia, affective psychosis and mental retardation. The presenting complaints of the psychiatrically 'ill' subjects were very similar to those of the total sample, the most common being weakness, dizziness, headache and abdominal pain (Harding *et al.*, 1980).

Leff (1981) suggests that the explanation of this tendency for peoples of 'non-Western' societies to use somatic rather than emotional representations of disease may reflect an evolutionary pattern in the development of words for unpleasant emotions. For example, in the earliest stages, single words reflect the somatic accompaniments of dysphoria; later, the same word comes to connote both a psychological and physical aspect of emotion, and finally, the word loses its physical associations entirely. In this view, 'psychologization' is a more recent phenomenon. He also presents evidence to suggest that unpleasant emotions seem to be less well differentiated in non-Indo-European cultures and suggests that 'languages with a restricted vocabulary of emotions do impair patients' ability to express emotions in a well-differentiated way' (Leff, 1981, p. 48). This formulation has been criticized both on empirical and conceptual grounds. Critics argue that the psychological and social significances of self-statements go deeper than the actual words used and can be understood only when their meaning within a particular society is taken into account. Therefore, the absence of specific words for emotion does not necessarily imply any lack of psychological sophistication; although an Iranian may refer to 'heart distress', he has no difficulty in conveying to others that he is distressed and the term probably conveys the same fundamental meaning as complaints of misery and tension do in the West (Good, 1977). Similarly, although Afghans with depression have no words to describe feelings of sadness and complain instead of a 'squeezing of the heart', they can differentiate this state from the grief felt for a deceased loved one, and indigenous mental health professionals have no difficulty in recognizing this as a synonym for depression (Waziri, 1973). Problems only arise when the patient is confronted by a 'Western' doctor, or where the popular concept of valid symptom presentation is very different from that held by the physician.

Regardless of the validity of Leff's theory, there is little doubt that an individual's expression of emotion is heavily influenced by the social context and the taboos against emotive expression. In impressive studies of neurasthenia in the Hunan Chinese, Kleinman (1986) utilized a Western semi-structured research interview schedule to interview 100 patients diagnosed as 'neurasthenic' by local doctors. Eighty-seven per cent of the patients fulfilled the criteria for major depressive disorder and a further 6% fulfilled DSM-III criteria for other forms of depression. All the patients had sought medical care for physical symptoms, with headaches, insomnia, dizziness and bodily pains being the most common. Fewer than 1 in 10 of these patients actually complained of depression although the majority experienced some dysphoric symptoms that could be ascertained if and when they were directly sought by the research interviewer. Kleinman pointed out that in the local social and cultural context, complaining of dysphoric symptoms came too close to admitting to highly stigmatized mental illness and to dissatisfaction with the way things were run by the state. Both patients and doctors shared this reserve of admitting to emotional illness; both utilized biological models to explain symptoms and both expected to give and receive physical medical treatments.

It is easy to dismiss these studies as interesting case histories from exotic cultures with little relevance to Western experience. However, studies of our own health care system show remarkably similar patterns. Recent large-scale epidemiological studies in the USA tend to confirm the ubiquity of somatization symptoms. In one such study Escobar *et al.* (1987) found that the most common symptoms included pains, palpitations, dizziness and faintness and the mean number of such symptoms was significantly related to the presence of psychiatric disorder as elicited by a structured psychiatric interview. Similar findings have been reported in UK studies carried out in primary care settings, where the majority of emotional disorders present with somatic symptoms (Boardman, 1987; Bridges & Goldberg, 1985; Hesbacher *et al.*, 1975; Marks *et al.*, 1979).

Our own research group has recently completed a study of affective disorder in general practice. In this study we were particularly interested in people who were presenting symptoms for the first time during a current episode of illness. Of 1220 consecutive consultations with 19 local general practitioners, 247 were first ever presentations of new episodes of illness. Of these, 85 had a primary or secondary diagnosis of affective disorder according to research diagnostic criteria. But very few of these psychiatric cases presented a straightforward story of depression or anxiety. When we analysed videotape recordings of their consultations with their family doctor we found that three-quarters had initial complaints which involved physical symptoms only (predominantly complaints of pain). Half the subjects made no direct mention of depression throughout the entire interview with their GP, even though the majority had no difficulty discussing their mood state with our researcher after the consultation. These patients presented bodily rather than emotional symptoms for much the same reasons as the Hunan Chinese — the stigma of psychological disorder; their belief that doctors were there only to treat physical illness (and the doctors' tacit agreement with this); and the belief in the virtue of stoicism (Craig *et al.*, in preparation).

### Life events, stress and secondary pain

There is now a large body of evidence attesting to the fact that emotional disorders can be brought about by the experience of severely threatening life events, particularly those which involve the loss or threatened loss of close emotional ties (Brown & Harris, 1978; Finlay-Jones & Brown, 1980; Paykel *et al.*, 1969). If, as we have argued, emotional disorder lies behind many presentations of acute and subacute somatization in primary care, then studies should detect links between somatization and the patient's experience of prior life events and other environmental stressors. Several studies support this; severely threatening life events, mainly involving losses, precede some functional disorders (Craig, 1989; Creed, 1981; Kellner, 1983). Furthermore, patients with somatization syndromes have not only a higher incidence of recent bereavement than patients with 'organic' illnesses (Burns & Nichols, 1972), but also the symptoms they report resemble those experienced during the terminal illness of the deceased (Parkes, 1965; Zisook & DeVaul, 1977).

Earlier, we presented evidence that the choice between somatization or psychologization is largely determined by the extent to which expressions of mental distress are condoned or condemned by culture and immediate social networks. In this formulation, there is nothing specific about the role of stressors, as they are important only in so far as they initiate distress. However, in addition to a general tendency to respond somatically, it is also possible that responses are determined by the nature of the stressful experience. In our own culture, for example, it may be reasonable to admit to mental distress after a bereavement and to expect sympathy and support from close friends and family. But this support is less likely to be forthcoming for a threatened break-up of a romance or a transfer to an undesirable task at work. Furthermore, misery is unlikely to stop a lover leaving or to prevent a work transfer taking place, while a physical illness may achieve just this and gain sympathy and support as well. Physical illness can also extricate people from undesirable commitments or from circumstances where failure would be painful and demoralizing. This idea, that somatization represents blame avoidance coupled with some personal gain, is hardly new. It runs as a major thread through most of the literature reviewed in preparing this chapter. However, there are virtually no studies which have specifically set out to test this hypothesis and it is still very much a notion based on clinical impression. In one of the very few studies of relevance, House and Andrews (1988) observed that the onset of 'functional' dysphonia was strongly associated with the prior occurrence of life events and chronic difficulties which involved a 'conflict over speaking out'. They defined this conflict as a situation in which on the one hand a person might wish to protest or complain, or to intervene verbally in some way, but on the other one in which such forthrightness would lead to adverse social consequences or difficulties.

### The effect of medical consultation on the course of somatization

Most discussions of somatization acknowledge that inappropriate physical and laboratory investigations can intensify a patient's conviction that he/she is physically ill, and most place a high priority on the early detection and treatment of mood disorders as a means of limiting chronicity. But this course is more easily prescribed than followed. Emotional disorders are misdiagnosed because patients present with somatic rather than emotional complaints or because of inadequate psychiatric knowledge and skill on the part of physicians. Even when they are detected, mood disorders may be dismissed as irrelevant or even 'trivial' (Cartwright, 1967; Cooperstock, 1971; Mechanic, 1970). For example, depression in women is sometimes thought to be a 'normal' reaction at a particular age and stage in life, or seen as a reaction to physical disease. These attitudes are bound to reinforce any tendency to somatize. In a study of consultation patterns of depressed women, Ginsberg and Brown (1982) found that the chances of depression being detected remained constant at 1 in 4 until the patient had made at least four visits, or the depression had lasted 12 months or longer. Only one in four presented their depression in a straightforward way (with complaints such as bad nerves, violence to children or worries). The women perceived depression as an inappropriate complaint to take to doctors. Half the women interviewed thought that doctors were there to deal with physical symptoms only and two-thirds said that doctors did not have enough time to talk. Finally, three-quarters of the women who were given drugs for their depression saw this as a rejection. All were looking for an opportunity to to talk about their feelings.

Obviously, we cannot wait for a change in attitudes to mental illness, or expect that educational campaigns will necessarily make all patients more willing to discuss emotions with doctors. If detection is to be improved we will have to look to the skills of the physician. A psychologically orientated doctor, with an interest and knowledge about psychiatry, detects more emotional disorder than one who is not knowledgeable or interested (Goldberg & Huxley, 1980; Shepherd *et al.*, 1966). This is not only a matter of asking the right questions, but also attending to a host of verbal and non-verbal cues emitted by the emotionally distressed patient.

In our current study of somatization of affect in primary care, we noted that 79% of first presentations with a mood disorder were couched in somatic terms only. This had a profound effect on the likelihood of detection. Only about half of these emotional disorders were detected by the GP compared with over 80% of disorders which presented with emotional or psychosocial complaints. Detection also depended on the skill of the doctor. In Figure 4.1, doctors are divided according to their 'identification index' (ii — a measure of the doctor's ability to identify symptomatic cases). Doctors with high-ii have been shown to display an interest in psychiatry, to look at their patients and to be good at dealing with interruptions to the interview (Goldberg & Huxley, 1980). Figure 4.1 shows the proportion of psychiatric cases correctly detected by low-ii and high-ii GPs by whether the patient presented with a physical or emotional complaint. While both high- and low-ii GPs do not differ in their ability to identify cases that present with emotional symptoms, the high-ii GPs are less likely to be misled by complaints of physical symptoms.

This data suggests an interaction between doctor's skills and cues emitted by patients. Davenport *et al.* (1987) have taken this a stage further. They examined videotapes of consultations of high- and low-ii doctors, measuring verbal and non-verbal cues emitted by the patients during consultation. Although verbal and non-verbal cues are strongly related to emotional disorder, there was a striking difference between the total number of cues

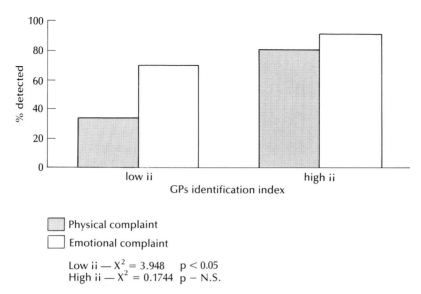

**Fig. 4.1.** Effect of identification index (ii) and presenting complaint on detection.

given by patients with emotional disorder which depended on the identification index of the doctor. Patients seeing high-ii doctors displayed, on average, 19.2 emotional cues compared with an average of only 10.8 cues in patients who attended low-ii doctors. For both total cues and vocal cues, there was a significant interaction on the two-way analyses of variance, indicating that although there was little effect of the identification index on patients without emotional disorder, there was a significant effect among those with emotional symptoms. In short, the high-ii doctor seems to encourage emotionally disordered patients to exhibit more cues; and this in turn increases the likelihood that the emotional disorder will be accurately detected.

It is still unclear whether it is these disorders which eventually become chronic, or whether the chronic somatizer represents the outcome of a process that does not involve undetected mood disorder. What one can say is that most theories of chronic somatization do involve a presumption that various psychosocial stressors, early life experiences and the effects of the social network are more important factors in symptom formation than any fundamental disorder of organ function. These presumptions are now being broadly supported by research across many fields of endeavour. It is also highly likely that mood disorder accentuates the perception of somatic symptoms and promotes help seeking so that even if it is not central to the 'cause' of the chronic disorder, it almost certainly plays a part in the timing and intensity of new episodes or relapses. We can bring some anecdotal evidence from our current study to bear on this issue in the form of two case histories with very different outcomes.

The first concerns a 40-year-old married woman who had presented to her GP complaining of head and back pain. Her depressive symptoms went undetected though she was able to discuss these with us and was rated as a mixed case of anxiety and depression at interview (Bedford College criteria — see Brown & Harris, 1978). During the subsequent 18 months, her depression and pains persisted. She believed that the two symptom clusters were unrelated and continued to seek medical help for the pain. Although her regular GP was by that time in no doubt that the headaches were 'functional', she managed to attract the attentions of a deputizing service one evening and was admitted to the local general hospital with suspected meningitis. Following discharge the next day, her resentment and symptoms intensified. She developed diplopia, weakness and eventually paralysis. She was admitted eventually to the local psychiatric hospital with a diagnosis of conversion hysteria in a hypochondriacal personality.

Our second case concerns a woman who became depressed when she lost her part-time job in her younger sister's hairdressing firm. For years she had been committed to caring for another older sister who suffered from multiple sclerosis which had been undetected for 10 years. Our subject had developed a number of hypochondriacal concerns at the time of her older sister's diagnosis and at one time had a bulging record of consultations. However, in more recent years, as her children grew older, her hypochondriacal concerns had abated and before our index episode she had not consulted her doctor for over a year. Shortly after losing her job, she and her younger sister had an argument that concerned their mutual commitments and some resentment was expressed about what she considered to be the unfair load she had to bear in looking after their sibling. She became mildly depressed and simultaneously noticed that her axilla felt uncomfortable. Close examination showed that the skin was 'more shiny and tense' and she immediately became alarmed by the thought of cancer. Her doctor reassured her but she was unconvinced. In the 6 months following the onset of her symptoms she consulted her doctor on innumerable occasions, and persuaded him to perform three cervical smears (the first two revealing slightly abnormal findings that were not seen on the last test). Shortly before our follow-up interview, her family started relieving her of the burden of caring for her sister and she found herself another job. Both her depression and her hypochondriacal concerns resolved although she still complained to the interviewer of her peculiar axillary sensation, for which she now had no explanation.

## Summary and synthesis

Although there are many questions still to be answered about the genesis and course of somatization, enough is known to provide a theoretical model which includes most of the major steps along the way. In this model (Fig. 4.2) somatization is seen as one result of an individual's attempt to come to terms with his/her environment (psychologization is the other). The process begins with an appraisal of the situation in which the individual finds him/herself. In this scheme of things, appraisal stands as a shorthand expression for the complex, intrapsychic processes through which people come to ascribe meaning to their experiences. Meaning is determined by past experience of similar events, by the threat that crises pose to current plans or goals and by a general awareness of what such events mean to others in similar situations. Crises lead us to brood on what our lives have been about, what we have achieved and what will become of us; and by their very nature, they trigger strong emotion (Brown & Harris, 1978). As Leventhal (1980) points out, perceptions are automatically referred to memories of previous emotions and the circumstances which elicited these. In most instances the links between emotion and its environmental triggers (past and present) are conscious. But sometimes emotional responses seem to occur in the absence of any aware-ness of their original basis, as for example when fear and resentment are elicited in response to persons in authority with no conscious link to the earlier experience which first shaped this antipathy. In this case, it is often the occurrence of the strong emotion which drives the individual to seek its source and to bring this to conscious awareness by an effort of will (Epstein, 1983).

Returning to our theoretical model, strong emotion (dysphoria) is the immediate precursor of most somatization. How these dysphoric states come to be expressed, however, depends both on individual response styles and on the cultural context. At an individual level it appears that any of four

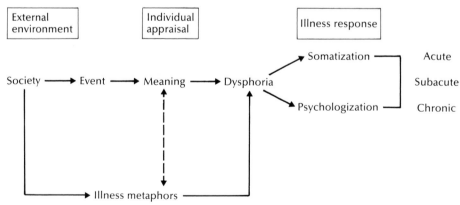

**Fig. 4.2.**  Theoretical model for somatization.

mechanisms may or                                              amplify the bodily signals that
accompany d··                                                  ective component of psychophysiological                                                  c components of arousal and
attribute these                                                to use a particular type of
coping style in v                                              e—somatic components of
arousal are height.                                            level, somatization rather than
psychologization o.                      where bodily disease is seen as a valid
consequence of stre.            .e there is a high level of stigma and taboo
associated with men    .usease. Of course, these culturally determined
attitudes to illness affect not only patients, but also their kin and their
therapists, so that everyone colludes to produce a biological theory of disease
in which personal responsibility for illness is minimized and in which disability associated with physical illness is more acceptable than 'bad nerves' or
mental illness.

Kleinman (1986) summarizes the essence of this theoretical model as
follows: '(somatization is) ... the presentation of personal and interpersonal
distress in an idiom of physical complaints together with a coping pattern of
medical help seeking .... Loss, injustice, failure, conflict — all are trans-
formed into discourse about pain and disability that is a metaphor for disease
and action about the self and the social world' (Kleinman, 1986, p. 51).

## Management and treatment

Viewed in the light of this causal model, the most obvious therapeutic task is
the identification of dysphoria and its symptomatic relief (with drug treatment if necessary). As our illustrative case histories showed, the failure to
recognize this can lead to inappropriate investigations, ambiguous diagnoses
and unhelpful treatments, which only serve to reinforce the patient's conviction that organic disease must be present and may even make matters
worse by introducing real organ damage or the side-effects of medication.
However, identifying emotional problems involves more than simply
checking off a list of symptoms of depression. A comprehension management strategy includes: locating the personal and environmental factors that
initiate and maintain the patterns of inappropriate illness behaviour; getting
the patient to accept a revised causal model which places these, rather than
disease, as the source of the discomfort; and persuading the patient to change
his/her behaviour to lessen their impact. David Goldberg and his colleagues
have recently produced a persuasive analysis of the tasks which must be
successfully accomplished in treating these disorders. They outline a model
of treatment which involves three stages of a reattribution process — making
the patient feel understood, changing the agenda and making the links

between physical symptoms and psychosocial difficulties (Goldberg *et al.,*
1989; Gask *et al.,* 1989).

*Making the patient feel understood*

Patients enter consultations with certain beliefs about the function of their
bodies and the signals which represent disease. They also carry resistances to
non-organic explanations which are part cultural and part personally determined. Finally, they enter with a number of expectations of treatment and of
their doctors' competence. This includes the expectation that the doctor will
be able to get to the bottom of the disorder provided he/she asks the right
questions and carries out the most appropriate examination and investigation. Against this background it is clear that the patient is likely to feel
rejected and not taken seriously if the doctor quickly attributes complaints to
depression, tension, or 'stress', without first taking a careful history.

The most important determinant of a patient's views on the competence
of his/her physician is the quality of the consultation. Competent doctors are
seen as taking more time enquiring about symptoms, avoiding repetitive
questioning, seeking clarification and displaying an empathic and open
attitude to emotional material. Measures of competence also correlate with
how well key complaints are elicited — imprecise or vague questioning leads
patients to feel that the doctor has missed important facts (Thompson &
Anderson, 1982). And there is little doubt that the explanations and treatments of a doctor who is judged to be incompetent are less likely to be
accepted than one who is viewed positively.

Of course, good history taking is also necessary if the doctor is to come to
an adequate understanding of the somatizing process. But beliefs cannot be
changed without attention to resistances and expectations. However good the
questioning, most patients with physical symptoms expect to be examined
and may have wondered about the possibility of a laboratory investigation. If
these are not indicated, the doctor must take the time to explain why they are
unnecessary. In the treatment of chronic somatization it is now accepted that
patients do best if they continue to see a single doctor who knows them, their
histories, and family situation in some detail. It is argued that this guards
against potentially dangerous but unindicated invasive diagnostic interventions (e.g. Ford, 1983; and Chapter 12). The same is certainly true of
acute somatization. Balint (1964) put forward the 'collusion of anonymity' in
which no one doctor took responsibility for difficult patients as one of the
major drawbacks of primary care of the period. But, despite the current
emphasis on personal care and personalized registers in general practice
(Pereira Gray, 1979) it is still a common phenomenon today — the patients in

our study of somatization universally decried the system where no one was given their 'own' doctor but saw whoever was available on the day.

## Changing the agenda

The purpose of this vital task is to shift the basis of the consultation towards a consideration of psychosocial factors that cause or aggravate the symptoms. A complete history, even for clear cut 'organic' disorders, ought to include information on personal and environmental factors which aggravate symptom severity or disability. For somatization disorders however, it is a particularly important step as this may be the entire basis of treatment intervention. With careful guidance, anyone can be led to discuss work, family and personal relationships and most see the relevance of their social context to their illness. Even chronic somatizers are not wholly resistant to the notion that psychosocial factors contribute to illness (they just resent the imputation that this is the most important factor). From this discussion, the patient is steered towards re-framing their problems. Open exploratory questions are often enough, such as 'I wonder if these symptoms are worse when you are tense/angry/depressed/at work/etc.'. When evidence that this may be the case is already to hand, simply reflecting this back to the patient can be useful (e.g. 'It seems that the symptoms are worse since you changed jobs. Is this right?').

## Making the link

Several strategies can be used to encourage patients to make the link between somatic symptoms and the psychosocial factors which lie behind these. It is never sufficient to state a medical belief that 'stress causes these symptoms' but, having an armamentarium of typical explanations is very useful — for example, that depression lowers pain thresholds or that anxiety increases attention to bodily sensations. These general explanations may need to be supplemented by more specific education about physiological processes and how these are influenced by 'stress'. We have found it helpful for example, in treating people with functional gastrointestinal disorder, to spend some time explaining how bowel motility is controlled and the reasons why normal motility can be impaired by environmental factors; similarly, patients with symptoms of hyperventilation will make efforts to change breathing behaviour one they grasp the biological basis for their symptoms. Often, these explanations can be reinforced by demonstrations such as showing that overbreathing does indeed produce light-headedness and paraesthesia (see Chapter 7, p. 192).

Health diaries, kept over a relatively short period of time, can form the

basis of a later, fruitful consultation linking patterns of symptoms to environmental stress. One patient, for example, noticed that his headaches and
bowel symptoms were aggravated on days when he had to travel to his head
office for a meeting with his boss. To make the appointment, he had to cross
the city and always seemed to get stuck in traffic jams. Although he put this
down to factors beyond his control (increased road transport use in London),
it was clear that he never allowed himself enough time for the journey. This
was related to his belief that he was 'laid back' by nature as well as to a
resented sense of obligation since marriage and parenthood. His anger
stemmed from outrage that he had been threatened with dismissal for poor
time keeping, coupled with his need for a steady income now that he was a
father of three. His symptoms cleared up after he was transferred to duties
which no longer required his visits to head office, even though he complained bitterly that this was, in effect, a demotion. Another young man
entirely lost his cardiac symptoms once he was persuaded to give up medita-
tion. In a very real sense, his search for his self had backfired when he noticed
irregularities in his cardiac rhythm and later found it impossible to deflect his
attention from these.

   The stages dealt with here are only a framework to approach the
somatizing patient. They will often extend over more than one consultation
and need to be covered again and again. All require quite sophisticated interviewing skills, though little in the way of specialized psychotherapy technique. A variety of training methods aimed at enhancing communication
skills have been developed, and those based on individual or small group
teaching using feedback linked to video or audiotaped consultations with real
and simulated patients seem particularly promising vehicles for improving
clinical detection and management skills. There is evidence to suggest that
doctors can radically alter their interviewing techniques following such
training (e.g. Goldberg *et al.*, 1980a, b; Lesser, 1985) and that this modification actually improves the accuracy of case detection (Goldberg *et al.*, 1980b).
Trainees with the poorest interview skills stand to gain the most from such
training but even experienced, psychologically orientated doctors show
improvements (Gask *et al.*, 1987a, b). Improvements in skills have been
shown to persist for up to 18 months (the longest follow-up period examined
to date) and to be appreciated by the clients of the trained doctors (D.
Goldberg, 1989 — personal communication).

   In addition to improved detection and better communication, several
studies of 'supportive' psychotherapy have shown good results of treatment
though adequately controlled trials are few and far between (Cohen & White,
1951; Melson *et al.*, 1982; Svedlund *et al.*, 1983; see also Chapter 6, p. 164).
Good results have also been reported for simple relaxation procedures in

muscle tension pains (Blanchard *et al.*, 1980) and simple behavioural psycho-therapy techniques for a wide range of mild hypochondriacal states (Kumar & Wilkinson, 1971). These and other specific therapies of functional disorders are discussed in more detail in the relevant chapters of this volume. But whatever the approach, a major component in all is their ability to get the patients to revise their views of the seriousness of their physical symptoms, to locate causal and maintaining factors, and to change their behaviour to lessen the impact of these.

The prognosis of these disorders, whether treated or untreated, is widely regarded as poor. In fact, the literature does not bear this out. A large proportion of patients with acute and subacute somatization recover and the results of treatment can be gratifying (e.g. Kellner, 1982). Even studies of the chronic forms of the disorder are less pessimistic than one might think. For example, it has been estimated that up to two-thirds of people with chronic hypochondriasis make a substantial recovery — to the extent that they no longer believe they have a physical disease and are able to return to a more normal social and occupational performance (Kellner, 1983; Pilowsky, 1968).

To conclude, although there are important unanswered questions about the evolution and management of these disorders there is little doubt that, in the acute form at least, they are amongst the most frequently encountered problems in primary care settings. Most will respond to quite simple interventions that lie at the heart of good medical care. It may not be too far from the truth to suggest that the detection and management of somatization is a good indicator of the skill base of a clinic.

# References

American Psychiatric Association (1987). *Diagnostic and Statistical Manual of Mental Disorders* (DSM-III-R) 3rd edn, revised, Washington, DC.

Anderson, R., Francis, A., Lion, J. *et al.* (1977). Psychologically related illness and health services utilization, *Medical Care*, **15**, 59–73.

Apley, J. (1958). Common denominators in the recurrent pains of childhood, *Proceedings of the Royal Society of Medicine*, **51**, 1023–1027.

Apley, J. & Hale, B. (1973). Children with recurrent abdominal pain: How do they grow up? *British Medical Journal*, **3**, 7–9.

Apple, D. (1960). How laymen define illness, *Journal of Health and Human Behavior*, **1**, 219–225.

Bain, D.J.G. & Philip, A.E. (1975). Going to the doctor — attendances by members of 100 families in their first year in a new town, *Journal of the Royal College of General Practitioners*, **25**, 821–827.

Balint, E. (1964). *The Doctor, His Patient and the Illness* (2nd edn), Pitman, London.

Banks, M.H., Beresford, S.A.A., Morrell, D.C., Waller, J.J. & Watkins, C.J. (1975). Factors influencing demand for primary medical care in women aged 20–44 years: A preliminary report, *International Journal of Epidemiology*, **4**, 189–195.

Barsky, A.J. (1979). Patients who amplify bodily symptoms, *Annals of Internal Medicine*, **91**, 63–70.

Bass, C. & Gardner, W. (1985). Emotional influences on breathing and breathlessness, *Journal of Psychosomatic Research*, **29**, 599–609.

Bass, C. & Wade, C. (1984). Chest pain with normal coronary arteries: a comparative study of psychiatric and social morbidity, *Psychological Medicine*, **14**, 51–61.

Baumann, B. (1961). Diversities in conceptions of health and physical fitness, *Journal of Health and Human Behavior*, **2**, 39–46.

Bianchi, G.N. (1973). Patterns of hypochondriasis: a principal components analysis, *British Journal of Psychiatry*, **122**, 541–548.

Blanchard, E.B., Andrasik, F., Ahles, T.A., Teders, S.J. & O'Keefe, D. (1980). Migraine and tension headache: A meta-analytic review, *Behaviour Therapy*, **11**, 613–631.

Boardman, A.P. (1987). The General Health Questionnaire and the detection of emotional disorder by general practitioners: a replicated study, *The British Journal of Psychiatry*, **151**, 373–381.

Bradley, J.J. (1963). Severe localized pain associated with the depressive syndrome, *British Journal of Psychiatry*, **109**, 741–745.

Bridges, R.N. & Goldberg, D.P. (1985). Somatic presentation of DSM-III psychiatric disorders in primary care, *Journal of Psychosomatic Research*, **29**, 563–569.

Brown, G.W. & Harris, T.O. (1978). *Social Origins of Depression: A study of psychiatric disorder in women*, Tavistock Press, London.

Burns, B.H. & Nichols, M.A. (1972). Factors related to the localisation of symptoms to the chest in depression, *British Journal of Psychiatry*, **121**, 405–409.

Burvill, P.W. & Knuiman, M.W. (1983). The influence of minor psychiatric morbidity on consulting rates to general practitioners, *Psychological Medicine*, **13**, 635–643.

Cartwright, A. (1967). *Patients and their Doctors*, Routledge and Kegan Paul, London.

Cay, E.L., Vetter, N.J., Philip, A.E. & Dugard, P. (1973). Return to work after a heart attack, *Journal of Psychosomatic Research*, **17**, 231–243.

Christensen, M.F. & Mortensen, O. (1975). Long term prognosis in children with recurrent abdominal pain, *Archives of Disease in Childhood*, **50**, 110–114.

Cloninger, C.R., Sigvardsson, S., von Knorring, A.L. & Bohman, M. (1984). An adoption study of somatoform disorders: II. Identification of two discrete somatoform disorders, *Archives of General Psychiatry*, **41**, 863–871.

Cohen, F. & Lazarus, R.S. (1973). Active coping processes, coping dispositions and recovery from surgery, *Psychosomatic Medicine*, **35**, 375–387.

Cohen, M.I. & White, P.D. (1951). Life situations, emotions and neurocirculatory asthenia, *Psychosomatic Medicine*, **13**, 335–337.

Cooperstock, R. (1971). Sex differences in the use of mood modifying drugs: an explanatory model, *Journal of Health and Social Behavior*, **12**, 238–244.

Craig, T.K.J. (1989). Abdominal pain, in *Life Events and Illness* (Eds. Brown, G.W. & Harris, T.O.), Guilford Pres, New York.

Craig, T.K.J. & Brown, G.W. (1985). Goal frustration and life events in the aetiology of painful gastrointestinal disorder, *Journal of Psychosomatic Research*, **28**, 411–421.

Creed, F. (1981). Life events and appendicectomy, *Lancet*, **i**, 1381–1385.

Dalrymple, D.G., Parbrook, G.D. and Steel, D.F. (1973). Factors predisposing to postoperative pain and pulmonary complications, *British Journal of Anaesthesia*, **45**, 21–32, 589–598.

Davenport, S., Goldberg, D. & Millar, T. (1987). How psychiatric disorders are missed during medical consultations, *Lancet*, **i**, 439–440.

Davidson, M. & Wasserman, R. (1966). The irritable colon of childhood, *Journal of Pediatrics*, **69**, 1027–1038.

Deighton, C.M. & Nicol, A.R. (1985). Abnormal illness behaviour in young women in a primary care setting: is Briquets syndrome a useful category? *Psychological Medicine*, **15**, 515–520.

Demers, R., Altamore, R., Mustin, H., Kleinman, A. & Leonardi, D. (1980). An exploration of the depth and dimensions of illness behavior, *Journal of Family Practice*, **11**, 1085–1092.

Dunnell, K. & Cartwright, A. (1972). *Medicine Takers, Prescribers and Hoarders*, Routledge and Kegan Paul, London.

Epstein, S. (1983). The unconscious, the preconscious, and the self-concept, in *Psychological Perspectives on the Self* (Eds. Suls, J. & Greenwald, A.G.), Erlbaum, New Jersey.

Escobar, J.I., Burnan, M.A., Karno, M. *et al.* (1987). Somatisation in the community, *Archives of General Psychiatry*, **44**, 713–718.

Finlay-Jones, R. & Brown, G.W. (1981). Types of stressful life events and the onset of anxiety and depressive disorders, *Psychological Medicine*, **11**, 801–815.

Ford, C.V. (1983). *The Somatizing Disorders: Illness as a way of Life*, Elsevier, New York.

Friedson, E. (1970). *Profession of Medicine: A study in the Sociology of Applied Knowledge*, Dodd Mead, New York.

Gask, L., Goldberg, D., Lesser, A. & Millar, T. (1987a). Improving the skills of the general practitioner trainee: evaluation of group training course, *Medical Education*, **22**, 132–138.

Gask, L., Goldberg, D., Porter, R. & Creed, F. (1989). Treatment of somatisation: evaluation of a teaching package with general practice trainees, *Journal of Psychosomatic Research*, **33**, 697–703.

Gask, L., McGrath, G., Goldberg, D. & Millar, T. (1987b). Improving the psychiatric skills of established general practitioners: evaluation of group teaching, *Medical Education*, **21**, 362–368.

Ginsberg, S.M. & Brown, G.W. (1982). No time for depression: A study of help-seeking among mothers of preschool children, in *Symptoms, Illness Behavior and Help Seeking* (Ed. Mechanic, D.), Prodist, New York.

Goldberg, D. (1970). A psychiatric study of patients with diseases of the small intestine, *Gut*, **11**, 459–465.

Goldberg, D., Gask, L. & O'Dowd, T. (1989). Treatment of somatisation: teaching techniques of reattribution, *Journal of Psychosomatic Research*, **33**, 689–695.

Goldberg, D. & Huxley, P. (1980). *Mental Illness in the Community: The Pathway to Psychiatric Care*, Tavistock, London.

Goldberg, D., Kay, G. & Thompson, L. (1976). Psychiatric morbidity in general practice and the community, *Psychological Medicine*, **6**, 565–569.

Goldberg, D., Steele, J. & Smith, C. (1980a). Teaching psychiatric interview techniques to family doctors, *Acta Psychiatrica Scandanavica*, **62**, 41–47.

Goldberg, D., Steele, J., Smith, C. & Spivey, L. (1980b). Training family doctors to recognise psychiatric illness with increased accuracy, *Lancet*, **ii**, 521–523.

Good, B.J. (1977). The heart of what's the matter: the semantics of illness in Iran, *Culture, Medicine and Society*, **1**, 25–58.

Greenley, J.R. & Mechanic, D. (1976). Social selection in seeking help for psychological problems, *Journal of Health and Social Behaviour*, **17**, 249–262.

Grings, W.W. & Dawson, M.E. (1978). *Emotions and Bodily Responses: A psychophysiological Approach*, Academic Press, New York.

Hanback, J.W. & Revelle, W. (1978). Arousal and perceptual sensitivity in hypochondriasis, *Journal of Abnormal Psychology*, **87**, 523–530.

Hannay, D. (1980). The 'Iceberg' of illness and 'trivial' consultations, *Journal of the Royal College of General Practitioners*, **30**, 551–554.

Harding, T.W., De Arango, M.V., Baltazar, J. *et al.* (1980). Mental disorders in primary health care: A study of their frequency and diagnosis in four developing countries, *Psychological Medicine*, **10**, 231–241.

Hartvig, P. & Sterner, G. (1985). Childhood psychologic environmental exposure in women with diagnosed somatoform disorders, *Scandinavian Journal of Social Medicine*, **13**, 153–157.

Hesbacher, P.T., Rickels, K. & Goldberg, D. (1975). Social factors and neurotic symptoms in family practice, *American Journal of Public Health*, **65**, 148–155.

Hoeper, E.W., Nycz, G.R., Cleary, P.D., Regier, D.A. & Goldberg, D. (1979). Estimated prevalence of RDC mental disorder in primary care, *International Journal of Mental Health*, **8**, 6–15.

House, A. & Andrews, H. (1988). Life events and difficulties preceding the onset of functional dysphonia, *Journal of Psychosomatic Research*, **32**, 319–331.

Ingham, J. (1980). Neurosis: Disease or distress? in *What is a Case?* (Eds. Wing, J.K., Bebbington, P.E. & Robbins, L.N.), Grant McIntyre, London.

Ingham, J. & Miller, P. (1982). Consulting with mild symptoms in general practice, *Social Psychiatry*, **17**, 77–78.

Johnston, M. & Carpenter, L. (1980). Relationship between pre-operative anxiety and post-operative state, *Psychological Medicine*, **10**, 361–367.

Katon, W., Kleinman, A. & Rosen, G. (1982). Depression and somatization: A review, *American Journal of Medicine*, **72**, 127–135.

Kellner, R. (1966). Neurotic symptoms in women: Attendances in a general practice, *British Journal of Psychiatry*, **112**, 75–77.

Kellner, R. (1982). Psychotherapeutic strategies in hypochondriasis: A clinical study, *American Journal of Psychotherapy*, **36**, 146–157.

Kellner, R. (1983). The prognosis of treated hypochondriasis: A clinical study, *Acta Psychiatrica Scandinavica*, **67**, 69–79.

Kenyon, F.E. (1964). Hypochondriasis: a clinical study, *British Journal of Psychiatry*, **110**, 478–488.

Kleinman, A. (1986). *Social Origins of Distress and Disease: Depression, Neurasthenia and Pain in Modern China*, Yale University Press, New Haven.

Kriechman, A.M. (1987). Siblings with somatoform disorders in childhood and adolescence, *Journal of the American Academy of Child and Adolescent Psychiatry*, **26**, 226–231.

Kumar, K. & Wilkinson, J.C.M. (1971). Thought stopping: A useful treatment in phobias of internal stimuli, *British Journal of Psychiatry*, **119**, 305–307.

Lacey, J.I., Bateman, D.E. & VanLehn, R. (1953). Autonomic response specificity: an experimental study, *Psychosomatic Medicine*, **15**, 8–21.

Lacey, J.I. & Lacey, B.C. (1958). Verification and extension of the principle of autonomic response-stereotypy, *American Journal of Psychology*, **71**, 50–73.

Ladee, G.A. (1966). *Hypochondriacal Syndromes*, North Holland Publishing Co., Amsterdam.

Lader, M. & Marks, I.M. (1971). *Clinical Anxiety*, Grune & Stratton, New York.

Last, J. (1963). The iceberg: completing the clinical picture in general practice, *Lancet*, **ii**, 28–31.

Leff, J. (1981). *Psychiatry around the Globe*, Marcel Dekker, New York.

Lesser, A.L. (1985). Problem-based interviewing in general practice: a model, *Medical Education*, **19**, 299–304.

Leventhal, H. (1980). Towards a comprehensive theory of emotion, in *Advances in Experimental Social Psychology* (Ed. Berkowitz, L.), **13**, 139–206, Academic Press, New York.

Lindsay, P.G. & Wyckoff, M. (1981). The depression pain syndrome and its response to anti-depressants, *Psychosomatics*, **22**, 571–577.

Lipowski, Z.J. (1988). Somatization: the concept and its clinical application, *American Journal of Psychiatry*, **145**, 1358–1368.

MacDonald, A.J. & Bouchier, I.A.D. (1980). Non-organic gastrointestinal illness, *British Journal of Psychiatry*, **136**, 276–283.

MacFarland, B.H., Freeborn, D.K., Mullooly, J.P. et al. (1985). Utilization patterns among long-term enrollees in a prepaid group practice health maintenance organization, *Medical Care*, **23**, 1211–1233.

MacKinlay, J.B. (1973). Social networks, lay consultation, and health-seeking behaviour, *Social Forces*, **51**, 255–292.

Maddox, G.L. (1962). Some correlates of differences in self-assessment of health status among the elderly, *Journal of Gerontology*, **17**, 180–185.

Malmo, R.B. & Shagass, C. (1949). Physiologic study of symptom mechanisms in psychiatric patients under stress, *Psychosomatic Medicine*, **11**, 25–29.

Marks, J.N., Goldberg, D.P. & Hillier, V.F. (1979). Determinants of the ability of general practitioners to detect psychiatric illness, *Psychological Medicine*, **9**, 337–353.

Marsella, A.J. (1979). Cross-cultural studies of mental disorders, in *Perspectives on Cross-cultural Psychology* (Eds. Marsella, A.J., Tharp, R. & Ciborowski, T.), Academic Press, New York.

Marsella, A.J. (1980). Depressive affect and disorder across cultures, in *Handbook of Cross-cultural Psychology* (Eds. Triands, H. & Draguns, J.), Alleyn & Bacon, Boston.

Marsh, G.N. & McNay, R.A. (1974). Factors affecting workload in a general practice, *British Medical Journal*, **i**, 319–321.

Mathews, A. & Ridgeway, V. (1981). Personality and surgical recovery: a review, *British Journal of Clinical Psychology*, **20**, 243–260.

Mayou, R. (1973). Psychological morbidity in the cardiac clinic. *Journal of Psychosomatic Research*, **17**, 353–357.

Mechanic, D. (1961). The concept of illness behavior, *Journal of Chronic Diseases*, **15**, 189–194.

Mechanic, D. (1964). The influence of mothers on their children's health attitudes and behaviour, *Pediatrics*, **33**, 444–453.

Mechanic, D. (1969). Illness and cure, in *Poverty and Health* (Eds. Kosa, J., Antonowsky, A. & Zola, I.), Harvard University Press, Cambridge, Massachusetts.

Mechanic, D. (1970). Frustration among British practitioners, *Journal of Health and Social Behavior*, **11**, 87–104.

Mechanic, D. (1976). Sex, illness, illness behavior and the use of health services, *Journal of Human Stress*, **2**, 2–6.

Mechanic, D. (1979). Development of psychological distress among young adults, *Archives of General Psychiatry*, **36**, 1233–1239.

Mechanic, D. (1980). The experience and reporting of common physical complaints, *Journal of Health and Social Behavior*, **21**, 146–155.

Mechanic, D. (1982). The epidemiology of illness behaviour and its relationship to physical and psychological distress, in *Symptoms, Illness Behaviour and Help-seeking* (Ed. Mechanic, D.), Prodist, New York.

Mechanic, D. (1983). Adolescent health and illness behaviour: hypotheses for the study of diseases in youth, *Journal of Human Stress*, **9**, 4–13.

Mechanic, D. (1986). The concept of illness behaviour: culture, situation and personal predisposition, *Psychological Medicine*, **16**, 1–7.

Melson, S.J., Rynearson, E.K., Dortzbach, J., Clark, R.D. & Snyder, A.L. (1982). Short term intensive group psychotherapy for patients with 'functional' complaints, *Psychosomatics*, **23**, 689–695.

Melzack, R. (1973). *The Puzzle of Pain*. Basic Books, New York.

Menninger, W.C. (1947). Psychosomatic medicine: somatization reactions, *Psychosomatic Medicine*, **9**, 92–97.

Mersky, H.A. & Evans, P.R. (1975). Variations in pain complaint threshold in psychiatric and neurological patients with pain, *Pain*, **1**, 59–72.

Miller, P. McC., Ingham, J.G. & Davidson, S. (1976). Life events, symptoms and social support, *Journal Psychiatric Research*, **20**, 515–522.

Morrell, D.C., Gage, H.G. & Robinson, N.R. (1970). Patterns of demand in general practice, *Journal of the Royal College of General Practitioners*, **19**, 331–342.

Morrell, D. & Wale, C. (1976). Symptoms perceived and recorded by patients, *Journal of the Royal College of General Practitioners*, **31**, 746–750.

Murphy, E. & Brown, G.W. (1980). Life events, psychiatric disturbance and physical illness, *British Journal of Psychiatry*, **136**, 326–338.

Oster, J. (1972). Recurrent abdominal pain, headache and limb pains in children and adolescents, *Pediatrics*, **50**, 429–435.

Parbrook, G.C., Steel, D.F. & Dalrymple, D.G. (1973). Factors predisposing to post-operative pain and pulmonary complications, *British Journal of Anaesthesia*, **45**, 21–32, 589–598.

Parkes, C.M. (1965). Bereavement and mental illness: A clinical study of the grief of bereaved psychiatric patients, *British Journal of Medical Psychology*, **38**, 1–26.

Paykel, E.S., Myers, J.K., Diendelt, M.N., Klerman, G.L., Lindenthal, J.J. & Pepper, M.P. (1969). Life events and depression: A controlled study, *Archives of General Psychiatry*, **21**, 753–760.

Pereira Gray, D.J. (1979). The key to personal care, *Journal of the Royal College of General Practitioners*, **29**, 666–678.

Petrie, A. (1967). *Individuality in pain and suffering*, University of Chicago Press, Chicago.

Pilowsky, I. (1968). The response to treatment in hypochondriacal disorders, *Australia & New Zealand Journal of Psychiatry*, **2**, 88–94.

Pilowsky, I. (1970). Primary and secondary hypochondriasis, *Acta Psychiatrica Scandinavica*, **46**, 273–285.

Querido, A. (1959). Forecast and follow-up, *British Journal of Preventive Social Medicine*, **13**, 13–49.

Racy, J. (1980). Somatization in Saudi women, *British Journal of Psychiatry*, **137**, 212–216.

Rosen, G., Kleinman, A. & Katon, W. (1982). Somatization in family practice, *Journal of Family Practice*, **14**, 493–502.

Roughmann, K.J. & Haggerty, R.J. (1972). Family stress and the use of health services, *International Journal of Epidemiology*, **1**, 279–286.

Rutter, B.M. (1979). The prognostic significance of psychological factors in the management of chronic bronchitis, *Psychological Medicine*, **9**, 63–70.

Rutter, M. (1963). Psychosocial factors in the short-term prognosis of physical disease: I. Peptic Ulcer, *Journal of Psychosomatic Research*, **7**, 45–60.

Sainsbury, P. & Gibson, J.G. (1954). Symptoms of anxiety and tension and the accompanying physiological changes in the muscular system, *Journal of Neurology, Neurosurgery and Psychiatry*, **17**, 216–224.

Scambler, A., Scambler, G. & Craig, D. (1981). Kinship and friendship networks and women's demand for primary care, *Journal of the Royal College of General Practitioners*, **26**, 746–750.

Shapiro, E.G. & Rosenfeld, A.A. (1986). *The Somatizing Child*, Springer-Verlag, New York.

Sheehan, D.V., Ballenger, J. & Jacobsen, G. (1980). Treatment of endogenous anxiety with phobic, hysterical and hypochondriacal symptoms, *Archives of General Psychiatry*, **37**, 51–59.

Shepherd, M., Cooper, B., Brown, A.C. & Kalton, G. (1966). *Psychiatric Illness in General Practice*, Oxford University Press, London.

Sime, M. (1976). Relationship of pre-operative fear, type of coping and information received about surgery to recovery from surgery, *Journal of Personality and Social Psychology*, **34**, 716–724.

Sims, A. (1973). Mortality in neurosis, *Lancet*, **ii**, 1072–1076.

Skuse, D. & Williams, P. (1984). Screening for psychiatric disorder in general practice, *Psychological Medicine*, **14**, 365–377.

Sternbach, R.A. (1974). Pain and depression, in *Somatic Manifestations of Depressive Disorders* (Ed. Sternbach, R.A.), North Holland Publishing Co., Amsterdam.

Suchman, E.A. (1964). Sociomedical variations among ethnic groups, *American Journal of Sociology*, **70**, 319–331.

Surtees, P.G., Sashidharan, S.P. & Dean, C. (1986). Affective disorder amongst women in the general population: a longitudinal study, *British Journal of Psychiatry*, **148**, 176–186.

Svedlund, J., Ottosson, J., Sjodin, I. & Dotevall, G. (1983). Controlled study of psychotherapy in irritable bowel syndrome, *Lancet*, **i**, 589–592.

Swartz, M., Blazer, D., George, L. & Landerman, R. (1986). Somatization disorder in a community population, *American Journal of Psychiatry*, **143**, 1403–1408.

Tessler, R. (1980). Birth order, family size, and children's use of medical services: a research note, *Journal of Health Services Research*, **15**, 55–62.

Tessler, R., Mechanic, D. & Dimond, M. (1976). The effect of psychological distress on physician utilization: a prospective study, *Journal of Health and Social Behavior*, **17**, 353–364.

Thompson, J.A. & Anderson, J.L. (1982). Patient preferences and the bedside manner, *Medical Education*, **16**, 17–21.

Tyrer, P., Fowler-Dixon, R. & Ferguson, B. (1990). The justification for the diagnosis of hypochondriacal personality disorder, *Journal of Psychosomatic Research* (in press).

Tyrer, P., Lee, I. & Alexander, J. (1980). Awareness of cardiac function in anxious, phobic and hypochondriacal patients, *Psychological Medicine*, **10**, 171–174.

von Knorring, L. (1975). The experience of pain in depressed patients: a clinical and experimental study, *Neuropsychobiology*, **1**, 155–165.

Waldron, I. (1983). Sex differences in illness incidence, prognosis and mortality. Issues and evidence, *Social Science and Medicine*, **17**, 1107–1123.

Watkins, G., Tarnopolsky, A. & Jenkins, L.M. (1981). Aircraft noise and mental health: II. Use of medicines and health care services, *Psychological Medicine*, **11**, 155–168.

Waziri, R. (1973). Symptomatology of depressive illness in Afghanistan, *American Journal of Psychiatry*, **136**, 213–217.

White, K., Andjelkovic, D., Pearson, J., Mabry, J., Ross, A. & Sagen, O. (1967). International comparisons of medical care utilization, *New England Journal of Medicine*, **277**, 516–524.

Wing, J.K., Cooper, J.E. & Sartorius, N. (1974). *The Measurement and Classification of Psychiatric Symptoms*, Cambridge University Press, Cambridge.

Wolfer, J. & Davis, C. (1970). Assessment of surgical patients: pre-operative emotional condition and post-operative welfare, *Nursing Research*, **19**, 402–414.

World Health Organization (1987). Mental, behavioural and developmental disorders, in *International Classification of Diseases* (10th revision) Draft chapter V(F). Division of Mental Health, World Health Organization, Geneva (copyright reserved).

Zborowski, M. (1952). Cultural components in response to pain, *Journal of Social Issues*, **8**, 16–30.

Zisook, S. & DeVaul, R.A. (1977). Grief-related facsimile illness, *International Journal of Psychiatric Medicine*, **7**, 329–336.

Zola, I.K. (1973). Pathways to the doctor: from person to patient, *Social Science and Medicine*, **7**, 677–689.

# 5

# Fatigue and Chronic Fatigue Syndromes

P.D. WHITE

## Introduction

Medical conditions characterized by excessive fatigue for which no simple explanation can be found have attracted intense public interest in the last 10 years. These fatigue syndromes have been given many names including myalgic encephalomyelitis (ME), Royal Free disease, postviral and postinfectious fatigue syndromes, neurocirculatory asthenia, fibromyalgia, and more recently chronic fatigue syndrome or CFS. They comprise a heterogeneous collection of disorders which have in common the cardinal symptoms of fatigue and fatigability, and all may be regarded as examples of a chronic fatigue syndrome.

Muscle physiologists describe both fatigue and fatigability as the inability to sustain a muscle contraction with a repeated stimulus (CIBA Foundation, 1981). Psychologists describe fatigue as the inability to sustain mental attention. Patients may describe fatigue as the subjective awareness of weakness or pain in the muscles, reduced ability to concentrate, reduced motivation, or drowsiness, whereas by fatigability they may mean the sensations caused by excessive effort. It is therefore important to understand exactly what patients mean when they complain of fatigue.

### Historical note

Clinical syndromes of fatigue have been described for at least two centuries. An early description was provided by the Scottish physician John Brown (Brown, 1780), who gave it the name of neurasthenia. But it was the American psychiatrist George Beard who first made the term popular (Beard, 1869). He described an 'exhaustion of the nervous system' with 'general malaise, debility of all the functions, poor appetite, abiding weakness in the back and spine, fugitive neuralgic pains, hysteria, insomnia, hypochondriases, disinclination for consecutive mental labor, severe and weakening attacks

104

of sick headache, and other analogous symptoms ...'. Two months before this description, van Deusen (1869), another American psychiatrist, described neurasthenia more narrowly and incidentally noted the chronic sequela of melancholia.

Initially, Beard thought that the condition was confined to white-collar American workers and ascribed it to the fast pace of modern life in the industrialized USA. The condition soon became a fashionable diagnosis among both doctors and patients; it spread rapidly throughout the USA and then on to Europe. This may have been due in part to the popular rest-cure of 'Doctor Diet and Doctor Quiet' described by Silas Weir Mitchell, the American neurologist (Mitchell, 1884). This consisted of a healthy diet, absolute rest, isolation from the family, and daily massage.

Neurasthenia became one of the most frequently diagnosed illnesses of the last century; Charles Darwin and Florence Nightingale were said to have suffered from the disorder. But by the turn of the century the diagnosis had become overinclusive and meaningless. Freud separated the neurosis of anxiety, and Janet separated hysteria from the main body of neurasthenia (Macmillan, 1976; Ellenberger, 1970). By the 1920s the diagnosis had fallen into disuse (Chatel & Peele, 1970). It is clear on reading the original case reports (Beard & Rockwell, 1905) that most patients would now be diagnosed as suffering from depressive and/or anxiety disorders. The links between neurasthenia, described a century ago, and current fatigue syndromes have been outlined elsewhere (White, 1989; Wessely, 1990).

### Definition of chronic fatigue syndrome

Holmes *et al.* (1988) reported a working definition of the chronic fatigue syndrome (see Table 5.1) with the cardinal symptom of 'persistent or relapsing, debilitating fatigue or easy fatigability ... that does not resolve with bedrest, and is severe enough to reduce or impair average daily activity below 50 percent of a patient's premorbid activity level for a period of at least six months' (Holmes *et al.*, 1988). These authors were trying to define a homogeneous group of patients for research purposes. The criteria are therefore more strict than those required for clinical purposes.

Lloyd *et al.* (1988c) defined it in a different way. They require the first criterion plus either the second or third: (i) 'generalised, chronic persisting or relapsing fatigue, exacerbated by very minor exercise, causing significant disruption of usual daily activities, and of over 6 months duration; (ii) neuropsychiatric dysfunction including impairment of concentration ... and/or onset of short-term memory impairment; ... (iii) abnormal cell-mediated immunity ...'. These are obviously less strict criteria than those of Holmes

**Table 5.1.** Chronic fatigue syndrome criteria.* Both major criteria are required, plus six minor symptoms and two physical signs, or eight minor symptoms.

**Major criteria**
Fatigue or easy fatigability for longer than 6 months (see text)
Exclusion of medical and psychiatric disorders likely to cause fatigue
 such as chronic infections or alcohol abuse

**Minor criteria**
*Symptoms*
 Mild fever
 Sore throat
 Painful cervical or axillary lymph nodes
 Unexplained generalized muscle weakness
 Muscle discomfort
 Unusually prolonged fatigue (>24 hours) after normal exercise
 Headaches
 Migratory arthralgia
 Neuropsychological symptoms (including poor concentration and
  depression)
 Hypersomnia or insomnia
 Acute onset

*Objective physical signs*
 Low-grade fever (<38.6 C)
 Non-exudative pharyngitis
 Palpable or tender cervical or axillary lymph nodes

* Adapted, with permission, from Holmes *et al.* (1988).

*et al.* It is interesting to note that these physicians, in attempting to define the syndrome, are confronting difficulties that are familiar to psychiatrists; i.e. having to provide an operational definition of a disorder that does not have a diagnostic test. It is not surprising therefore that the two best definitions that are currently available share little in common.

## Measurement of fatigue

Fatigue has proved difficult to measure because it lacks a precise definition. Observer-rated scales do exist, but have limited application (Kashiwagi, 1971). Those scales which concentrate on measuring one particular facet of fatigue are the most useful, such as the Stanford Sleepiness Scale (Hoddes *et al.*, 1973), but Broadbent (1979) concluded correctly that there is no single comprehensive measure of fatigue. Biochemical measures of fatigue have been unable to differentiate cause from effect (Poteliakhoff, 1981).

Muscle fatigue is easier to measure. In humans repeated exercise, enough to use greater than 40% of the maximum oxygen uptake by a muscle, will be sufficient to guarantee fatigue within a reasonable time. However, any repetitive muscle activity will eventually induce fatigue. Measurement of physiological muscle weakness and fatigability is straightforward and needs no further discussion in this chapter, apart from noting that individuals can be quite accurate in judging physical fatigue on exercise. This correlates closely with the physical load involved (Hueting & Sarphati, 1966).

## Validity of a fatigue syndrome

Surprisingly little research has addressed the validity and reliability of a fatigue syndrome. Hobbs *et al.* (1983) surveyed 1517 women in the community using the General Health Questionnaire (GHQ). The authors identified three main factors, namely 'debility', 'depression', and 'somatic' factors. The 'debility' factor explained the largest proportion of the variance. It consisted of items related to lack of pleasure (anhedonia), lack of energy, not coping, and feeling in need of a tonic. In a subsequent analysis they compared this factor to psychiatric diagnoses, derived from the Clinical Interview Schedule (CIS), and suggested that 'debility' was mainly associated with diagnoses of mild anxiety neurosis and, to a lesser extent, mild depressive illness.

Goldberg *et al.* (1987) examined patients attending their general practitioner. In an attempt to examine the underlying dimensions of distress and illness, psychiatric symptoms were entered into a latent trait analysis. The authors found that the main dimensions were represented by anxiety and depression. They also found a much smaller dimension which included tiredness, lack of energy, sleep symptoms and self-pity.

Verhaest and Pierloot (1980) examined psychiatric outpatients and entered their symptoms into a cluster analysis. This produced a cluster of fatigue, exhaustion, and various somatic symptoms especially involving the head. This was separate from depression and agitation. McNair and Lorr (1964) also examined psychiatric outpatients. A factor analysis of symptoms produced one factor with fatigue which was reliable over three studies. Associated symptoms included weariness, sluggishness, being worn out and sleepy.

These studies provide evidence both for and against the existence of a discrete fatigue syndrome. More recently White (1988) (see below) has suggested there is a discrete fatigue syndrome which may follow certain infections.

Psychiatric glossaries have never found fatigue syndromes easy to accommodate. Neurasthenia was included in the 9th edition of the International Classification of Diseases (ICD-9, World Health Organization, 1978) whereas the 3rd edition of the Diagnostic and Statistical Manual (DSM-III, American Psychiatric Association, 1980) deleted it. The draft version of ICD-10 (WHO, 1988) has retained the concept, which is based on a narrow definition provided by Kraepelin (1907). Symptoms include easy fatigability after physical effort or a feeling of mental fatigue, insomnia or hypersomnia, poor concentration, anhedonia and irritability. The authors make the point that any accompanying anxiety or depression should *not* be sufficient to meet the criteria for a generalized anxiety or depressive disorder.

## Prevalence of fatigue and chronic fatigue syndromes

In a large community study carried out in the USA Chen (1986) found that 20% of adults reported fatigue as a current symptom of more than 1 month's duration. In a UK community sample of nearly 9000 people, Cox *et al.* (1987) found that 19% of men and 30% of women 'always feel tired'.

Chronic fatigue is also common in primary care settings: 24% of consecutive patients attending a primary care clinic complained of fatigue as a 'major problem' and 72% of these had experienced the complaint for at least 1 year (Kroenke *et al.*, 1988). In another survey Buchwald *et al.* (1987) reported that 21% of primary care patients in the USA complained of 'severe loss of energy or easy fatigability either constantly or recurrently for at least the past 6 months'. These findings suggest that, in both general practice and the community, between a fifth and a quarter of the population report significant fatigue.

Studies of the prevalence of fatigue syndromes are almost unknown. Western psychiatrists rarely establish a diagnosis of neurasthenia (Chatel & Peele, 1970), and general practitioners vary greatly in the frequency with which they record this diagnosis. In the second National Morbidity Survey (1971/2) 20% of general practitioners reported the diagnosis more than 10 times per year for every 1000 patients seen (D. Crombie, personal communication). There is therefore considerable discrepancy between the prevalence of the symptom of fatigue (20%) and the frequency with which a specific diagnosis is established (less than 1%). Reasons for this will be discussed below.

### Fatigue and gender

Every study which has examined the effect of gender on reported fatigue has found an excess of females. In both acute and chronic fatigue the ratio varies from 4:1 in general practice (Jerrett, 1981) to 3:2 in large community studies (Chen, 1986; Cox *et al.*, 1987). No definite explanation for this has been made. It is known that women report more physical and more psychological symptoms than men (Cox *et al.* 1987), although with regard to physical symptoms this difference is not always significant (Hannay, 1978). Jenkins (1985) found no sex differences in minor psychiatric morbidity once differences in social, educational, and occupational factors were controlled. The same factors could help to explain the gender differences in the prevalence of fatigue. For instance, 46% of women in the UK have dual responsibilities of home-care and a job. The sleep deprivation caused by childbirth and child-care is another possible explanation for chronic fatigue, along with the well recognized fatigue of pregnancy, breast-feeding, and the menopause (for review see Riddle, 1982). It may be that premenstrual symptoms are in part responsible for differences in the prevalence of acute fatigue, although this would not explain differences in chronic fatigue. Finally, Gendel (1973) has presented some evidence for the importance of reduced physical fitness as an explanation of unexplained fatigue in women.

## Clinical syndromes

There are several syndromes which all share the cardinal symptoms of fatigue or fatigability induced by physical or mental effort.

### Postinfectious fatigue syndrome

The best recognized fatigue syndrome following an infection was that associated with encephalitis lethargica. Von Economo described 'headaches, fatigue, feelings of strangeness, hypochondriacal complaints of every variety ... states of abulia (lack of motivation), irritable weakness, generally linked up with a peculiar subjective feeling of unrest and irritability' (von Economo, 1931). There have been more recent studies of fatigue syndromes following encephalitis (Lawton *et al.*, 1970) as well as after other infections, not necessarily viral, such as hepatitis (Benjamin & Hoyt, 1945; Martini & Strohmeyer, 1974), brucellosis (Calder, 1939), and toxoplasmosis (Kotrlik *et al.*, 1968). Because some of these infections are treatable, doctors should be careful to consider them (Ladee *et al.*, (1966), as the following case illustrates:

> A 30-year-old journalist presented with a 6 month history of fatigue and lack of energy. This started with a 'flu-like' illness of sore throat, headache, generalized aching, fever, and sweating which lasted for 1 week. After this she complained of headaches every second day, and aching in her limbs, which were exacerbated by her baths and exercise. She had also noticed emotional lability, which never amounted to a depressive illness, and difficulty with her short term memory. She was less 'jolly' than before and more irritable, needing more sleep and

gaining weight.

There was no past psychiatric history, but 8 years previously she had suffered from a glandular fever-like illness (with a negative Paul–Bunnell test), had needed 4 months off work to recover, and suffered two further relapses of similar symptoms in the following year. She visited the family farm regularly and had two healthy cats. Her brother had had toxoplasmosis a year previously and her flatmate was still suffering from the after-effects of a Parvovirus infection. She had been a keen and accomplished sportswoman until her illness.

Mental state examination was unremarkable. Physical examination showed a single firm but non-tender lymph node in the posterior triangle. Her VP1 antigen test was positive a month before presentation to the hospital. The toxoplasma dye test was positive (a reciprocal titre of 1000) and the toxoplasma IgM was also positive. Her total IgM concentration was twice the upper limit of normal. She was successfully treated for toxoplasmosis, and her fatigue syndrome remitted.

Some infections may be more likely to lead to fatigue than others. Isaacs (1948) described 'chronic infectious mononucleosis' in a quarter of patients 3 months after onset. As well as weakness patients reported depression, nervousness, ease of perspiration and dizziness. Straus *et al.* (1988) recently reviewed the 'chronic mononucleosis syndrome' and noted the similarity to neurasthenia.

White (1988) has presented his preliminary findings on patients studied prospectively after infectious mononucleosis. He carried out a principal components analysis of symptoms measured by a standardized interview. At 2 months one-third of patients had a fatigue syndrome distinct from depressive illness, but this had fallen to 10% by 6 months. Muller *et al.* (1958) described a similar fatigue syndrome following 'primary aseptic meningo-encephalitis' (mainly caused by enteroviruses such as Coxsackie virus).

### Myalgic encephalomyelitis ('ME')

Descriptions of postinfectious fatigue syndromes and myalgic encephalomyelitis are similar. Behan *et al.* (1985) reported fatigue at rest and after exercise, depression, difficulty in concentrating, change in sleep pattern, tinnitus, disequilibrium, and hot and cold flushes. The obvious differences between 'ME' and accounts of fatigue following proven infectious illnesses are the different frequencies of physical symptoms such as myalgia and dizziness. The prevalence of different physical symptoms varies considerably according to the patients studied, although the importance of myalgia is stressed by most authors. However, the neuropsychological symptoms, along with physical fatigue and weakness, are common to descriptions of both 'ME' and postinfectious fatigue syndromes.

Similar symptoms are recorded in epidemic outbreaks of 'ME'. Henderson and Shelokov (1959) reviewed 23 outbreaks. The most common symptoms were malaise and fatigability, headache and muscle ache. Muscle weakness or paralysis was common, but without enhanced or absent reflexes and without atrophy. Shifting paraesthesiae were also common but without anaesthesia, and the authors made the following important observations: 'Depression, tension, and emotional instability have been impressive and among the most incapacitating and persistent symptoms . . . persons tending to be emotionally labile before illness have appeared to be most severely afflicted'. Cognitive problems were also common. Sweating, pallor or flushing were 'noted in several epidemics' and menstrual disturbances were 'repeatedly noted'.

Acheson (1959) reviewed 14 epidemics, especially those where patients reported paralyses. He noted similar symptoms to those reported by Henderson and Shelokov. An absence of objective neurological signs was evident but Acheson remarked on the intensity of the myalgia in three outbreaks. Lymphadenopathy was common in only one outbreak, at the Royal Free Hospital in 1955. Recovery occurred in most patients within 1 or 2 months but in various individuals relapses occurred, although these involved diverse symptoms (general, neurological, and psychological).

All three authors considered that the evidence of signs or symptoms of an infection at the onset of the illnesses was impressive, although the infections themselves were usually transient. In contrast to the endemic forms, the paralyses and paraesthesiae in the epidemic forms were notable. Other symptoms, such as fatigue and difficulty in concentration were similar.

Myalgic encephalomyelitis is an unsatisfactory name for this syndrome because it implies an aetiological role for inflammation of the brain which has never been confirmed. The evidence for an organic basis for the disorder has been reviewed elsewhere (David *et al.*, 1988; Bannister, 1988). In summary, there is intriguing evidence of abnormal immune function, persistence of viral immune response, and even viral antigen persistence in the blood, muscle, and faeces of highly selected patients. The specificity and sensitivity of these abnormalities are uncertain. It is also uncertain whether these findings are aetiologically relevant or merely represent epiphenomena.

## Fibromyalgia

Fibromyalgia is another controversial diagnosis with so many similarities to a chronic fatigue syndrome that in all probability they are one and the same. Goldenberg (1987) has provided a comprehensive review and described 118 patients. Criteria include chronic generalized aches, pains or stiffness, plus minor criteria of 'disturbed sleep, generalised fatigue or tiredness, subjective swelling or numbness, pain in the neck or shoulders, headaches, and irritable bowel symptoms' (Goldenberg, 1987). Goldenberg noted links with a past history of depressive illness and a current link with insomnia. The allegedly diagnostic 'tender points' have also been reported in 'myalgic encephalo-myelitis' (Ramsay, 1986).

Interesting work by Moldofsky and colleagues has demonstrated the role of specific sleep deprivation in causing fatigue, muscle aches and tenderness. Those healthy subjects deprived of Stage 4 sleep (the deepest slow-wave form of sleep) developed not only fatigue and muscle aches but also muscle tender-ness significantly more often than those deprived of rapid eye movement (REM) sleep (Moldofsky & Scarisbrick, 1976). The same research group pre-sented evidence to support their hypothesis that the fatigue, insomnia, mus-cle pain and tenderness, reported by patients with 'fibrositis' (fibromyalgia), was related to a specific anomaly of alpha rhythm non-REM sleep (Saskin *et al.*, 1986). The normal pattern of deep non-REM sleep was interrupted by episodes of alpha wave (Stage 1) sleep, thus giving the patient a 'restless' sleep. Goldenberg's review concluded that amitriptyline was superior to both non-steroidal anti-inflammatory drugs and placebo, but often at quite a low dose. The drug's efficacy may therefore be related as much to its hypnotic and an-algesic properties as to its antidepressant properties. The work by Moldofsky and his colleagues on alpha wave sleep disturbance has implications for other disorders characterized by chronic fatigue and muscle pain, in particular 'myalgic encephalomyelitis'.

**Neurocirculatory asthenia**

In 1950 this disorder was thought to affect 5% of the population (Wheeler *et al.*, 1950). It has many synonyms, including effort syndrome, irritable heart, da Costa's syndrome, soldier's heart, and more recently cardiac neurosis or more simply anxiety neurosis (see Chapter 7, p. 171). It resembles neuras-thenia but cardiac and respiratory symptoms predominate and coexist with anxiety. A 20 year follow-up study demonstrated its cardinal symptoms, benign prognosis, and close link with anxiety (Wheeler *et al.*, 1950). At one time a possible causal link with mitral valve prolapse (MVP) was considered (Hickey *et al.*, 1983) but this has since been thought to be a chance association.

The link between this syndrome and hyperventilation has been known for many years (Friedman, 1947). Gardner *et al.* (1986) have demonstrated that some patients have chronic hyperventilation or hypocapnia, confirmed by continuous measurement of end-tidal $PCO_2$. The fatigue felt by patients with hyperventilation has been shown to be a central rather than peripheral phenomenon (Folgering & Snik, 1988). Folgering and Snik found that hyper-

ventilators had less evidence of objective muscle fatigue than normal controls, although these authors suggested that this may have been a consequence
of suboptimal effort by the hyperventilators. This underlines the importance
of *central* mechanisms in the subjective fatigue of these patients.

It is also important to note the association between reduced physical
fitness and individuals with 'effort syndrome'. This is presumably a consequence of the avoidance of exercise which patients find aggravates their
symptoms. It is probably a crucial illness-maintaining factor (Benjamin &
Hoyt, 1945; Jones *et al.*, 1946) (see section on physical fitness).

## Fatigue and the 'mind–body problem'

It is not fruitful to consider fatigue as being of either organic or psychological
origin. In clinical practice both factors normally make contributions, although
some clinical characteristics may help to differentiate between fatigue of
predominantly 'organic' or 'psychological' origin. For example, fatigue which
is worse in the morning (Solberg, 1984), associated with poor sleep (Jerrett,
1981), anxiety or depression (Chen, 1986), and which lasts more than 4 months
(Morrison, 1980) is more likely to be associated with psychiatric disorder.
Morrison's finding that prolonged fatigue is associated with psychiatric disorder is reminiscent of Lishman's conclusions in the 'post-concussional
syndrome' (Lishman, 1988). In a review of the factors that contribute to continued neuropsychiatric symptoms following mild or moderate head injury,
Lishman concluded that 'organic' factors are chiefly relevant in the earlier
stages, but that persistent symptoms are perpetuated by psychological factors
interacting in a complex way with neurological factors.

But differentiation between either 'organic' or 'psychological' causes is
based on an outmoded and illogical Cartesian dualism. In clinical practice
both 'organic' and 'psychological' contributions often occur in the same patient
(Morrison, 1980; Archer, 1987; David *et al.*, 1988), and it is the interactions
between these variables that give fatigue syndromes their clinical complexity.

The American philosopher John Searle (1989) offers a solution to the mind–
body problem. He has remarked that 'conscious states are caused by neurophysiological processes and are realised in neurophysiological systems'. It is
therefore impossible to have a 'psychological' event without an 'organic'
brain event.

## Fatigue and 'physical' illnesses

Although this chapter is principally concerned with chronic unexplained
fatigue, it is important to know about the physical illnesses that can cause

fatigue. The diagnosis is usually evident from the history, examination, and appropriate investigations.

Allan (1944) described 300 patients presenting to an American primary care physician complaining of 'weakness, fatigue, or weak spells' as their chief complaint. Twenty per cent had physical illnesses, the commonest being neurological (5%), chronic infection (4%), and either diabetes or myxoedema in a further 4%.

In a similar study, Ffrench (1960) described 1200 outpatients who presented to a medical specialist. He examined them in two ways. Firstly, he asked all his patients, whatever their diagnosis, whether they suffered any fatigue. He found that one-third or more of the patients with either hypothyroidism, anaemia, liver disease, infectious mononucleosis or hyperthyroidism, suffered from fatigue of some degree. Secondly, he described the prevalence of different diagnoses in the 9% of his patients who suffered 'tiredness, lassitude, or exhaustion as either primary or major secondary symptoms'. The commonest diagnoses are shown in Table 5.2. Even though Ffrench was a hospital specialist, it is clear that a psychiatric illness was the most common cause of fatigue, but cardiac, hepatic, endocrine, and viral diseases, as well as anaemia, are worth while excluding.

Studies of fatigued patients in general practice report a higher percentage of psychiatric diagnoses, mainly depression or anxiety. Of the 'physical' diagnoses the most common are viral syndromes or infectious mononucleosis, which comprise 40% of the total 'physical' diagnoses, especially in the young (Morrison, 1980). Other diagnoses are similar to those described by Ffrench (1960). Rockwell and Burr (1974) have published a comprehensive list of all possible diagnoses associated with 'physiological', acute, and chronic fatigue.

**Table 5.2.**   Percentage diagnoses in fatigued patients

| Diagnosis | Percentage |
|---|---|
| Anxiety state/tension | 25 |
| Cirrhosis/hepatitis | 9 |
| Heart disease | 9 |
| Anaemia | 6 |
| Infectious mononucleosis | 6 |
| Thyrotoxicosis | 5 |
| Diabetes mellitus | 4 |
| Duodenal ulcer | 4 |
| Hypothyroidism | 3 |
| Others | 29 |

From French (1960).

The section on 'postinfectious fatigue syndromes' (see above) has already emphasized the importance of excluding treatable infections. Table 5.3 summarizes those studies which noted an association with fatigue. The link between fatigue and cytokines deserves more comment. Treatment with interferons causes fatigue, poor concentration, irritability and hypersomnia. This is dose-related and associated with generalized slow-waves on the electroencephalogram, suggesting an encephalopathy (Horning *et al.*, 1982; Mattson *et al.*, 1983; Smedley *et al.*, 1983). Macdonald *et al.* (1987) have suggested that postinfectious fatigue syndromes might be caused by cytokines, although studies to date have not provided significant support (Ho-Yen *et al.*,

**Table 5.3.** Diagnoses associated with chronic fatigue

| Diagnoses | Specific comments | Reference |
|---|---|---|
| Infections & their sequelae | See text (postinfectious fatigue syndrome) | See text |
| Multiple Sclerosis | Noted by 78%. Worse in afternoon and evening, after exercise and with heat | Freal *et al.*, 1984 |
| Parkinson's disease | Fatigue very common, relieved by L-dopa | Parkes, 1983 |
| Minor head injury | Cognitive symptoms most prominent. Only 5% at 3 months had neurasthenia | Wrightson & Gronwall, 1981 |
| Post-concussion syndrome | Physiological and psychological factors interact depending on how long after injury the patient was seen | Lishman, 1988 |
| Diabetes mellitus | Reported by 62% as main symptom. Considerable impairment in 40%. Worse in the evening. Associated with depressed mood but no patient had a depressive illness | Surridge *et al.*, 1984 |
| Hyperparathyroidism | Calcium concentration related to progression from neurasthenia, or depression, to delirium | Petersen, 1968 |
| Cancer | 40–72% of patients. Many secondary associations | Bruera & Macdonald, 1988 |
| Lymphoma | Lack of energy and tiredness, most common symptoms 1 year after diagnosis, accompanied by cognitive problems | Devlen *et al.*, 1987 |
| Iron-deficient anaemia | Easy fatigability and reduced concentration. Iron therapy reversed the symptoms and cognitive tasks improved | Mehta, 1984 |
| Reserpine | Re-evaluation of Reserpine induced depression suggested the majority were 'pseudo-depression' of a similar description to neurasthenia | Ayd, 1958, Goodwin & Bunney, 1971 |
| Cytokines | See text | See text |

**Table 5.3.**   cont'd

| Diagnoses | Specific comments | Reference |
|---|---|---|
| Post-abdominal operation | Not related to preoperative anxiety state or trait | Christensen *et al.*, 1986 |
| Postoperative | Bedrest is an intervening variable | Rose & King, 1978 |
| Localized x-radiation | Total dose related, physical symptoms most prominent. It may last several months | Haylock & Hart, 1979. Hughson *et al.*, 1987 |
| Industrial gases e.g. chlorine, $SO_2$ | 40% neurasthenia after acute exposure (but small study) | Wessel-Aas *et al.*, 1968 |
| Hot climate | Reduced by air conditioning | Mallows, 1970 |
| High altitude | Associated with EEG changes and cognitive difficulties, occurring after 2 days at 3500 metres | Ryn, 1979 |

1988; Morte *et al.*, 1988; Lloyd *et al.*, 1988b). Interleukin-1 does induce sleep (Krueger *et al.*, 1985) and is particularly associated with slow-wave sleep (Moldofsky *et al.*, 1986).

## Fatigue and 'psychiatric' disorders

Most patients with chronic fatigue will fulfil criteria for a psychiatric disorder. The most important illnesses are shown in Table 5.4.

**Table 5.4**   Psychiatric disorders with fatigue as a prominent symptom

Depressive illness
Anxiety disorders
Adjustment disorder
Alcoholism
Drug abuse
Eating disorders
Somatization disorder
Schizophrenia

### Fatigue and affective disorders

The most important associations are with self-reported anxiety and depression. After excluding patients with either known significant medical disorder or those currently attending a psychiatrist, Kroenke *et al.* (1988) found that

80% of primary care attenders with fatigue lasting a month or more reported significant 'depression' or 'somatic anxiety' on standardized questionnaires. This compared with 12% of control patients without fatigue.

Studies of hospital samples have revealed high rates of psychiatric morbidity in patients with chronic fatigue. Taerk *et al.* (1987) found that, of 24 patients wth postinfectious 'neuromyasthenia' (weakness or exhaustion, with no significant physical signs, for a mean of 18 months duration, following an apparent infection), 16 (67%) had 'depression' on the Beck depressive self-report inventory, compared with 17% of an age and sex matched healthy volunteer group. Fifty per cent of the patients with 'neuromyasthenia' reported a premorbid episode of DSM-III major depression compared with 12% of the controls. Regrettably, the depressive inventory used in this study included measures of somatic complaints and fatigue, symptoms which could be caused as much by an independent 'fatigue syndrome' as by depressive illness.

In four recent studies standardized interviews have been used to measure psychiatric morbidity. In the first, Hickie *et al.* (1990) reported the findings on 48 selected patients with 'chronic fatigue syndrome' (not all postinfectious) diagnosed according to the criteria of Lloyd *et al.* (1988c) (*vide supra*). Forty-six per cent had satisfied the DSM-III criteria for major depressive illness at some time during their illness, and 21% satisfied current criteria for major depressive illness. In this study only 12.5% reported a premorbid depressive illness, a proportion similar to that in the general population, but much lower than that reported by Taerk *et al.* (1987). The authors concluded that the psychiatric illness was the consequence rather than the cause of the fatigue.

In the second study of 100 self-referred patients with chronic fatigue (average duration of 13 years and not necessarily postinfectious), Manu *et al.* (1988) found high rates of psychiatric illness. Using the Diagnostic Interview Schedule (DIS) the authors attributed the fatigue to DSM-III psychiatric illness in 66 patients. Forty-seven had mood disorders, 12 somatization disorder, and 9 anxiety disorders (some patients had more than one diagnosis). In a subsequent publication, Manu *et al.* (1989) reported a close correlation between current mood disorder and fatigue, as well as a temporal relationship between the two. The time of onset of depressive disorder was significantly associated with onset of fatigue ($r = 0.61$) in those reporting depression within the last 6 months. The first episode of depression preceded fatigue in 23 of those 44 patients. The authors concluded that the fatigue was caused by the psychiatric illness in two-thirds of patients.

In the third study Wessely and Powell (1989) examined 47 patients with unexplained fatigue referred to a specialist neurological hospital in the UK. Their findings bore a striking resemblance to those of Manu *et al.* (1988):

psychiatric illness was diagnosed in 72% (using Research Diagnostic Criteria (RDC)) even when fatigue was excluded as a symptom. Furthermore, 47% had probable or definite major depression and 15% somatization disorder. Wessely and Powell compared their patients with two control groups: one with a peripheral neuromuscular disorder and another with major depressive illness. Rates of psychiatric disorder were significantly more common in the fatigue group compared with the neuromuscular group (72% versus 36%). This suggests that the psychiatric disorder was more than simply an understandable reaction to a fatiguing illness. The most striking difference between the fatigue group and the depressed controls was in *illness attribution*: the fatigued patients ascribed their symptoms to *physical* causes whereas the depressed group cited *psychological* causes.

In the fourth study, Kruesi *et al.* (1989) examined 28 patients who met the criteria of Holmes *et al.* (1988) for the chronic fatigue syndrome. All patients were selected for abnormal Epstein–Barr virus antibody profiles. Using the DIS the authors found that 75% had had a psychiatric illness during their lifetime: 2 reported that fatigue began before the psychiatric illness and 10 that it came afterwards. Unfortunately current diagnoses were not given.

There are three main criticisms of these four studies. Firstly, the diagnostic criteria used for the 'fatigue syndrome' varied between studies; secondly, many of the patients were self-referred or from highly selected populations; and thirdly, study designs were retrospective. These shortcomings make it difficult to draw firm conclusions about aetiological mechanisms. Apart from the small group with somatization disorder, it is difficult to establish whether the psychiatric disorder was a cause or consequence of fatigue. The finding of a high prevalence of premorbid depressive illness in three out of four of the studies suggests that either: (i) an independent factor predisposed some individuals to develop both depressive illness and a fatigue syndrome as a response to different physical and psychological stresses, or (ii) the fatigue syndrome was the somatic presentation of a depressive illness in some patients.

## The nature of the relationship between fatigue and depression

The link between depressive illness and fatigue deserves further examination. Some authors have suggested that a mild form of depressive illness is characterized by anhedonia (lack of interest or pleasure) (Snaith, 1987). This is similar to Kraupl Taylor's 'hypothymic condition' and 'hypomelancholia' (Kraupl Taylor, 1966), the former being the milder form of the latter. He described 'a decrease in mental and physical activity, in self-confidence and in the enjoyment of pleasure. The patient lacks energy and initiative in general ...'. Myerson (1922) describes anhedonia as a 'dropping out from consciousness of desire and satisfaction ...'. He noted 'in anhedonia the feeling of energy is low so that effort is painful, fatigue following rapidly upon exertion and having a peculiar painful component not present in ordinary fatigue'. Myerson made acute infection, 'typically influenza', the first cause of 'anhedonia' and noted the similarity of his description to that of neurasthenia, describing 'loss of appetite, loss of sleep, a lowered energy feeling, a loss of desire and satisfaction in everything in life, feelings of unreality and the increased reaction to excitement ...' (Myerson, 1922). By the latter he meant inability to cope with too many stimuli at once, leading to avoidance.

Importantly, these latter three authors believed the symptoms were part of, or led to, a depressive illness even though such patients *denied* depressed mood. Recent research supports these views. Anhedonia has been shown to be useful in discriminating depressive illness from physical illness (Zigmond & Snaith, 1983), and somatic symptoms, including fatigue, were found to be common early symptoms of a developing depressive illness (Wilson *et al.*, 1983). These descriptions are reminiscent of the vegetative form of 'atypical' depressive illness (Davidson *et al.*, 1982). This depressive illness is characterized by anergia, hypersomnia, reactivity of mood, hyperphagia, and sensitivity to rejection. Some of these patients may not report feeling sad but are more aware of anhedonia.

### Fatigue and somatoform disorders

Studies of patients with chronic fatigue have revealed a small but important association with somatization disorder. In two separate studies 15% of those with chronic fatigue were assigned a diagnosis of somatization disorder (Manu *et al.*, 1988; Wessely & Powell, 1989). Kirmayer *et al.* (1988) studied patients with fibromyalgia (the syndrome with fatigue and muscle pain described above), and found the symptoms fitted the description of a somatoform disorder better than a depressive illness.

Smith *et al.* (1986) described 41 patients who met DSM-III criteria for somatization disorder (see Chapter 12, p. 322). In this sample weakness was reported by 83%, dizziness by 83%, headache by 78%, and fatigue by 76%. Most patients were female, in their forties, with past history of psychological ill health. They perceived themselves as more disabled, with worse physical and mental health, than did people with chronic obstructive lung disease or diabetes mellitus.

In a well-known study McEvedy and Beard (1970a) re-investigated the case notes of some of the patients involved in the epidemic at the Royal Free Hospital in 1955 (Ramsay, 1986). They ascribed the symptoms to 'mass hysteria'. They noted the high attack rate in females, the normal investigations, the intensity of malaise compared with the slight pyrexia, and the similarity of the symptoms to those brought on by overbreathing. In fact, they produced evidence to support the hypothesis that anxiety and secondary hyperventilation (rather than a conversion disorder) produced the symptoms of the Royal Free epidemic. Their findings did not account for the high prevalence of lymphadenopathy at the start of the illnesses nor the prominent muscle pain reported by so many. Furthermore, McEvedy and Beard reviewed only 20 case notes of the most severely affected patients.

### Fatigue and other psychological explanations

In a second paper McEvedy and Beard (1970b) reviewed other outbreaks. They suggested that altered medical perception, particularly in endemic cases, might be a second aetiological mechanism. They noted that, of 52 cases of sporadic disorder reviewed by Acheson (1959), 49 were reported by physicians who had previously reported hospital outbreaks. They suggested that physicians, believing in the existence of the syndrome, might ascribe similar groups of symptoms to the same syndrome, even when the symptoms could equally well be ascribed to other disorders. Their hypothesis is difficult to refute or prove.

A final psychiatric 'disorder' to consider is 'burn-out'. The concept was introduced by Freudenberger (1974) who described 'a feeling of exhaustion and fatigue, being unable to shake a lingering cold, suffering from frequent headaches and gastrointestinal disturbances, sleeplessness and shortness of breath': in other words a chronic fatigue state with prominent somatic complaints. The behavioural signs are irritation, inflexible cynical thinking, and appearing depressed. Although the syndrome was first described in mental health care workers it has now been described in other 'helping' professionals such as teachers (Roberts, 1986). It is caused allegedly by high sustained levels of work-related stress and it is said to occur in people with unrealistic work-related goals (Roberts, 1986). It is reminiscent of the 'chronic nervous exhaustion' described by Allan (1945). The current nosological status of 'burn-out' is uncertain, but the similarity to the anhedonic forms of depressive illness, described above, is clear.

## Pathogenesis

Predisposing, precipitating and perpetuating factors must always be considered in every patient with a chronic fatigue syndrome. In this section the most important of these factors will be discussed.

## Predisposing factors

### *Personality*

In their survey of fatigued primary care attenders, Kroenke *et al.* (1988) noted associations with several personality dimensions. Fatigued patients were more sensitive, less sociable, and more inhibited. They also noted an association with premorbid pessimism, although this was closely correlated with the Beck depressive inventory score and may therefore have represented a state-dependent finding rather than a premorbid trait.

Montgomery (1983) studied a sample of 99 American college undergraduates who described themselves as 'uncommonly tired' compared to their fellow students. Tired students scored themselves as more introverted and less emotionally stable. Similar findings were reported by May *et al.* (1980) in a study of schoolgirls with 'benign myalgic encephalomyelitis', although this finding only held good for those under 14 years of age who had no objective infection.

In these studies assessments of personality were made retrospectively, after the onset of fatigue. This methodological shortcoming can be overcome in prospective studies using measures which do not contaminate trait with state (Kendell & Discipio, 1968). One such study was reported by Lindegard and Nystrom (1970), who found that symptoms which predicted later attendance to a psychiatrist for patients with 'neurasthenia' included habitual morning fatigue, general irritability, absent-mindedness, forgetfulness, and habitual or occasional uncontrolled behaviour. These results are interesting, but it is inadvisable to generalize to patients not attending a psychiatrist. Secondly, some of these predictive complaints may have represented early symptoms of 'neurasthenia' rather than true personality traits.

In a well known prospective study Imboden *et al.* (1961) used the Cornell Medical Index (CMI) and the Minnesota Multiphasic Personality Inventory (MMPI) to predict postinfectious tiredness and weakness in 600 USA service personnel before a predicted epidemic of Asian influenza. Twenty-six personnel later reported infections (19 serologically proven), of whom 12 took longer than three weeks to recover. Compared to the others, these 12 had higher CMI scores and had higher 'morale loss' and 'depression-proneness' scores on the MMPI. Interestingly, they were no more hypochondriacal or hysterical on the MMPI. Severity of the initial illness had no influence on convalescence, but older patients took longer to recover.

Later analysis of the same experiment by Cluff *et al.* (1966) revealed that 'psychologically vulnerable' individuals were three times more likely than the non-vulnerable to report their illness to the dispensary. A significant rise in antibody titres to the appropriate virus occurred in 106 of individuals. Seroconversion occurred in 41.5% of the psychologically vulnerable, compared to 33.5% of the non-vulnerable, a statistically insignificant difference. We can therefore conclude that psychological vulnerability did not affect infection rates, but did increase rates of reporting sick.

In another prospective experiment, this time with tularaemia, the same group of scientists inoculated volunteers with tularaemia and found that psychologically vulnerable subjects not only reported more symptoms but also had longer duration of independently measured fever (Canter, 1972). Totman *et al.* (1980) replicated this with the common cold: introverted subjects reported more severe symptoms but also had increased nasal virus shedding, once premorbid antibody titres were controlled for. These findings suggest that personality and psychological vulnerability can lead to both higher rates of symptom-reporting as well as more severe illnesses.

*Psychosocial stressors*

Many patients with chronic fatigue syndromes report that the precipitating infection occurred at a time of significant life stress. White (1990) has reviewed the ways in which stress may influence the onset and course of infectious illnesses.

## Precipitating factors

*Infections*

Most patients with chronic fatigue date their illness to an acute infective episode. Factors such as 'effort after meaning' (Creed, 1985) and recall bias will make it difficult to draw firm conclusions about such retrospective information, but the patient's account of a putative infective agent must always be very carefully considered. However, it is important to realize that not all patients with CFS have an infective cause.

There are regrettably few longitudinal studies of the outcome of defined infections. Two important studies have already been mentioned in the section on 'postinfectious fatigue syndromes' (see above). In a follow-up study Muller *et al.* (1958) concluded that the infection did not contribute substantially to the risk of persistent neurasthenia. White (1988) followed up a large number of patients after infectious mononucleosis. Preliminary analysis suggests that whereas at 2 months fatigue was associated with several virological abnormalities, no such association was found at 6 months. Moreover, there was an association between a persistent fatigue syndrome and psychological variables 6 months after infection. These findings suggest that precipitating and perpetuating factors differ in chronic fatigue syndromes.

## Perpetuating factors

### Sleep

Sleep deprivation causes irritability, malaise, reduced attention span and poor work performance (Rubin & Poland, 1977). Sleep deprivation of greater than 48 hours causes an increase in perceived physical exertion over and above the physiological muscle fatigue noted with exercise (Myles, 1985). Studies of mental performance after sleep deprivation show objective reductions in vigilance, attention span, and cognitive performance (Mackie, 1977).

The seminal work of Moldofsky and his colleagues on the effects of specific slow-wave sleep deprivation has already been mentioned in the section on fibromyalgia (see above). There are several other sleep disorders which may give rise to sleepiness or fatigue during the day (Guilleminault & Mondini, 1984). One of the most treatable diagnoses to exclude is sleep apnoea. Any middle-aged or older man with a history of snoring, particularly if hypertensive or overweight, is at risk (Lancet, 1985). Less common disorders such as narcolepsy and the Kleine–Levin syndrome have been well described by Parkes (1985).

In a study of 12 patients with daytime sleepiness following infectious mononucleosis Guilleminault and Mondini (1986) confirmed objectively excess total sleep time and reduced sleep latency, but found no difference in sleep architecture (i.e. proportion of REM sleep). Interestingly, reduced performance in cognitive tasks was associated with stage 1 non-REM 'micro-sleeps' occurring during the day.

Hypersomnia may occur in patients with depressive illness (Hawkins *et al.*, 1985). It is one of the features of 'atypical' depression, and the accompanying symptoms of overeating and fatigue make this an important differential diagnosis in any fatigue state (Davidson *et al.*, 1982).

Paradoxically, too much sleep may lead to a fatigue state. Globus (1970) studied 49 nursing students who reported feeling worse after excess sleep. After such a night they reported symptoms including feeling sleepy, less full of pep, worn out, tired, weary and exhausted. Another group of symptoms included cognitive difficulties, irritability, and muscle aches: therefore the whole 'syndrome' is reminiscent of neurasthenia.

In summary, because both insufficient and excess sleep are associated with fatigue states it is important to take a detailed history of sleep pattern in all patients with chronic unexplained fatigue.

*Muscle function*

The disabling symptoms of chronic fatigue are often ascribed to abnormalities in muscle function, but there is little objective evidence to support this claim.

In a prospective study Friman and colleagues (1985) examined the effects of the viral illness Sandfly fever on muscle function. They found both reduced isometric and dynamic (isotonic) muscle performance during fever compared with pre-illness levels. However, this was related to subjective perception of the severity of symptoms rather than to objective signs of illness such as duration and severity of fever. Unlike others (e.g. Astrom *et al.*, 1976), these authors found no associated reduction in serum or muscle enzyme nor any unexplained alteration of muscle ultrastructure. Although there were small numbers in this study, the results suggest that subjective perception is as important as any peripheral mechanism in mediating fatigue in acute infections.

Turning now to chronic fatigue, Stokes *et al.* (1988) showed that, after controlling for body weight, maximal isometric force was within the normal range in most patients with more than 1 year of excessive general and muscular fatigue. They used a twitch interpolation technique to show that the minority of patients with reduced maximal isometric force were using a sub-maximal effort. This technique interpolates a direct electrical stimulus onto the tested muscle as the patient is asked to make a maximal effort. If maximal force is being applied by the patient a direct stimulation of the muscle will have little effect. However, in the minority of the patients who were below the normal range of maximal force, stimulation boosted the force recorded by the muscle to within normal range. The failure to exert maximal force in these patients was therefore caused by central mechanisms rather than muscular pathology. The authors went on to examine physiological fatigability over time and found no differences between patients and controls.

Using their own criteria Lloyd and colleagues studied 20 patients with chronic fatigue syndrome (of greater than 10 months), excluding patients with obvious evidence of sub-maximal effort on muscle testing (Lloyd *et al.*, 1988a; 1988c). They compared these patients with age and height matched controls. There were no significant differences between the two groups on maximal isometric muscle strength and endurance, apart from an impairment of recovery of maximal isometric strength following endurance testing. However, these authors did not use a twitch interpolation technique. They acknowledged that the excess fatigability shown in the patients could have resulted from failure to recruit motorneurones (a consequence of reduced central nervous system command).

These findings are supported by those of Byrne and Trounce (1987), who found normal concentrations of muscle enzymes, including mitochondrial enzyme, in 11 patients with 'chronic asthenia and myalgia of obscure aetiology'.

A single case report of a patient with fatigue following chickenpox suggested that such patients might have abnormal metabolism on exercise, demonstrated by early and sustained fall in pH measured by phosphorus nuclear magnetic resonance (NMR) (Arnold *et al.*, 1984). However, later studies by the same group revealed inconsistent findings in patients diagnosed as having postviral fatigue syndrome (Yonge, 1988). Furthermore, these studies did not control for the important effects of disuse which result from enforced rest. Therefore it is possible that these inconsistent abnormalities may have been the consequence rather than the cause of muscle disuse.

In summary, the muscle findings are as follows:
1   A reduction in isometric force has been found in acute viral illnesses. This is probably due to both central and peripheral mechanisms.
2   No physiological weakness or fatigability has been demonstrated in patients with chronic fatigue which could not be explained by central mechanisms.

## Physical fitness

Can a peripheral basis for fatigue be demonstrated objectively? There is evidence that being physically unfit is associated with increased reports of subjective fatigue after exercise. In his large community study, Chen (1986) found an association between complaints of fatigue and physical inactivity. Similar associations were reported by Kroenke *et al.* (1988) and Valdini *et al.* (1987) in fatigued primary care attenders. In a study of middle-aged men at risk of coronary heart disease Hughes *et al.* (1984) exercised men on a treadmill until they achieved their appropriate target heart rate. Those who were generally physically inactive reported excess perceived exertion during the test and during recovery.

Jones and colleagues (1946) measured physical fitness by *mean* oxygen uptake after dynamic exercise on a bicycle ergometer. Patients with 'effort syndrome' needed a greater oxygen uptake, compared with healthy controls, after the same amount of exercise (i.e. they were more unfit).

One possible explanation for being unfit after infections is muscle disuse because of bedrest or general inactivity. This explanation was supported by an important prospective study of 5 healthy young men who were assessed before and after 20 days of bedrest (Saltin *et al.*, 1968). Bedrest caused a mean reduction of 28% of *maximal* oxygen uptake during dynamic exercise (probably the best estimate of general muscle fitness).

Of course, associations can work in two ways. Physical inactivity may cause or predispose towards fatigue, or the fatigue itself may cause the physical inactivity. One important question is: does return to physical fitness eradicate the fatigue? Edwards and colleagues demonstrated the benefit, as well as objective improvement, with physical retraining on an individual basis (Newham & Edwards, 1979; Edwards, 1986). In a placebo controlled study of physical fitness training in patients with fibromyalgia, those who trained achieved a 29% increase in peak work capacity (on a bicycle ergometer) compared with a 4% reduction in controls. This was accompanied by significantly less general pain and myalgia, as well as fewer psychological symptoms on a standard questionnaire (McCain, 1986) (see section on management).

## Management

It is important to recall that chronic fatigue can be caused by a variety of treatable physical disorders. The history and examination will usually point to the important investigations to undertake (see section on physical causes of fatigue).

There is no current consensus about the appropriate treatment of a cryptogenic chronic fatigue state. Many claims have been made about a large number of treatments, but most are anecdotal and none have been shown to be of benefit in double-blind placebo controlled trials. The guiding principles of treatment therefore must be flexibility, open-mindedness, and *'primum non nocere'*.

### Diagnostic labelling

As in all unexplained syndromes, the patient's illness attributions are of great importance and must be enquired into (see Chapter 3, p. 50). Once a thorough history, examination, and relevant investigations have been performed, it is important for patients to be reassured that they have no potentially fatal or serious illness, such as cancer or multiple sclerosis. Regrettably, many patients may have seen other professionals and have been given the explanation that 'there is nothing seriously wrong' or 'it's all in your mind', or worse still 'in your imagination'. I believe it is this scenario that has led many patients to reject psychological explanations and, more seriously, psychiatric treatments. The pejorative description of the Royal

Free disease outbreak of 1955 as 'mass hysteria' has added to this suspicion (McEvedy & Beard, 1970a).


**Typical explanation of illness**

An adequate and comprehensive explanation for the symptoms is essential. An example might be as follows:

> You are suffering from a chronic fatigue syndrome which, in your case, was precipitated by glandular fever: in other words, a postviral fatigue syndrome. This is an illness which we do not understand properly, although a lot of research is being undertaken at the moment.
>
> Your continued symptoms are caused by several factors acting together. As you say yourself, you were unfit when you caught the virus. The 6 weeks in bed caused a further weakening of your muscles because they weren't being exercised. This means that whenever you now try to exert yourself you feel weak, tired, and have aching muscles. Understandably, this causes you to rest, which in turn makes you more unfit; thus the cycle repeats itself.
>
> Added to this you returned to work and found it difficult to cope; your boss criticized your work which put you under pressure and made you feel anxious. This disturbed your sleep which made you more tired in the morning and less able to cope with the demands of work.
>
> Your doctors told you they could find nothing wrong, so you began to wonder whether it was you after all, yet you knew you could not cope, and that there was something seriously wrong. This led to low self-confidence, low self-esteem, and depression. Your symptoms had gone on for so long that you could not see how you were ever going to get better.
>
> Then the next infection you met found you already run down and therefore you were unable to shake it off. This caused more fatigue, so the cycle repeated itself.
>
> We can work together to help you to tackle several things at the same time. So long as there are no active signs of infection, we must try to increase your muscular fitness in a gradual way. I can also help you to learn to cope better with the stress you are under. We do this by teaching you how to relax and by breaking large tasks down into smaller ones that you feel you can manage. I can also help you with the very understandable depressive illness you have at the moment.

This sort of explanation seems to be acceptable to patients and leads on logically to the appropriate treatments. Handouts can also be very helpful.

**Cognitive–behavioural treatment**

The treatment proposed by Wessely and his colleagues (1990) is based on the following premise: the patient experiences genuine symptoms, learns that carrying on aggravates them, then attributes the symptoms to a persistent viral infection. Because he/she assumes that they are a warning of damage, activity is avoided. This may have been adaptive initially but is no longer so. Avoidance of activity leads to more *inactivity*, which in turn perpetuates the fatigue. As a consequence symptoms occur at progressively lower levels of exertion and the patient becomes convinced that his/her own explanations are accurate. Demoralization, fear and depression compound the problem. Because fear of symptoms provokes and maintains avoidance behaviour (Philips, 1987), the cornerstone of treatment involves mutually agreed behavioural targets between patient and therapist, which are then practised between appointments. At no stage is intensive exercise training endorsed. The patient should agree to undertake the activity even when symptomatic, and not to abandon it if symptoms develop. Thus the patient is being asked to undertake the activity in response to an agreed timetable, and not the absence of symptoms.

The key to this approach is to abolish the handicapping stimulus-driven cycle seen so often in patients with postviral fatigue states, in which symptoms are always a signal to rest, and to replace sensitization with tolerance. After reassuring him/herself that an agreed goal can be attained, each patient is encouraged to cease using symptoms as a warning to stop, but to carry on to the agreed target. The overall aim, of course, is to increase the patient's sense of mastery and control over the disorder, i.e. improve self-efficacy.

This treatment can be quite time-consuming, and therefore it is fortunate that it may only be required for patients with the most severe and persistent symptoms. The results of an open study of cognitive–behavioural therapy, by Wessely and his colleagues, are awaited with interest.

**Exercise**

The programme of exercise in this treatment must start with minimal effort and only gradually increase in intensity. Patients should be advised to start with only a small effort on a daily basis, such that it causes no more than a minimal increase in fatigue. It may be disastrous to attempt too much too quickly; this can lead to increased muscular aching and fatigue (Lancet, 1987) which will discourage the patient from trying again. In some patients with severe symptoms it may be necessary to sanction only stretching exercises to start with, for 5 or less minutes daily. Once a week the patient, with or without the clinician, can judge his/her general level of fatigue. If he/she does not feel more fatigued, the level of exercise can be increased, keeping the duration the same. The next step is gradually, week by week, to increase the duration of exercise aiming at 20 minutes per day, fatigue allowing. Exercise should involve all muscle groups and be isotonic (i.e. dynamic) exercise. Newham and Edwards (1979) have described an exercise retraining programme which was successful in relieving symptoms in an open study. McCain (1986) found such a programme to be superior to placebo in patients with 'fibromyalgia'.

Encouraging the patient to persist with the treatment can be achieved in two ways. Firstly, the patient should be encouraged to keep a daily diary of exercise completed and its duration. The level of fatigue should also be recorded using a scale from 0–10. The patient can thus review exercise performed over the week as well as the level of fatigue; then the following week's level can be determined. Over the weeks the patient can readily judge the progress being made. The second method is by feedback from the clinician reviewing the diary and progress with the patient. For patients with severe symptoms it is very useful to involve a physiotherapist from the early stage. They can make a baseline assessment of fitness, design an appropriate exercise programme, and monitor progress, which they should reward with praise and encouragement.

## Return to normal activities

In many patients gradual return to general activities can be just as important as exercise. The same principles should be employed as those used with return to exercise, namely explanation, support, and feedback with a gradually increasing schedule. Sometimes it may be necessary to negotiate a gradual return to activity with employers or the family. Couple and/or family therapy is usually essential when chronic somatization is present.

## Treatment of affective illness

A significant proportion of patients with chronic fatigue may have a depressive illness (see above), and since suicide is the only cause of death (Ramsay, 1986), treatment of depressive illness can be particularly important. For this reason antidepressant drugs may have an important place, but they need to be chosen with care. Side-effects such as sedation and postural hypotension may exacerbate symptoms. It is worth remembering that these drugs are not simply 'antidepressant' but also have other properties which may be therapeutic in patients with fatigue, e.g. hypnotic, anxiolytic, and analgesic. The choice of antidepressant depends on the patient's associated symptoms. Table 5.5 outlines the principal choices.

To date there are no reported placebo controlled double-blind trials of antidepressants in patients with a chronic fatigue syndrome, apart from their successful use in patients with 'fibromyalgia' (see above). Jones and Straus (1987) reported 'clinical improvement' in 70% of patients with 'low doses of doxepin'. Manu *et al.* (1989) reported that 83% of 24 patients with chronic fatigue and depressive illness reported 'significant improvement of their symptoms of fatigue, as well as of their depressive disorder'. These authors most commonly used desipramine.

The similarities between the chronic fatigue syndrome and the vegetative form of atypical depressive illness have already been alluded to. A recent trial treating patients with this form of depressive illness has been reported by Quitkin and colleagues (1988) who compared imipramine, a tricyclic drug, with phenelzine (a monoamine oxidase inhibitor) and placebo. Phenelzine was significantly superior to both placebo and imipramine at 6 weeks and improvement was maintained after a further 6 weeks of treatment. These findings support Slater and Roth's clinical acumen that patients with 'chronic neurasthenia ... are frequently helped by monoamine oxidase inhibitors' (Slater & Roth, 1969).

All antidepressants should be started at a low dose and gradually increased to therapeutic levels, side-effects allowing (see Chapter 3, p. 60). This generally applicable advice is particularly true of patients with chronic fatigue who may be particularly sensitive to side effects. Monoamine oxidase

**Table 5.5.**   Selection of an antidepressant

---

*Atypical features (see text):*
Phenelzine, or another MAOI, if dietary exclusions and drug interactions are not a problem. Last dose by 4 pm, to avoid insomnia

*Mixed anxiety and depression:*
Anxiolytic tricyclics, e.g. imipramine or amitriptyline, in divided doses. Alternatively consider phenelzine

*Insomnia:*
A sedative tricyclic, given as one dose at night, e.g. dothiepin or amitriptyline

*Daytime hypersomnia:*
Non-sedative tricyclics, e.g. protriptyline or nortriptyline. Beware insomnia

*Prominent side-effects:*
New generation drugs, e.g. lofepramine or fluvoxamine

---

inhibitors such as phenelzine and the most stimulating tricyclics, such as protriptyline, should not be given after 4.00 pm in order to avoid insomnia. Tranylcypromine may be particularly effective with its stimulant properties but this may give rise to later problems of dependence. Some severe postviral depressive illnesses do not respond to antidepressant treatment but do respond to electroconvulsive treatment (Gould, 1957). This seems to be as true today as 30 years ago (White & Lewis, 1988).

Anxiety may also be a common accompaniment of chronic fatigue, and is amenable to conventional anxiety management techniques. These include relaxation therapy involving breathing control, muscle relaxation, and distraction through mental imagery. Graded exposure is recommended for avoidance behaviour and cognitive therapy can be helpful especially in episodic generalized anxiety states. Reducing caffeine-containing beverages (tea, coffee, and certain soft drinks) prevents caffeine-induced anxiety and insomnia. Therapeutic self-use of caffeine, however, does not seem to be too common with chronic fatigue. Beta-blockers are helpful for prominent somatic symptoms, but care should be taken to exclude the side-effect of cognitive retardation. When anxiety and depression coexist an antidepressant drug may ameliorate both problems (see Table 5.5). Many patients with chronic fatigue states report reduced tolerance to alcohol, therefore abuse is rarely a problem.

The following case vignette illustrates the need for a flexible approach to treatment:

> A 34-year-old married teacher presented in 1988 with a 7 year history of fatigue with a relapsing and remitting course. The illness started with typical infectious mononucleosis, with a positive Paul–Bunnell test, and she required 6 weeks of bedrest. Recovery was gradual and incomplete. Relapses were precipitated by work, exercise, mental stress, and infection. Symptoms included mild sore throat, painful cervical lymphadenopathy, arthralgia, headache, and nocturnal sweating. She also complained of profound physical and mental fatigue. Other symptoms included poor concentration, irritability, and an excess need for sleep but waking unrefreshed. Relapses lasted between 1 week and 4 months and occurred about three times a year.
>
> Since 1983 she had also experienced episodes of depressive illness and her social confidence had suffered. The depressive episodes usually lasted 6 weeks, although the first episode had lasted 12 months. Depressive episodes were precipitated by relapses of fatigue as well as concern over her marriage. She had not worked for more than a term without significant time off work, and was being considered for retirement on medical grounds. Housework was out of the question

because during a relapse she was barely able to climb the stairs. There was no relevant premorbid family psychiatric history. She had suffered from hepatitis in the past and had taken 3 months to recover from this.

On examination she looked pale with dark rings around her eyes. She had tender cervical lymphadenopathy but no pharyngitis. Almost all investigations were normal including computerized tomography (CT) scan, electroencephalogram (EEG), full blood count, erythrocyte sedimentation rate (ESR), thyroid function tests, immunoglobulins, blood sugar, and toxoplasma dye test. However, her Epstein–Barr virus (EBV) serology was abnormal compared with seropositive controls measured at the same laboratory. Her early antigen titre was grossly elevated and she had no antibody to nuclear antigen. The IgM and heterophil antibody tests were negative. These abnormalities had persisted over time.

She was treated in several ways. Phenelzine cured her depressive illness and ibuprofen helped her headaches and body aches. One session of couple therapy was enough to place the marriage on a firmer basis. Her husband was encouraged to act as a co-therapist and he prompted her to return to normal activities. Between severe relapses she undertook a programme of gradually increasing daily exercises, which made her more physically fit. A relaxation technique, combined with *in vivo* desensitization, led to reduction of her social anxiety. She is now working part time and about to start full time. She cycles 3 times a week and takes other exercise on a daily basis. Both she and her husband are much happier and making plans for the future. She has had no relapses in the last 6 months.

**Stimulants and psychic energizers**

Various stimulants have been found to help patients with fatigue of no obvious cause (Lucas *et al.*, 1966; Valle-Jones, 1978). These include amphetamine, dexamphetamine, methyl phenidate, prolintane and pemoline. Intriguingly, the dopamine agonist amantadine was superior to placebo in relieving fatigue secondary to multiple sclerosis (Canadian MS Research Group, 1987).

The main disadvantages of these drugs are those of dependence and tolerance when prescribed for any significant length of time. Insomnia is also a common side-effect. Finally, although patients admit their usefulness in increasing mental energy, they notice no reduction in the physical sensations of fatigue.

**Antiviral and immunological therapies**

Little work has been published in this area, although current trials of immunoglobulin therapy are awaited with interest. Bolden (1972) reported successful amelioration of acute infectious mononucleosis, as well as re-duced length of convalescence, with 12 days of prednisolone compared with an aspirin placebo. This has not been replicated and there are no reports of placebo controlled trials of steroids in chronic fatigue syndromes. Anecdotally, steroids, immunoglobulins, and immune-enhancing drugs such as inosine pranobex are not helpful (Behan *et al.*, 1984).

A well-designed study of anti-EBV agent, acyclovir, has recently been reported (Straus *et al.*, 1988). This was a double-blind crossover placebo con-trolled trial of 24 subjects with chronic fatigue syndrome (mean duration 7 years) and abnormal EBV serology. No difference in outcome was found between placebo and acyclovir, and there was a high placebo response (42%). The authors also found a significant relationship between reduction in psychological symptoms and overall clinical improvement. The investi-gators, who were virologists, concluded that 'affect plays an important part in the perception of illness severity in the chronic fatigue syndrome' (Straus *et al.*, 1988).

# Summary

Chronic fatigue is common and leads to considerable disability. The present evidence supports the existence of a fatigue syndrome, which is characterized by a constellation of both physical and psychological symptoms. The syndrome may be caused by many physical illnesses and several psychiatric illnesses, but often there is no obvious single cause.

When the cause is not obvious, the history and examination will often clarify the important factors which predispose an individual to develop a fatigue syndrome. Precipitating events and illnesses should be enquired into, as should the presence of maintaining factors. All three types of factor are often quite different, but interact to cause a chronic fatigue syndrome. Physical and psychosocial factors are often active at the same time, but will have different relative importance in different patients. Treatments that take account of both physical and psychological factors offer promise in patients with chronic unexplained fatigue.

# Acknowledgements

I am grateful to Drs S. Wessely and C. Bass for helpful discussions and drawing my attention to relevant studies. Dr D. Crombie provided un-reported data and Ms Janet Foster kindly typed the manuscript.

# References

Acheson, E.D. (1959). The clinical syndrome variously called benign myalgic encephalomyelitis, Iceland disease, and epidemic neuromyasthenia, *American Journal of Medicine*, **26**, 569–595.

Allan, F.N. (1944). The differential diagnosis of weakness and fatigue, *New England Journal of Medicine*, **231**, 414–418.

Allan, F.N. (1945). The clinical management of weakness and fatigue, *Journal of the American Medical Association*, **127**, 957–960.

American Psychiatric Association (1980). *Diagnostic and Statistical Manual of Mental Disorders* 3rd edn, (DSM-III), Washington DC.

Archer, M.I. (1987). The post-viral syndrome: a review, *Journal of the Royal College of General Practitioners*, **37**, 212–214.

Arnold, D.L., Bore, P.J., Radda, G.K., Styles, P. & Taylor, D.J. (1984). Excessive intracellular acidosis of skeletal muscle on exercise in a patient with post-viral exhaustion/fatigue syndrome, *Lancet*, **i**, 1367–1369.

Astrom, A.E., Friman, G. & Pilstrom, L. (1976). Effects of viral and mycoplasma infections on ultrastructure and enzyme activities in human skeletal muscle, *Acta Pathologica Microbiologica Scandinavica (A)*, **84**, 113–122.

Ayd, F.J. (1958). Drug-induced depression — fact or fallacy, *New York State Journal of Medicine*, **58**, 354–356.

Bannister, B.A. (1988). Post-infectious disease syndrome, *Postgraduate Medical Journal*, **64**, 559–567.

Beard, G.M. (1869). Neurasthenia, or nervous exhaustion, *Boston Medical and Surgical Journal*, **3**, 217–221.

Beard, G.M. & Rockwell, A.D. (1905). *A Practical Treatise on Nervous Exhaustion (Neurasthenia), its Symptoms, Nature, Sequences, Treatment*, E.B. Treat & Co., New York. Reprinted by Kraus Reprint Co., New York, 1971.

Behan, P.O. & Behan, W.M.H. (1984). Immunological observations in chronic muscular disorders of presumed viral etiology, with a note on therapy, in *Neuroimmunology* (Eds. Behan, P. & Spreafico, F.), pp. 359–369, Raven Press, New York.

Behan, P.O., Behan, W.M.H. & Bell, E.J. (1985). The postviral fatigue syndrome — an analysis of the findings in 50 cases, *Journal of Infection*, **10**, 211–222.

Benjamin, J.E. & Hoyt, R.C. (1945). Disability following post-vaccinal (yellow fever) hepatitis. A study of 200 patients manifesting delayed convalescence, *Journal of the American Medical Association*, **128**, 319–324.

Bolden, K.J. (1972). Corticosteroids in the treatment of infectious mononucleosis, *Journal of the Royal College of General Practitioners*, **22**, 87–95.

Broadbent, D.E. (1979). Is a fatigue test now possible? *Ergonomics*, **22**, 1277–1290.

Brown, J. (1780). *Elementa Medicinae*, Edinburgh.

Bruera, E. & Macdonald, R.N. (1988). Overwhelming fatigue in advanced cancer, *American Journal of Nursing*, **88**, 99–100.

Buchwald, D., Sullivan, J.L. & Komaroff, A.L. (1987). Frequency of 'chronic active Epstein–Barr virus infection' in a general medical practice, *Journal of the American Medical Association*, **257**, 2303–2307.

Byrne, E. & Trounce, I. (1987). Chronic fatigue and myalgia syndrome: mitochondrial and glycolytic studies in skeletal muscle, *Journal of Neurology, Neurosurgery and Psychiatry*, **50**, 743–746.

Calder, R.M. (1939). Chronic Brucellosis, *Southern Medical Journal*, **32**, 451–460.

Canadian MS Research Group (1987). A randomised controlled trial of Amatadine in fatigue associated with multiple sclerosis, *Canadian Journal of Neurological Sciences*, **14**, 273–278.

Canter, A. (1972). Changes in mood during incubation of acute febrile disease and the effects of pre-exposure psychologic status, *Psychosomatic Medicine*, **34**, 424–430.

Chatel, J.C. & Peele, R. (1970). The concept of neurasthenia, *International Journal of Psychiatry in Medicine*, **9**, 36–49.

Chen, M.K. (1986). The epidemiology of self-perceived fatigue among adults, *Preventive Medicine*, **15**, 74–81.

Christensen, T., Hjortso, N.C., Mortensen, E., Riis-Hansen, M., Kehlet, H. (1986). Fatigue and anxiety in surgical patients, *Acta Psychiatrica Scandinavica*, **73**, 76–79.

Ciba Foundation (1981). *Human Muscle Function: Physiological Mechanisms*, Symposium no. 82, Pitman Medical, London.

Cluff, L.E., Canter, A. & Imboden, J.B. (1966). Asian influenza: infection, disease, and psychological factors, *Archives of Internal Medicine*, **117**, 159–163.

Cox, B.D., Blaxter, M., Buckle, A.L.J. *et al.* (1987). *The Health and Lifestyle Survey*, Health Promotion Research Trust, Cambridge.

Creed, F. (1985). Life events and physical illness, *Journal of Psychosomatic Research*, **29**, 113–123.

David, A.J., Wesseley, S. & Pelosi, A.J. (1988). Post-viral syndrome: time for a new approach, *British Medical Journal*, **296**, 696–699.

Davidson, J.R.T., Miller, R.D., Turnbull, C.D. & Sullivan, J.L. (1982). Atypical depression, *Archives of General Psychiatry*, **39**, 527–534.

Devlen, J., Maguire, P., Phillips, P., Crowther, D., Chambers, H. (1987). Psychological problems associated with diagnosis and treatment of lymphomas, *British Medical Journal*, **295**, 953–957.

Edwards, R.H.T. (1981). Human muscle function and fatigue, in *Human Muscle Function: Physiological Mechanisms*, the Ciba Foundation, Symposium no. 82, pp. 1–18, Pitman Medical, London.

Edwards, R.H.T. (1986). Muscle function and pain, *Acta Medica Scandinavica* (Suppl.), **711**, 179–188.

Ellenberger, H.R. (1970). *The discovery of the unconscious. The History and Evolution of Dynamic Psychiatry*, Allen Lane, Penguin Press, London.

Ffrench, G. (1960). The clinical significance of tiredness, *Canadian Medical Association Journal*, **82**, 665–671.

Folgering, H. & Snik, A. (1988). Hyperventilation syndrome and muscle fatigue, *Journal of Psychosomatic Research*, **32**, 165–171.

Freal, J.E., Kraft, G.H. & Coryell, J.K. (1984). Symptomatic fatigue in multiple sclerosis, *Archives of Physical Medicine and Rehabilitation*, **65**, 135–138.

Freudenberger, H.J. (1974). Staff burn-out, *Journal of Social Issues*, **30**, 159–165.

Friedman, M. (1947). Studies concerning the etiology and pathogenesis of neurocirculatory asthenia. V. The introduction of a new test for the diagnosis and assessment of the syndrome, *Psychosomatic Medicine*, **9**, 233–241.

Friman, G., Wright, J.E., Ilback, N.G. *et al.* (1985) Does fever or myalgia indicate reduced physical performance capacity in viral infections? *Acta Medica Scandinavica*, **217**, 353–361.

Gardner, W.N., Meah, M. & Bass, C. (1986). Controlled study of respiratory responses during prolonged measurement in patients with chronic hyperventilation, *Lancet*, **ii**, 826–830.

Gendel, E.S. (1973). Women: fitness and fatigue, *West Virginia Medical Journal*, **69**, 112–118.

Globus, G.G. (1970). Sleep duration and feeling state, *International Psychiatry Clinics*, **7**, 78–84

Goldberg, D.P., Bridges, K., Duncan-Jones, P. & Grayson, D.A. (1987). Dimensions of neuroses seen in primary care settings, *Psychological Medicine*, **17**, 461–470.

Goldenberg, D.L. (1987). Fibromyalgia syndrome: an emerging but controversial condition, *Journal of the American Medical Association*, **257**, 2782–2787.

Goodwin, F.K. & Bunney, W.E. (1971). Depressions following Reserpine: a re-evaluation, *Seminars in Psychiatry*, **3**, 435–448.

Gould, J. (1957). Virus disease and psychiatric ill-health, *British Journal of Clinical Practice*, **11**, 918–922.

Guilleminault, C. & Mondini, S. (1984). Sleep disorders, in *Recent Advances in Clinical Neurology* (Number 4) (Eds. Matthews, W.B. & Glaser, G.H.), Churchill Livingstone, Edinburgh and New York.

Guilleminault, C. & Mondini, S. (1986). Mononucleosis and chronic daytime sleepiness: a long-term follow-up study, *Archives of Internal Medicine*, **146**, 1333–1335.

Hannay, D.R. (1978). Symptom prevalence in the community, *Journal of the Royal College of General Practitioners*, **28**, 492–499.

Hawkins, D.R., Taub, J.M. & Van de Castle, R.L. (1985). Extended sleep (hypersomnia) in young depressed patients, *American Journal of Psychiatry*, **142**, 905–910.

Haylock, P.J. & Hart, L.K. (1979). Fatigue in patients receiving localised radiation, *Cancer Nursing*, **2**, 461–467.

Henderson, D.A. & Shelokov, A. (1959). Epidemic neuromyasthenia — clinical syndrome? *New England Journal of Medicine*, **260**, 757–764.

Hickey, A.J., Andrews, G. & Wilcken, D.E.L. (1983). Independence of mitral valve prolapse and neurosis, *British Heart Journal*, **50**, 333–336.

Hickie, I., Lloyd, A., Wakefield, D. & Parker, G. (1990). The psychiatric status of patients with chronic fatigue syndrome, *British Journal of Psychiatry*, **156**, 534–540.

Hobbs, P., Ballinger, C.B. & Smith, A.H.W. (1983). Factor analysis and validation of the general health questionnaire in women: a general practice survey, *British Journal of Psychiatry*, **142**, 257–264.

Hoddes, E., Zarcone, V., Smythe, H., Phillips, R. & Dement, W.C. (1973). Quantification of sleepiness: a new approach, *Psychophysiology*, **10**, 431–436.

Holmes, G.P., Kaplan, J.E., Gantz, N.M. *et al.* (1988). Chronic fatigue syndrome: a working case definition, *Annals of Internal Medicine*, **108**, 387–389.

Horning, S.J., Levine, J.F., Miller, R.A., Rosenberg, S.A. & Merigan, T.C. (1982). Clinical and immunologic effects of recombinant leukocyte interferon in eight patients with advanced cancer, *Journal of the American Medical Association*, **247**, 1718–1722.

Ho-Yen, D.O., Carrington, D. & Armstrong, A.A. (1988). Myalgic encephalomyelitis and alpha-interferon, *Lancet*, **i**, 125.

Hueting, J.E. & Sarphati, H.R. (1966). Measuring fatigue, *Journal of Applied Psychology*, **50**, 535–538.

Hughes, J.R., Crow, R.S., Jacobs, D.R., Mittelmark, M.B. & Lean, A.S. (1984). Physical activity, smoking and exercise induced fatigue, *Journal of Behavioural Medicine*, **7**, 217–230.

Hughson, A.V.M., Cooper, A.F., McArdle, C.S. & Smith, D.C. (1987). Psychosocial effects of radiotherapy after mastectomy, *British Medical Journal*, **294**, 1515–1518.

Imboden, J.B., Canter, A. & Cluff, L.E. (1961). Convalescence from influenza: a study of the psychological and clinical determinants, *Archives of Internal Medicine*, **108**, 393–399.

Isaacs, R. (1948). Chronic infectious mononucleosis, *Blood*, **3**, 858–861.

Jerrett, W.A. (1981). Lethargy in general practice, *Practitioner*, **225**, 731–737.

Jenkins, R. (1985). Sex differences in minor psychiatric morbidity, *Psychological Medicine* (Monograph Suppl. 7), Cambridge University Press, Cambridge.

Jones, J.F. & Straus, S.E. (1987). Chronic Epstein–Barr virus infection, *Annual Reviews of Medicine*, **38**, 195–209.

Jones, M., Mellersh, V. & Musgrave, M. (1946). A comparison of the exercise response in anxiety states and normal controls, *Psychosomatic Medicine*, **8**, 180–187.

Kashiwagi, S. (1971). Psychological rating of human fatigue, *Ergonomics*, **14**, 17–21.

Kendell, R.E. & Discipio, W.J. (1968). Eysenck personality inventory scores of patients with depressive illnesses, *British Journal of Psychiatry*, **114**, 767–770.

Kirmayer, L.J., Robbins, J.M. & Kapusta, M.A. (1988). Somatization and depression in fibromyalgia syndrome, *American Journal of Psychiatry*, **145**, 950–954.

Kotrlik, J., Peychl, L. & Zastera, M. (1968). Pseudoneurasthenic syndrome in lymph node toxoplasmosis, *Sbornik Vedeckych Praci Lekarske Fakulty Karlovy University*, **11**, 393–395.

Kraepelin, E. (1907). Acquired neurasthenia: chronic nervous exhaustion, in *Clinical Psychiatry* (2nd edn.) (Transl. Diefendorf, A.R.), pp. 146–158, Scholars' Facsimilies and Reprints, New York, Delmar (1981).

Kraupl Taylor, F. (1966). The psychopathology of affect — functional psychoses, in *Psychopathology: its Causes and Symptoms*, pp. 136–150, Butterworth, London.

Kroenke, K., Wood, D.R., Mangelsdorff, A.D., Meier, N.J. & Powell, J.B. (1988). Chronic fatigue in primary care: prevalence, patient characteristics, and outcome, *Journal of the American Medical Association*, **260**, 929–934.

Krueger, J.M., Walter, J., Dinarello, C.A. & Chedid, L. (1985). Induction of slow-wave sleep by Interleukin-1 in *The Physiologic, Metabolic, and Immunologic Actions of Interleukin-1* (Eds. Kluger, M.J., Oppenheim, J.J. & Powenda, M.C.), pp. 161–170, Alan R. Liss Inc., London.

Kruesi, M.J.P., Dale, J. & Straus, S.E. (1989). Psychiatric diagnoses in patients who have chronic fatigue syndrome, *Journal of Clinical Psychiatry*, **50**, 53–56.

Ladee, G.A., Scholten, J.M. & Meyes, F.E.P. (1966). Diagnostic problems in psychiatry with regard to acquired toxoplasmosis, *Psychiatria Neurologia Neurochirurgia*, **69**, 65–82.

Lancet (1985). Snoring and sleepiness, *Lancet*, **ii**, 925–926.

Lancet (1987). Aching muscles after exercise, *Lancet*, **ii**, 1123–1124.

Lawton, A.H., Rich, T.A., McKendon, S., Gates, E.H. & Bond, J.O. (1970). Follow-up studies of St. Louis encephalitis in Florida: reevaluation of the emotional and health status of the survivors five years after acute illness, *Southern Medical Journal*, **63**, 66–71.

Lindegard, B. & Nystrom, S. (1970). Predisposition for mental illness: a prospective study of adult male psychiatric in- and out-patients in a Swedish urban population, *Acta Socio-medica Scandinavica*, **1**, 1–22.

Lishman, W.A. (1988). Physiogenesis and psychogenesis in the post-concussional syndrome, *British Journal of Psychiatry*, **153**, 460–469.

Lloyd, A.R., Hales, J.R. & Gandevia, S.C. (1988a). Muscle strength, endurance and recovery in the post-infection fatigue syndrome, *Journal of Neurology, Neurosurgery and Psychiatry*, **51**, 1316–1322.

Lloyd, A.R., Hanna, D.A. & Wakefield, D. (1988b). Interferon and myalgic encephalomyelitis, *Lancet*, **i**, 471.

Lloyd, A.R., Wakefield, D., Boughton, C. & Dwyer, J. (1988c). What is myalgic encephalomyelitis? *Lancet*, **i**, 1286–1287.

Lucas, C.J., Linken, A. & Knowles, J.B. (1966). A trial of prolintane in the treatment of fatigue, *Practitioner*, **197**, 801–805.

McCain, G.A. (1986). Role of physical fitness training in the fibrositis/fibromyalgia syndrome, *The American Journal of Medicine* (Suppl. 3a), **81**, 73–77.

Macdonald, E.M., Mann, A.H. & Thomas, H.C. (1987). Interferons as mediators of psychiatric morbidity. An investigation in a trial of recombinant alpha-interferon in hepatitis-B carriers, *Lancet*, **ii**, 1175–1178.

McEvedy, C.P. & Beard, A.W. (1970a). Royal Free epidemic of 1955: a reconsideration, *British Medical Journal*, **1**, 7–11.

McEvedy, C.P. & Beard, A.W. (1970b). Concept of benign myalgic encephalomyelitis, *British Medical Journal*, **1**, 11–15.

Mackie, R.R. (1977). *Vigilance, Theory, Operational Performance, and Physiological Correlates*, Plenum Press, New York and London.

Macmillan, M.B. (1976). Beard's concept of neurasthenia and Freud's concept of the actual neuroses, *Journal of the History of the Behavioural Sciences*, **12**, 376–390.

McNair, D.M. & Lorr, M. (1964). An analysis of mood in neurotics, *Journal of Abnormal and Social Psychology*, **69**, 620–627.

Mallows, H.R. (1970). Hot-climate fatigue in the far east fleet 1966–1968. Surveys of lay opinion, *Journal of the Royal Naval Medical Service*, **56**, 186–191.

Manu, P., Matthews, D.A. & Lane, T.J. (1988). The mental health of patients with a chief complaint of chronic fatigue: prospective evaluation and follow-up, *Archives of Internal Medicine*, **148**, 2213–2217.

Manu, P., Matthews, D.A., Lane, T.J. *et al.* (1989). Depression among patients with a chief complaint of chronic fatigue, *Journal of Affective Disorders*, **17**, 165–172.

Martini, G.A. & Strohmeyer, G. (1974). Posthepatitis syndrome, *Clinics in Gastroenterology*, **3**, 377–390.

Mattson, K., Niiranen, A., Iivanainen, M. *et al.* (1983). Neurotoxicity of interferon, *Cancer Treatment Reports*, **67**, 958–961.

May, P.G.R., Donnan, S.P.B., Ashton, J.R., Oglivie, M.M. & Rolles, C.J. (1980). Personality and medical perception in Benign Myalgic Encephalomyelitis, *Lancet*, **ii**, 1122–1124.

Mehta, B.C. (1984). Effects of iron deficiency — an iceberg phenomenon, *Journal of the Association of Physicians of India*, **32**, 895–900.

Mitchell, S.W. (1884). *Fat and Blood: An Essay on the Treatment of Certain Forms of Neurasthenia and Hysteria*, (3rd edn.), J.B. Lippincott, Philadelphia.

Moldofsky, H., Lue, F.A., Eisen, J., Keystone, E. & Gorczynski, R.M. (1986). The relationship of Interleukin-1 and immune functions to sleep in humans, *Psychosomatic Medicine*, **48**, 309–318.

Moldofsky, H. & Scarisbrick, P. (1976). Induction of neurasthenic musculoskeletal pain syndrome by selective sleep stage deprivation, *Psychosomatic Medicine*, **38**, 35–44.

Montomergy, G.K. (1983). Uncommon tiredness among college undergraduates, *Journal of Consulting and Clinical Psychology*, **51**, 517–525.

Morrison, J.D. (1980). Fatigue as a presenting complaint in family practice, *Journal of Family Practice*, **10**, 795–801.

Morte, S., Castilla, A., Civeira, M.P., Serrano, M. & Prieto, J. (1988). Gamma-interferon and chronic fatigue syndrome, *Lancet*, **ii**, 623–624.

Muller, R., Nylander, I., Larsson, L.E., Widen, L. & Frankenhaeuser, M. (1958). Sequelae of primary aseptic meningo-encephalitis, *Acta Psychiatrica et Neurologica Scandinavica* (Suppl. 126), **33**, 1–117.

Myerson, A. (1922). Anhedonia, *American Journal of Psychiatry*, **2**, 87–103.

Myles, W.A. (1985). Sleep deprivation, physical fatigue, and the perception of exercise intensity, *Medicine and Science in Sports and Medicine*, **17**, 580–584.

Newham, D. & Edwards, R.H.T. (1979). Effort syndromes, *Physiotherapy*, **65**, 52–56.

Parkes, J.D. (1983). Variability in Parkinson's disease; clinical aspects, causes and treatment, *Acta Neurologica Scandinavica* (Suppl.), **95**, 27–35.

Parkes, J.D. (1985). *Sleep and its Disorders*, W.B. Saunders, Eastbourne.

Petersen, P. (1968). Psychiatric disorders in primary hyperparathyroidism, *Journal of Clinical Endocrinology and Metabolism*, **28**, 1491–1495.

Philips, C. (1987). Avoidance behaviour and its role in sustaining chronic pain, *Behaviour Research and Therapy*, **25**, 273–279.

Poteliakhoff, A. (1981). Adrenocortical activity and some clinical findings in acute and chronic fatigue, *Journal of Psychosomatic Research*, **25**, 91–95.

Quitkin, F.M., Stewart, J.W., McGrath, P.J. *et al.* (1988). Phenelzine versus imipramine in the treatment of probable atypical depressive illness; defining syndrome boundaries of selective MAOI responders, *American Journal of Psychiatry*, **145**, 306–311.

Ramsay, M.A. (1986). *Post-viral Fatigue Syndrome: The Saga of Royal Free Disease*, Gower Medical Publishing, London.

Riddle, P.K. (1982). Chronic fatigue and women: a description and suggested treatment, *Women and Health*, **7**, 37–47.

Roberts, G.A. (1986). Burnout: psychobabble or valuable concept? *British Journal of Hospital Medicine*, **36**, 194–197.

Rockwell, D.A. & Burr, B.D. (1974). The tired patient, *Journal of Family Practice*, **1**, 62–65.

Rose, E.A. & King, T.C. (1978). Understanding postoperative fatigue, *Surgery, Gynaecology and Obstetrics*, **147**, 97–102.

Rubin, R.T. & Poland, R.E. (1977). Human sleep: basic mechanisms and pathologic patterns, in *Biological Bases of Psychiatric Disorders* (Eds. Frazer, A. & Winokur, A.), Spectrum Public Inc., New York and London.

Ryn, Z. (1979). Nervous system and altitude syndrome of high altitude asthenia, *Acta Medica Polona*, **20**, 155–169.

Saltin, B., Blomqvist, G., Mitchell, J.H., Johnson, R.L., Wikdenthal, K. & Chapman, C.B. (1968). Response to exercise after bed rest and after training, *Circulation* (Suppl. 7), **38**, 1–78.

Saskin, P., Moldofsky, H. & Lue, F.A. (1986). Sleep and post-traumatic rheumatic pain modulation disorder (fibrositis syndrome), *Psychosomatic Medicine*, **48**, 319–323.

Searle, J.R. (1989). *The Mind Body Problem*, 3rd Jacobson Lecture, 16 May, University of London.

Slater, E. & Roth, M. (1969). Personality deviations and neurotic reactions, in *Clinical Psychiatry* (3rd edn.) (Eds. Slater, E. & Roth, M.), pp. 81–85, Balliere Tindall and Cassell, London.

Smedley, H., Katrak, M., Sikora, K. & Wheeler, T. (1983). Neurological effects of recombinant human interferon, *British Medical Journal*, **286**, 262–264.

Smith, G.R., Monson, R.A. & Ray, D.C. (1986). Patients with multiple unexplained symptoms: their characteristics, functional health, and health care utilization, *Archives of Internal Medicine*, **146**, 69–72.

Snaith, R.P. (1987). The concepts of mild depression, *British Journal of Psychiatry*, **150**, 387–393.

Solberg, L.I. (1984). Lassitude: a primary care evaluation, *Journal of the American Medical Association*, **251**, 3272–3276.

Stokes, M.J., Cooper, R.G. & Edwards, R.H.T. (1988). Normal muscle strength and fatigability in patients with effort syndromes, *British Medical Journal*, **297**, 1014–1017.

Straus, S.E., Dale, J.K., Tobi, M. *et al.* (1988). Acyclovir treatment of the chronic fatigue syndrome. Lack of efficacy in a placebo-controlled trial, *New England Journal of Medicine*, **319**, 1692–1698.

Surridge, D.H.E., Williams Erdahl, D.L., Lawson, J.S. *et al.* (1984). Psychiatric aspects of diabetes mellitus, *British Journal of Psychiatry*, **145**, 269–276.

Taerk, G.S., Toner, B.B., Salit, I.E., Garfinkel, P.E. & Ozersky, S. (1987). Depression in patients with neuromyasthenia (benign myalgic encephalomyelitis), *International Journal of Psychiatry in Medicine*, **17**, 49–56.

Totman, R., Kiff, J., Reed, S.E. & Craig, J.W. (1980). Predicting experimental colds in volunteers from different measures of recent life stress, *Journal of Psychosomatic Research*, **24**, 155–163.

Valdini, A.F., Steinhardt, S.I. & Jaffe, A.S. (1987). Dermographic correlates of fatigue in a university family health center, *Family Practice*, **4**, 103–107.

Valle-Jones, J.C. (1978). Pemoline in the treatment of psychogenic fatigue in general practice, *Practitioner*, **221**, 425–427.

Van Deusen, E.H. (1869). Observations on a form of nervous prostration (Neurasthenia) culminating in insanity, *American Journal of Insanity*, **25**, 445–461.

Verhaest, S. & Pierloot, R. (1980). An attempt at an empirical delimitation of neurasthenic neurosis and its relation with some character traits, *Acta Psychiatrica Scandinavica*, **62**, 166–176.

von Economo, C. (1931). *Encephalitis Lethargica; its sequelae and treatment* (Transl. Newman, K.O.), Oxford University Press, London.

Wessel-Aas, T., Vale, J.R. & Schaaming, J. (1968). Occupational disease caused by gas inhalation. Pulmonary functional impairment and neurasthenic symptoms following industrial gas injury, *Scandinavian Journal of Respiratory Diseases* (Suppl.), **63**, 95–99.

Wessely, S. (1990). Old wine in new bottles: Neurasthenia and 'ME', *Psychological Medicine*, **20**, 35–53.

Wessely, S., Butler, S., Chalder, T. & David, A. (1990). The cognitive behavioural management of the postviral fatigue syndrome, in *The Postviral Fatigue Syndrome* (Eds. Jenkins, R. & Mowbray, J.), John Wiley, Chichester, (in press).

Wessely, S. & Powell, R. (1989). Fatigue syndromes: a comparison of chronic 'postviral' fatigue with neuromuscular and affective disorder, *Journal of Neurology Neurosurgery and Psychiatry*, **52**, 940–948.

Wheeler, E.O., White, P.D., Reed, E.W. & Cohen, M.E. (1950). Neurocirculatory asthenia (anxiety neurosis, effort syndrome, neurasthenia). A twenty year follow-up study of one hundred and seventy three patients, *Journal of the American Medical Association*, **142**, 878–889.

White, P.D. (1988). Psychiatric illness after glandular fever, *Society for Psychosomatic Research Annual Conference*, November 14th, London (abstract).

White, P.D. (1989). Fatigue syndrome: neurasthenia revived, *British Medical Journal*, **298**, 1199–1200.

White, P.D. (1990). Psychoimmunology, in *Principles and Practice of Biological Psychiatry* (Ed. Dinan, T.), Clinical Neuroscience Publishers, London (in press).

White, P.D. & Lewis, S.W. (1988). Delusional depression after infectious mononucleosis, *British Medical Journal*, **295**, 97–98.

Wilson, D.R., Widmer, R.B., Cadoret, R.J. & Judiesch, K. (1983). Somatic symptoms: a major feature of depression in a family practice, *Journal of Affective Disorders*, **5**, 199–207.

World Health Organization (1978). *Manual of the International Statistical Classification of Diseases, Injuries, and Causes of Death* (9th revision) World Health Organization, Geneva.

World Health Organization (1988). Mental, behavioural and developmental disorders, in *International Classifications of Disease* (10th revision) Draft chapter V(F), Division of Mental Health, World Health Organization, Geneva (copyright reserved).

Wrightson, P. & Gronwall, D. (1981). Time off work and symptoms after minor head injury, *Injury*, **12**, 445–454.

Yonge, R.P. (1988). Magnetic resonance muscle studies: implications for psychiatry, *Journal of the Royal Society of Medicine*, **81**, 322–326.

Zigmond, A.S. & Snaith, R.P. (1983). The hospital anxiety and depression scale, *Acta Psychiatrica Scandinavica*, **67**, 361–370.

# 6

# Functional Abdominal Pain

F.H. CREED

## Review of the disorder

### Historical introduction

Functional abdominal pain was described by Cummings in 1849 when he associated left hypochondriac or iliac pain with bowels which were 'at one time constipated at another lax in the same person'. These symptoms were accompanied by the discharge of a 'peculiar membranous matter' and the syndrome became known as 'membranous colitis'. This was much more common among females than males and often accompanied by dysmenorrhoea. The patient's personality was characterized by 'more or less nervousness ... with an expression of continence so striking that one can with tolerable certainty tell, without more minute examination, what the nature of the condition is'.

White (1905) described 60 cases of 'membranous colitis', of whom 51 were female. White observed that 'it is so frequently associated with many forms of neurosis that those who maintain that its cause lies in the nervous system cannot be regarded as unreasonable'. He noted the presence of pronounced illness behaviour in a few patients who did not recover: they belonged to 'the hopeless group of neurotic bedridden invalids, dwelling on their illness, interested in their motions, magnifying their aches and pains and apparently almost loving their complaint'.

The link between functional bowel symptoms and neurosis has remained to this day and will form a central theme of this chapter. Experimental evidence to support the link between the nervous system and the colon came from McEwan's (1904) observation that a man's exposed caecum contracted vigorously when he received bad news and Almy's et al. (1949) demonstration that colonic motility was altered by experimental stress. But experimental evidence to support a complete physiological explanation of functional abdominal complaints is still lacking, which is why we still rely on a series of clinical findings to describe the syndrome.

The syndrome was put on a secure footing by Chaudhury and Truelove's (1962) classic description of the disorder known then as the irritable colon. They recognized that a proportion of cases followed an episode of dysentery and that some were associated with psychological factors; these two aetiological agents could be related to prognosis.

Although much has been learned about bowel function over the subsequent 20 years, the clinical description given by Chaudhury and Truelove still holds, though it has been renamed irritable bowel syndrome because it affects the whole bowel, not just the colon. In his review, Thompson (1984) delineated five syndromes:

1  spastic colon
2  constipation — spastic, — atonic/painless
3  painless diarrhoea
4  gas
5  chronic abdomen

### Definition of the syndrome

Definition of terms has been imprecise in this field of medicine, reflecting our poor understanding of pathophysiology and lack of any definite clinical criteria to delineate meaningful subgroups of patients. Early definitions relied solely on the absence of organic disease and the term functional gastrointestinal disorder has recently been used to describe 'a variable combination of chronic or recurrent gastrointestinal symptoms which cannot be explained by structural or by chemical abnormalities' (IBS Working Team Report, 1988). But the largest group of patients with functional gastrointestinal disorder is that with the irritable bowel syndrome, and this chapter will use this syndrome (IBS) as a model for understanding functional bowel disorder.

There is no clear agreement about how widely the term should be used. Some authors include all of the syndromes listed by Thompson (see above) and include, in addition, oesophageal spasm, hepatic flexure syndrome, flatulent or X-ray negative dyspepsia and proctalgia fugax (McCloy & McCloy, 1988). Others wish to limit the definition, especially for research purposes, and the IBS Working Team Report for the International Congress of Gastroenterology (1988) has recently defined IBS as continuous or recurrent symptoms of:

1  Abdominal pain, relieved with defaecation, or associated with change in frequency or consistency of stool, and/or
2  Disturbed defaecation (two or more of):
   (a)  altered stool frequency
   (b)  altered stool form (hard or loose/watery)

(c) altered stool passage (straining or urgency, feeling of incomplete evacuation)

(d) passage of mucus

Usually with:

**3** Bloating or feeling of upper abdominal distension.

Whatever the exact definition, there is widespread agreement that the irritable bowel syndrome affects all of the gut and not just the colon as originally thought. Patients with typical lower abdominal IBS symptoms have been shown to have abnormalities of oesophageal motility (Whorwell *et al.*, 1981) and often complain of belching, acid regurgitation, heartburn or nausea (Cann & Read, 1985). Although patients with upper abdominal symptoms — so-called 'functional dyspepsia', are sometimes regarded separately (Crean, 1985), they may also experience lower abdominal symptoms and are often eventually diagnosed as having IBS (Colgan *et al.*, 1988).

In this chapter no attempt will therefore be made to distinguish between these syndromes, especially as most research has included 'IBS patients' as a group without precisely defining the syndrome. It is likely that a model constructed on the evidence relating to IBS will be applicable to other syndromes of functional gastrointestinal disorders.

## Epidemiology

Approximately one-third of new outpatients seen in the gastroenterology clinics have functional bowel disorders, predominantly IBS (Table 6.1). These disorders therefore represent a major part of a gastroenterologist's workload, and a working party to assess the need for more gastroenterologists in the UK estimated that between 600 and 1000 new patients with functional bowel

**Table 6.1.** Proportion of patients attending a gastroenterology clinic who have functional complaints

| | Number of patients | IBS (%) | Total 'functional' (%) |
|---|---|---|---|
| Ferguson *et al.* (1977) | 88 | 26 | 31 |
| Sullivan (1983) | 1082 | 17 | |
| Switz *et al.* (1976) | 369 | | 23 |
| Manning (1980) | 1276 | 9 | 29 |
| MacDonald & Bouchier (1980) | 67 | | 48 |
| Harvey *et al.* (1983) | 2000 | 23 | 44 |
| Ford *et al.* (1987) | 134 | | 78 |
| Mitchell & Drossman (1987) (survey of gastroenterologists) | | 28 | 41 |

disorders were attending gastroenterology clinics each week (Royal College of Physicians, 1984).

Hospital discharge figures for the USA in 1984 indicated that 472 000 patients were discharged during that year with an ICD-9 diagnosis of 'other and unspecified noninfectious gastroenteritis and colitis'. The number of hospital days totalled 1 942 000 which was exceeded in the digestive diseases category only by ulcer and gall bladder disease. Those patients discharged with a diagnosis of 'undiagnosed abdominal pain' (ICD code 785.5) were studied in detail in Oxford (Rang *et al.*, 1970); young females predominated, the readmission rate was high and subsequent admissions to a psychiatric unit were 13 times the expected rate.

Information from general practice is limited, but functional complaints are probably twice as common as organic ones. Colic, appendicular pains, disorders of function of the stomach, constipation and other symptoms total 36.7 patients consulting per year, compared to 19 per year for peptic ulcer and other organic conditions (OPCS 1974). Bond (1987) identified a small sample of IBS sufferers in his practice and fewer than half had been referred to the hospital clinic.

Surveys in the community have yielded reasonably consistent results; their main disadvantage is reliance on questionnaires without physical examination. Six or more episodes of abdominal pain a year are reported by approximately 20% of the population but this pain is associated with con-comitant disturbed bowel function in only 12–14% of the population — the IBS group (Table 6.2). These symptoms are reported more often by females than by males, and females predominate in clinic samples. In India males used to predominate (Pimparkar, 1970; Bordie, 1972) but now females have higher rates there also (Kapoor *et al.*, 1985), reflecting the importance of changing consultation patterns.

A few community surveys have also examined psychosocial factors. In the large Tromso survey Johnsen *et al.* (1986) found that cramping abdominal pain together with bloating were closely associated with depression, sleeping difficulties and problems of coping. Sandler *et al.* (1984) found that those subjects in the community with IBS symptoms who had consulted a doctor for their bowel symptoms showed a generalized tendency to consult more frequently than those who reported IBS symptoms but who had not seen a doctor about them. This finding raised the possibility that it is only neurotic people who consult with IBS symptoms, but it is worth noting that the consulters also experienced more abdominal pain.

In a subsequent study Drossman *et al.* (1988) measured severity of bowel symptoms more accurately with a diary and confirmed that IBS consulters had more severe symptoms than non-consulters. But the consulters also had

**Table 6.2.** Community surveys of IBS, indicating the proportion of the general population who reported gastrointestinal symptoms (regular episodes of abdominal pain or a symptom complex amounting to IBS) and the proportion who were 'consulters'

|  | Number of subjects | Abdominal pain (%) | IBS syndrome (%) | % Who had consulted |
|---|---|---|---|---|
| Thompson & Heaton (1980) | 301 | 21 | 14 | 23[*] |
| Drossman *et al.* (1982) | 789 | 24 | 12 | 46[†] |
| Sandler *et al.* (1984) | 566 | — | 15 | 38[†] |
| Johnsen *et al.* (1986) | 14 000 | 14 | 11 | 23[†] |
| Whitehead *et al.* 1988 | 149 (not random) | | | 20[*] |

[*] Seen doctor during previous year for bowel complaints.
[†] Seen doctor ever for bowel complaints.

raised scores on several MMPI and IBQ scores. After controlling for severity of bowel symptoms some of these raised scores remained, and the authors concluded that it was the *interaction* of psychosocial factors and the degree of altered bowel physiology that determined the illness experience and treatment-seeking behaviour.

Whitehead *et al.* (1988) found raised scores on the Hopkins symptom checklist among two groups of women: attenders at a medical clinic with either organic or functional complaints, and those in the community who reported vague abdominal complaints but who had not consulted a doctor. Other women in the community who described specific attacks of abdominal pain associated with disturbance of bowel function (IBS) did not show evidence of neuroticism.

One last study examined health beliefs. Compared to non-consulters with dyspepsia, consulters at the general practice did not appear to have more severe symptoms, but had experienced more stressful life events and had more pronounced concerns that their dyspeptic symptoms might represent underlying serious or fatal disease. They also were much more likely to possess health-related literature and to read articles in newspapers or magazines about their symptoms (Lydeard & Jones, 1988).

## Model

Gastroenterologists have long searched for a specific physiological abnormality in the gut of those who experience IBS symptoms. This would elevate the syndrome to the status of an illness, which would then be recognized by all doctors (McCloy & McCloy, 1988). But motility studies have failed to distinguish IBS subjects from healthy controls (Greenbaum *et al.*, 1983), and there is evidence that the gut responds to stress in IBS patients and normal controls in a similar fashion (Chaudhury & Truelove, 1961; Sandler *et al.*, 1984).

The evidence from epidemiological studies indicates that a different model is required and Barsky (1987) has suggested that the disorder is better viewed as a dimensional disorder akin to depression or hypertension, disorders which form a continuum with normality. Thus severe states are associated with physiological or pathological abnormalities and only some sufferers in the community reach medical attention. Depression may follow severe life events but other factors including inherited constitutional factors and current social support modify the severity of the depression. It may well be the same with the gut response to stress — some subjects are constitutionally predisposed to develop very severe bowel symptoms, whereas in others the symptoms are milder. In either case, severity of symptoms is not the only factor that determines whether medical attention is sought.

It is possible to rate attenders at a clinic with IBS along these two continua:

| | | B | | A C | |
|---|---|---|---|---|---|
| Severity of bowel symptoms: | Mild | ———————————— | | | Severe |
| | | C | | A B | |
| Active psychosocial factors: | Absent/ mild | ———————————— | | | Present/ severe |

Patient A has severe bowel symptoms and is under severe stress. Patient B has mild bowl symptoms but is distressed about them and has attended the clinic because of severe stress (e.g. recent divorce). Patient C's bowel symptoms are sufficiently severe to merit medical attention in their own right even though there is no apparent stress.

In this model social stress is related to seeking medical treatment but the picture is complicated because stress may also be related to the causation of bowel symptoms. Chaudhury and Truelove (1962) described a middle-aged man whose symptoms occurred at the time of his marital separation and cleared once he had successfully remarried. A younger female patient with conflicts at home had severe bowel symptoms until she left home, but the younger age of this patient and the persistence of symptoms during her teenage years suggest that she was constitutionally predisposed to develop IBS symptoms to a greater extent than the first patient.

A *model* of the aetiology of IBS can therefore be constructed as follows:
**1** Constitutional tendency to develop bowel dysfunction (presumably reflected in family history)

**2** Current severity of bowel symptoms; related to social stress and/or concomitant anxiety/depression

**3** Tendency to seek treatment:
    (a) past learning from parental response to childhood abdominal pain
    (b) past or recent abdominal illness in family members, and
    (c) recent social stress

It can be seen from this model that the role of social stress (and any concomitant anxiety/depression) might be active in both exacerbating bowel symptoms *and* lowering the threshold for seeking treatment. Initial clinical assessment must therefore establish whether one or both of these is the case.

## Clinical features

The symptoms of the irritable bowel syndrome vary considerably, reflecting referral patterns. Patients generally present in the third and fourth decades by which time the symptoms have often been present for several years (Waller & Misiewicz, 1969; Harvey *et al.*, 1987). The patient may have undergone an appendicectomy some years before, which yielded a normal appendix (Chaudhury & Truelove, 1962; Lane, 1973; Keeling & Fielding, 1975). In retrospect this may have been the first manifestation of the disorder.

The diagnosis has often been made by the referring doctor who may request help for one of the following reasons: (i) for further reassurance that organic disease is not being missed, especially during an acute episode of pain; (ii) for further help with treatment; and (iii) for further help with those patients whom the GP cannot satisfy. A chronic neurotic problem may be suspected but referral occurs for some 'peace and quiet' (McCloy & McCloy, 1988).

Pain is most common across the lower abdomen or in the left iliac fossa but distension of the colon may lead to pain at any point in the abdomen (Swarbrick *et al.*, 1980). The disturbance of bowel function occurs in these proportions: diarrhoea 39%, constipation 36%, alternating diarrhoea and constipation 25% (Harvey *et al.*, 1987). Tenderness over the colon and reproduction of the pain by insufflation of air into the colon at sigmoidoscopy are the only common signs, and there has been much debate about the number of investigations required to exclude organic disease. The IBS Working Team Report (1988) recommended a physical examination to exclude other diseases which may coexist with IBS and a blood test for a full blood count and ESR. A sigmoidoscopy on a single occasion is recommended to exclude colitis or melanosis coli, but only if individual symptoms merit further investigations should these be contemplated.

**Table 6.3.** Prognosis of patients with IBS

| Authors | Number of subjects | Duration of follow-up (years) | % With organic diagnosis |
|---|---|---|---|
| Hawkins & Cockel (1971) | 163 | 2–20 | 2 |
| Holmes & Salter (1982) | 77 | 6+ | 2 |
| Svedsen *et al.* (1985) | 112 | 6 | 4 |

**Prognosis**

This recommendation to keep investigations to a minimum reflects increasing confidence in making a clinical diagnosis as well as evidence from follow-up studies that organic disease is rarely missed in IBS patients (Table 6.3). Even the detection of organic disease may be coincidental rather than aetiologically relevant; in at least one study (Holmes & Salter, 1982) the organic diagnosis was established only after fresh symptoms had emerged, which suggests a different disease process.

Chaudhury and Truelove addressed the other aspect of prognosis — which clinical features predict improvement in bowel symptoms? A history of dysentery at the onset of the disorder predicted a good prognosis whereas the presence of psychological factors predicted a poor one (Fig. 6.1). This aspect of the syndrome has been inadequately studied but three other studies have suggested that the presence of psychiatric symptoms indicates a poor prognosis (Macdonald & Bouchier, 1980; Lancaster-Smith *et al.*, 1982; Whorwell *et al.*, 1987).

Patients in the poor prognosis group were tertiary referrals to Kingham and Dawson (1985); 22 patients had seen 76 consultants for their functional abdominal pain and had undergone the investigations listed in Figure 6.2. The association with depression was clear from the Hamilton Rating Scale results; whether this depression was primary or secondary to the prolonged disability is not clear. There is an obvious need to prevent such overinvestigation.

## Pathophysiological mechanisms

*Site and origin of the pain*

Swarbrick *et al.* (1980) indicated that distension of the colon by a balloon could exactly reproduce the abdominal pain of IBS. They also noted that distension of a balloon in the colon could cause pain in many sites around the abdomen, particularly the iliac fossae. These findings explain why the site of pain in IBS may be so variable.

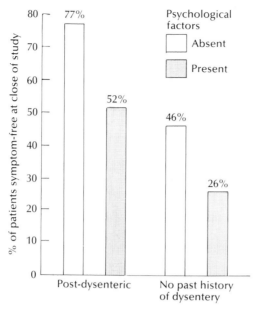

**Fig. 6.1.** The presence of identifiable psychological factors made the prognosis worse both in the post-dysenteric group and in the other patients (after Chaudhary & Truelove, 1962).

Ritchie (1973) had previously used a similar technique to demonstrate that IBS patients had a reduced pain threshold when their gut was distended. In normal subjects a balloon in the colon did not cause any real pain until it contained at least 80 ml of air whereas 60% of IBS patients experienced pain at 60 ml or less. This study is one of the few that has apparently demonstrated a clear difference between IBS patients and normal controls.

Further evidence that the abdominal pain in IBS originates in the colon was provided by Cann and Read (1985). They found a clear temporal relationship between the entry of a test meal into the colon and the onset of abdominal pain in IBS patients.

Although there seems to be reasonable agreement about the *site* of the pain the *mechanism* is much less well understood. Firstly, distension of the colon, to the degree which has been used experimentally, does not occur spontaneously. Nevertheless it has been suggested that increased tension in the bowel wall or compression of the mucosa and submucosa may occur, even though these structures are not normally sensitive to pain (Ritchie, 1985). Secondly, patients with anxiety show similar reduction of pain threshold in the absence of bowel dysfunction (Latimer *et al.*, 1981). Thirdly, Cook *et al.* (1987) have recently demonstrated that IBS subjects have *increased* pain threshold for cutaneous electrical stimuli. They concluded that IBS patients

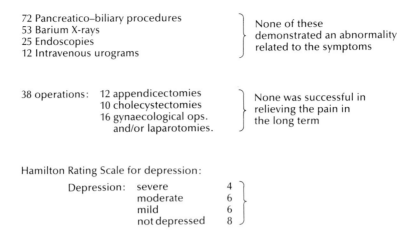

72 Pancreatico–biliary procedures
53 Barium X-rays
25 Endoscopies
12 Intravenous urograms
} None of these
demonstrated an abnormality
related to the symptoms

38 operations:    12 appendicectomies
                  10 cholecystectomies
                  16 gynaecological ops.
                      and/or laparotomies.
} None was successful in
relieving the pain in
the long term

Hamilton Rating Scale for depression:
            Depression:    severe            4
                           moderate          6
                           mild              6
                           not depressed     8

**Fig. 6.2.** Investigations and operations performed on 22 patients with functional abdominal pain reported by Kingham and Dawson (1984).

must have a pain experience comparable to those who have a structural abnormality of the bowel (Crohn's disease) rather than a generalized reduction in pain tolerance.

### Disturbed bowel function

Disturbed bowel function has been measured in several ways. Abnormalities of myoelectrical activity have been demonstrated, with a predominance of 3 cycles per minute activity in IBS subjects that is present even when the patient is in an asymptomatic phase (Snape *et al.*, 1977). Alteration of migrating motor complexes and abnormal contractile activity is altered by the stress of driving in London traffic to a greater extent in IBS patients than normal controls (Kumar & Wingate, 1985).

Reduced whole gut transit time is more common in constipation-prone than diarrhoea-prone IBS subjects, but both these groups have times that are within the normal range (Cann *et al.*, 1985). In patients with constipation, but not those with diarrhoea, transit time increased as symptoms improved but the predominant 3 cycle per minute electrical activity remained, suggesting some form of persistent abnormality (Taylor, 1985).

Increased air swallowing has been found in one study (Calloway & Fonagy, 1985) and was suggested as a possible cause of the bloating that is so common in IBS. But another study failed to demonstrate an increase in volume of gas in the gut; instead more gas tended to reflux back into the stomach of those with functional abdominal pain indicating disordered motility (Lasser *et al.*, 1975).

These experimental findings do not add up to a clear picture of abnormal motility in IBS subjects. Findings have been inconsistent because different techniques of measurement have been used on small groups of subjects with different symptomatology; comparison between IBS subjects and normals on the one hand, and IBS subjects with anxious subjects without bowel symptoms on the other, has failed to reveal any consistent differences (Latimer *et al.*, 1981).

## Psychological factors

The early observations of Cummings and White that the IBS was linked to nervousness was supported by studies using personality inventories and self-rated anxiety questionnaires (Palmer *et al.*, 1974; Esler & Goulston, 1973). But high scores on the Eysenck Personality Inventory or the IPAT may result from any chronic condition and so do not necessarily indicate premorbid neuroticism.

Structured interviews allow more satisfactory assessment, but need to be used with care. Two often quoted studies using such standardized instru-

**Table 6.4.** Proportion of patients with functional abdominal pain and organic disease who were classified as cases of psychiatric disorder

|  |  |  | % With psychiatric disorder | |
| --- | --- | --- | --- | --- |
|  | Number of subjects | Standardized psychiatric interview | Functional abdominal pain | Organic disease |
| McDonald & Bouchier (1980) | 32 | CIS | 53 | 20 |
| Colgan *et al.* (1988) | 37 | CIS | 57 | 6 |
| Kingham & Dawson (1985) | 22 | HRS | 64 | — |
| Craig & Brown (1984) | 79 | PSE | 42 (34) | 18 (16) |
| Ford *et al.* (1987) | 48 | PSE | 42 (31) | 6 (0) |

CIS = Clinical Interview Schedule, HRS = Hamilton Rating Scale for Depression, PSE = Present State Examination. Figures in parentheses represent those patients whose psychiatric disorder occurred before, or at the time of abdominal symptoms.

ments (Young *et al.*, 1976, and Liss *et al.*, 1973) diagnosed the majority of IBS patients as psychiatrically ill because they fulfilled the Feighner criteria for hysteria. That diagnosis rests on the presence of multiple somatic symptoms starting before the age of 30 years. But non-colonic symptoms such as urinary frequency, dyspareunia, back pain, headaches, tiredness, incomplete emptying of bladder, tremor are common in IBS (Whorwell *et al.*, 1986a) and do not by themselves provide adequate evidence of definite psychiatric disorder. Indeed some authors have interpreted these as evidence of a generalized smooth muscle disorder (Whorwell *et al.*, 1986b).

Subsequent studies have used standardized instruments to diagnose anxiety and depression and produced consistent results (Creed & Guthrie, 1987). Table 6.4 indicates that approximately half of IBS patients attending gastroenterology clinics have anxiety or depression by research criteria. In two of the studies (Craig & Brown, 1984; Ford *et al.*, 1987) the authors accurately dated the onset of the psychiatric disorder and the IBS — one-third of IBS patients had anxiety or depression that antedated or coincided with the onset of the bowel symptoms.

**Life events**

Two separate studies have been performed to examine the relationship between the onset of functional bowel symptoms and the experience of stressful life events (Creed, 1981; Craig & Brown, 1984). One study used patients undergoing appendicectomy comparing appendicitis patients with those whose appendix was not acutely inflamed. The second study used patients attending a gastroenterology clinic selecting only those patients whose abdominal symptoms had a clear onset during the previous year.

The results were strikingly similar (Fig. 6.3). Approximately two-thirds of each group with functional abdominal disorder had experienced a severely threatening life event during the previous 38 weeks, a proportion very similar to those presenting with depressive illness (Brown & Harris, 1978) or following an overdose (Farmer & Creed, 1989). These results held even for those subjects who did not have anxiety or depression, which indicates that for some the stressful life event led directly to presentation with abdominal symptomatology, whereas for others anxiety or depression was probably an important intervening variable.

Two similar life events studies have been performed. Ford *et al.* (1987) considered anxiety-provoking life events and found that two-thirds of patients with IBS had experienced either an anxiety-provoking life situation and/or had anxiety with or without depression. Canton *et al.* (1984) found that 48% of patients who had a normal appendix removed had experienced an

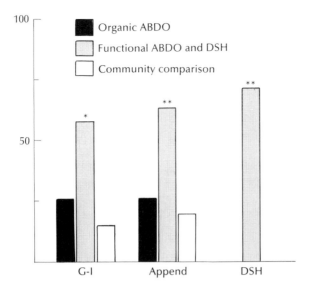

**Fig. 6.3.** Proportion of subjects (as %) experiencing a severe life event during 38 weeks prior to onset of abdominal pain, self-poisoning, or interview in the case of community subjects. (G-I = patients attending gastroenterology clinics; Append = patients undergoing appendicectomy; DSH = deliberate self harm.) $^*p < 0.01$ compared with community comparison group and organic gastrointestinal illness group; $^{**}p < 0.0001$ compared with community comparison group and acute appendicitis group.

'exit' event (loss of close person through death, broken relationship or move) compared to 56% of depressed patients and 16% of normal controls.

### Importance of life event studies to management

Patients attending the gastroenterology clinic with irritable bowel symptoms have often experienced symptoms for many years (Waller & Misiewicz, 1969; Harvey *et al.*, 1987; Sullivan, 1983). As a consequence they cannot be studied by the life event method without fear that the results become contaminated by life events which occurred *after* the onset of abdominal pain. Craig and Brown (1984) circumvented this problem by selecting only those patients whose bowel symptoms had either occurred for the first time, or recurred after a symptom-free period, during the 6 months before the clinic visit. Ford *et al.* (1987) appear to have included patients with chronic symptoms but were able to discern many patients whose anxiety-provoking situations and/ or psychiatric symptoms had preceded the onset of the abdominal symptoms.

It is of interest that chronic difficulties, especially interpersonal ones, have been shown to be present in an unusually high proportion of these patients *before* the onset of the abdominal symptoms. So, although many patients attribute their interpersonal difficulties to their abdominal symptoms (Bouchier & Mason, 1979), the experimental evidence contradicts this. Careful history-seeking is required to elicit the relationship between the onset of the disorder and emotional problems.

The first episode of functional abdominal pain may have led to a normal appendix being removed (Chaudhury & Truelove, 1962; Lane, 1973; Keeling & Fielding, 1975), usually without lasting resolution of the pain (Kingham & Dawson, 1985; Ingram *et al.*, 1965; Creed, 1981). The association with a severely threatening life event at that time might provide the first clear relationship between stress and abdominal pain.

## Illness behaviour

White's early description of illness behaviour among patients with functional abdominal pain has been borne out by more recent studies. In a series of telephone interviews Whitehead *et al.* (1982) elicited more minor illnesses, more childhood illness and more doctor visits among IBS patients than those with a peptic ulcer. Sandler *et al.* (1984) confirmed the frequency of minor ailments and doctor visits.

Two studies have used the Illness Behaviour Questionnaire (Pilowsky, 1981). Canton *et al.* (1984) compared patients who had had a normal appendix removed with depressed patients. Compared to those with depressive illness the appendicectomy patients scored lower on the scales measuring affective disturbance and phobic concern with health but significantly higher on those of disease conviction and somatic versus psychological scale, indicating their conviction that they had severe physical illness. They also denied life problems to a greater extent than the depressed patients even though their life events experience had been similar. These IBQ results were repeated by Joyce *et al.* (1986) who found that acute admissions to a surgical ward with 'non-organic' abdominal pain differed significantly from those with organic disorders; the former showed more affective disturbance, denied life problems and viewed their illness in somatic rather than psychological terms.

Colgan *et al.* (1988) showed that these differences on the IBQ in those with non-organic abdominal symptoms could be attributed to the 50% with psychiatric disorder. This finding may simply reflect the psychometric properties of the IBQ but it also suggests that there are some patients with functional abdominal symptoms who neither have psychiatric disorder nor demonstrate illness behaviour on a self-administered questionnaire.

The *model* of IBS can now be refined in the light of these life events and illness behaviour studies. Severe interpersonal problems, manifest as either discrete life events or chronic difficulties, are associated with the onset of functional bowel complaints irrespective of the presence of psychiatric disorder (anxiety/depression). Illness behaviour, in terms of doctor visits and numerous complaints, may be widespread among those seeking medical treatment for IBS, but in terms of the IBQ those subjects with anxiety and/or depression may play down these psychological symptoms, present somatic symptoms to the doctor and deny other problems in their lives.

# Management

## General principles

There are several aspects of management of patients with IBS. First line treatment for the majority who present to gastroenterologists (approximately 500 new patients each week in the UK — Royal College of Physicians, 1984) includes reassurance, an explanation of the symptoms together with an antispasmodic drug and a bulking agent. Harvey *et al.* (1987) found that up to 83% of patients may respond to such treatment in the short term and the psychological aspects of this management will be discussed below.

In the long term, 30% of Harvey's patients remained troubled by their symptoms; half of these patients were the same or worse as when they had first seen the gastroenterologist. It is this group of patients who are most at risk of becoming chronic clinic attenders and merit a second line of treatment. The aims of management for these patients are: (i) relief of symptoms, if possible; (ii) reduction of disability and secondary illness behaviours; and (iii) reduction of excessive investigations for organic disease. Since this group of patients is smaller than those requiring first line treatment it is reasonable to assess whether more extensive psychological treatments might improve symptoms and be cost-effective. The intensive psychological treatments that have been used — psychotropic drugs, psychotherapy, hypnotherapy, and behaviour therapy — will be reviewed in the second section followed by a brief discussion of our own treatment trial.

A recent survey of American gastroenterologists revealed that half the physicians in academic settings used personal psychosocial support at least three-quarters of the time to treat IBS patients (Mitchell *et al.*, 1987). The techniques that are outlined below can be used by all physicians and others involved in treatment of IBS patients.

## Reassurance and explanation

All doctors must develop the right kind of relationship with the patient if any treatment is to be successful. The correct approach is described elsewhere

(Chapter 3; Creed & Lennard-Jones, 1982). Thereafter some physicians (Sullivan, 1983; Hislop, 1980) rely on explanation and reassurance as the only treatment but most use it in conjunction with some form of medication (anti-spasmodic and bulking agent).

A rational approach to reassurance demands that the doctor first elicits the nature of the patient's worries. These often concern underlying serious physical disease causing the bowel symptoms. It is usually this fear that has led the patient to seek further investigations and treatment. Such fears may often be reinforced by the knowledge of friends or relatives whose serious bowel pathology had initially been regarded as a functional symptom. The question: 'most patients who come with these symptoms fear that they have some serious physical illness, is this the case with you?' will elicit these concerns more often than an open question. For some patients a negative series of investigations will be reassuring but for others they will reinforce doubts that organic disease may be present. The correct approach is to provide a positive explanation for the symptoms.

The first part of the *explanation* concerns the cause of the symptoms. The doctor should use whatever diagrams or models are available to indicate firstly the normal passage of faeces through the bowel by a sequence of contractions. If there is premature distal contraction the subsequent proximal contractions will simply cause a pocket of high pressure and pain. The bowel is not altered structurally, which is why there are no abnormalities on barium enema or sigmoidoscopy; it is simply that the bowel does not function normally. There are three ways that abnormal motility can be improved: (i) for some patients altering the contents of the gut by dietary manipulation or taking Fybogel Bran is sufficient; (ii) others require an antispasmodic drug to reduce the spasm of the bowel wall; and (iii) others require help to reduce the excessive nervous stimulation that occurs during tension and anxiety. Everyone develops butterflies in the stomach when they are anxious, but in those people who are constitutionally liable to develop bowel symptoms under stress the resulting contractions are painful and are often accompanied by bowel dysfunction. This constitutional tendency tends to run in families — a point with which many patients spontaneously concur.

Next, the patient's attention needs to be drawn towards the relation between symptoms and life stress. The symptoms may fluctuate with levels of stress but other factors, including diet, may be involved. Many patients deny that this occurs for them. For example, one of my patients pointed out that diet was more important; her recent episode of severe pain followed the consumption of chocolate and sherry, substances which she knew would upset her bowel. However, closer questioning revealed that she had con-sumed these in a moment of great anger with her mother, who had threatened to leave the patient's home if she did not get her own way. The emotional precipitant was admitted reluctantly by the patient.

Typically, this patient had agreed that her symptoms followed a fluctuating course but immediately denied that there was an emotional precipitant to the present episode. It is therefore best to enquire about previous episodes to determine whether they coincided with major trauma such as the break up of a close relationship, death of a relative, or a more minor problem such as stress at work or trouble with the children. This part of the exploration is very much more effective if the doctor has taken a detailed history which allows him/her to make the appropriate link between emotional stresses and exacerbation of symptoms. The doctor should remember that some patients tend to avoid admitting such a link between emotional stresses and bowel symptoms because they have difficulty facing up to their emotional problems.

*Techniques* which help to make the link between changes in bowel symptoms and emotional changes include:

1  correlation of these two in time, which is best achieved using a diary (see below).

2  commenting on the way that emotionally laden topics cause obvious tension in the patient's hands, posture, etc. during interview.

3  beneficial effect of relaxation either occurring naturally (e.g. on holiday) or induced by relaxation exercises.

It is not uncommon for patients to resist accepting this explanation of the relationship between emotional changes and bowel symptoms. Comments such as 'but everyone gets upsets in their family — that's nothing to do with my diarrhoea', are common. The doctor should not be put off by such statements. If the patient was openly admitting to emotional problems they would not be presenting in this somatic way. It is best to engage the patient in some joint detective work suggesting that the cause of the exacerbation of symptoms is as yet undiscovered and the doctor and patient must work together to look at possible reasons for the symptoms getting worse when they do. This is best done prospectively with a *diary* upon which the patient records the severity of bowel symptoms daily, together with his/her mood and any important life events.

## Keeping an open mind

The most difficult patients to manage are those who continue to express concern about the presence of organic disease in spite of normal investigations. Some persuasive and insistent patients can even arouse such anxieties in the doctor. In these circumstances it is reasonable to proceed along the following lines. Organic causes for the pain have been sought and not found.

The usual physical treatments have been tried and found useless. It is reasonable now to try a different approach to see if it improves the symptoms. Adopting such an approach *does not* mean that the doctors have closed their minds to the possibility of a physical illness *nor* that they are suggesting that the patient is imagining his/her symptoms, but a trial of psychological treatment is a logical next step in the ongoing search for cause and effective treatment. It is worth engaging the patient in discussion about his/her feelings regarding investigations. Most patients become hopeful before a new investigation which might yield the cause of their symptoms, but despondent when no such cause is found — they readily agree that repeated raising of hopes and subsequent disappointment saps the morale. Many feel the failure of the doctors to find a cause for their symptoms is the reason they are so depressed. One can point out at this stage that although they regard their depression as secondary to the bowel symptoms, it may further exacerbate pain by reducing the pain threshold and interfering with bowel function. For this reason alone it is appropriate to attempt some treatment for depression.

### Considering psychological treatments

It can be seen from the above description that patients vary in their readiness to accept that organic disease is not present and accept instead a psychological explanation for their symptoms. This is a crucial step as the psychological treatments that are to be described in the next section can only be utilized if the patient can be engaged in such a course of treatment. Marked resistance to this approach usually indicates that the patient will not comply with such a course of treatment and often drops out, searching once again for a fresh set of investigations.

## Physical treatments

### Tranquillizers and antidepressants

Many gastroenterologists use antidepressants and antidepressant/anxiolytic combinations for symptoms of IBS, though whether their effect is statistically greater than a placebo is disputed (Klein, 1988; Holdsworth, 1985).

Psychotropic drugs may improve IBS symptoms, especially diarrhoea and abdominal pain, partly because of a direct effect on bowel motility (Ritchie & Truelove, 1979; Heefner *et al.*, 1978; Lancaster-Smith *et al.*, 1982) but also possibly because of their known analgesic properties in painful conditions independent of their antidepressant action (Feinmann, 1985). Only two studies have suggested that relief of anxiety and depression are important in their mode of action (Dotevall & Groll, 1974; Greenbaum *et al.*, 1987); and only in the latter study was a tricyclic antidepressant used in a therapeutic dose. That study (Greenbaum *et al.*, 1987) was also the only one in which mood state was adequately measured. The raised Hamilton Rating Scale scores at the beginning of the study indicated that antidepressants would have been clinically indicated at least for a proportion of the patients. The use of psychotropic drugs has not been adequately evaluated but is clinically indicated in those patients who have been shown to have significant depression (see Table 6.4).

## Psychological treatments

### Psychotherapy

In an open trial Hislop (1980) found brief psychotherapy helped the majority of patients. His patients were unusual as they accepted an emotional basis for their IBS symptoms at the outset and were prepared to explore repressed emotions under Hislop's guidance; this alone apparently led to a resolution of bowel symptoms as no drugs were used. Those patients who could not express their feelings in this way did least well with Hislop's treatment.

The controlled study of Svedlund *et al.* (1983) has provided the best evidence for the efficacy of psychotherapy in IBS. Ten hours of dynamic psychotherapy, in addition to conventional medical treatment, led to significantly greater improvement in abdominal pain, bowel dysfunction and mental symptoms than the control group which received the drug treatment alone. The difference was apparent after 3 months' treatment but was maintained or increased at 1 year. The authors argued that this increasing difference between the groups during the follow-up year indicated the specific success of psychotherapy rather than a nonspecific effect of more doctor time; the latter only occurred during the initial 3 months treatment period.

Two other controlled studies using behaviour therapy rather than dynamic psychotherapy have also shown beneficial results. Bennett and Wilkinson (1985) treated first time attenders at a GI clinic with either an 8 week package of relaxation training or the medical regime of Ritchie and Truelove (1979) (Motival, Mebevrine and Fybogel). They found the psychological treatment was superior to the medical treatment in reducing anxiety, but there was no difference between the two treatments regarding IBS symptom reduction.

Blanchard *et al.* (1988) found progressive muscle relaxation, thermal biofeedback and training in cognitive stress coping led to an improvement in 73% of IBS patients measured in terms of a composite score involving change in abdominal pain, diarrhoea and/or constipation. These authors were able to correlate improvement in bowel symptoms with a reduction in anxiety, but, to the authors' surprise, the best result was obtained in those whose initial anxiety scores were low. Those with high initial anxiety were least likely to improve.

*Hypnotherapy*

Whorwell's (1984) controlled study of hypnotherapy involved patients who had not been helped by previous treatments for IBS — so-called 'refractory' patients. The treatment included standard hypnosis, relaxation, the use of a daily autohypnosis tape, and a specific technique which encouraged the subjects to believe they achieved control over intestinal motility. The patients who received this treatment did significantly better than those treated with some form of psychotherapy (to control for time spent with the patient). The psychotherapy would not have been as sophisticated as that of Svedlund *et al.* (1983) and results are most impressive because of the improvement that the patients made with hypnotherapy after their failure to respond to previous medical treatments.

The beneficial effects of hypnotherapy were evident 1 year later (Whorwell *et al.*, 1987), but with further experience of hypnosis the authors suggested that patients over 50 years of age, those with atypical IBS or with pronounced psychological symptoms did less well with this treatment.

*Group psychotherapy*

Wise *et al.* (1982) reported a small study of patients with IBS undergoing group therapy. Despite an intensive amount of educational work, discussion of life problems and individual relaxation most patients showed little improvement in bowel symptoms. But this study included patients with severe and chronic IBS symptoms which would be a severe test of any treatment. Interestingly, those patients with high anxiety felt they could not control their illness and greatly feared accidents resulting from incontinence. They also used enemas more frequently, were less satisfied with their sex lives and had experienced more hospitalizations than those with lower levels of anxiety. These factors might explain why patients with high anxiety levels in other studies did poorly with psychological treatments (Lancaster-Smith, 1982; Whorwell *et al.*, 1987; Blanchard *et al.*, 1988). By contrast, those patients who reported low levels of anxiety were able to identify stressors which were associated with their IBS symptoms and could modify their response to such stressors using relaxation techniques.

There are several common strands running through these reports of psychological treatments of IBS patients.

*Engagement in treatment*  It appears that Hislop and Whorwell treated selected patients who were prepared from the outset to accept psychological treatment. Bennett and Wilkinson (1985) found that they could only utilize behaviour therapy after an initial 'educational phase to change any misconceptions concerning bowel function and provide a rationale for psychological intervention'. Svedlund *et al.* (1983) engaged patients in a study to explore social and psychological conditions that might be of relevance to the disorder because they recognized that inviting patients to take part in a trial of psychotherapy would reduce recruitment to a minority of patients with IBS. Psychological treatment is only possible if the person engages with it and in most cases this preliminary phase is required to engage the patient.

*Education/reorientation*  Three studies used a preliminary explanation of gut physiology at the start of the psychological treatment (Whorwell *et al.*, 1987; Bennett and Wilkinson, 1985; Wise *et al.*, 1982). Such a theoretical explanation is necessary if the person is to accept that their bowel symptoms are linked to emotions and can be exacerbated by stressful situations. Compliance with a more intensive psychological therapy requires that the patient accepts, at least to some extent, that psychological factors are related to bowel symptomatology. Such acceptance of the importance of psychological factors appears to be an important ingredient in all the psychological treatments and reflects a 'reversal' of the somatization process.

*Relaxation*  Daily relaxation was employed in several studies (Whorwell *et al.*, 1984; Bennett & Wilkinson, 1985; Blanchard *et al.*, 1988; Wise *et al.*, 1982). It is an obvious way to reduce somatic symptoms of anxiety and also enables the patient to accept that such symptoms can be brought under voluntary control. However, the psychotherapy used in both the Svedlund and Hislop studies could apparently achieve good results without this technique.

*Close doctor–patient relationship*  It is clear from reading the descriptions of these treatments that a close doctor–patient relationship developed and this may form an important aspect of effective treatment. One study attempted to administer a drug treatment with minimal discussion but found that the patients initiated communication about their complaints and the need to take a psychotropic drug; the beneficial effect of this communication appeared to be greater than that attributable to the specific therapies offered (Schonecke & Schuffel, 1975). Two elements of the doctor–patient relationship appear to have been important:

**1** *the doctor as an 'expert'*   To some extent all doctors enhance the doctor–patient relationship by taking such an intense interest in their patients' symptoms and showing concern towards their suffering. This increases the doctor's ability to reassure the patient that no serious physical illness is present and to convince him/her that effective treatment can be provided.

**2** *the doctor as therapist*   In the more intensive psychological therapies the doctor–patient relationship is greatly enhanced by designating more time and prescribing specific therapeutic tasks. In the case of hypnotherapy the role of doctor as expert is initially enhanced, but control later given to the patient in the form of autohypnosis. In the dynamic therapy of Svedlund the doctor and patient work together to solve the patient's personal fears and conflicts. Since so many IBS patients have marital or family conflicts (Creed *et al.*, 1988) the opportunity to share these concerns and discuss ways of coping may make the person feel better in themselves and in turn reduce bowel dysfunction.

There is evidence to support the view that the symptoms of diarrhoea and abdominal pain are the most responsive to psychological therapies. In addition, those patients whose symptoms can readily be linked to exacerbation and relief by environmental stressors also appear to do well, presumably because they can make the link between psychological factors and changes in bowel function. By contrast, those patients with more chronic symptoms, 'atypical IBS' (severe and constant abdominal pain without pronounced bowel symptoms — Whorwell *et al.*, 1987) and those with severe anxiety do poorly with these treatments.

### Investigating the efficacy of psychological treatment

A treatment trial is currently assessing the efficacy of psychological treatment in patients with severe and persistent IBS (Guthrie *et al.*, 1990). The trial is designed to compare psychotherapy plus conventional medical treatment (bulking agent and antispasmodic) with medical treatment alone. Patients have been selected only if they have had current IBS symptoms for over 1 year and attended the clinic for over 6 months without improvement, i.e. a chronic, treatment-resistant group. Many of these patients had seen previous consultant gastroenterologists, as had the patients described by Kingham and Dawson (1985). The prevalence of psychiatric disorder was similar to previous studies (approximately half could be given a DSM-III psychiatric diagnosis of major depression or anxiety states).

These patients provide a severe test of the efficacy of psychological treatment because they represent patients whose symptoms have not responded to conventional medical treatment. They therefore resemble the 'refractory' patients treated with hypnosis by Whorwell *et al.* (1984). The difference is that Whorwell's patients were self-selected for hypnosis whereas the present series represents a consecutive series of treatment-resistant patients attending a teaching hospital clinic. In terms of a cost-benefit approach to efficacy of treatment these are the patients who can best be helped by psychological treatment: potential savings could be made if repeated expensive investigations were avoided in this group.

A surprisingly high proportion of patients have been engaged in this study considering that it only includes chronically ill patients whose symptoms had not responded to first-line treatment. Three factors could explain this high recruitment; first, the sympathetic approach of the gastroenterologist; second, the research psychiatrist was present at each clinic and met patients as soon as the gastroenterologist suggested entry into the trial; and third, the method of psychotherapy was modified to suit patients presenting with somatic symptoms to a gastroenterologist and *not* requesting help with a psychological problem.

*Sympathetic approach of the gastroenterologist*   There is a great danger that the gastroenterologist who refers an IBS patient to a psychiatrist is perceived as dismissing the complaint as 'all in the mind'. In order to overcome this problem the gastroenterologist discussed briefly with the patient the implications of the negative investigations (all patients had been extensively investigated at previous hospitals as well as at our own), the failure of usual treatments, and our increasing knowledge relating gut function to stress. He then suggested that the patient be involved in a trial that 'assessed in detail whether stress affects IBS symptoms'. Many patients were initially reluctant to accept that psychological factors might be partly responsible for their symptoms but were prepared to engage in a treatment plan that might alleviate their persistent and troublesome symptoms.

*The approach of the psychiatrist*   The gastroenterologist introduced the research psychiatrist in the clinic but later sessions took place in the psychiatry department. The initial interview was long (up to 3 hours). It began with the patient being asked to discuss in detail her symptoms and the way these had affected her life, aspirations and personal relationships. The patient was asked specifically about fears of cancer — many patients had such fears but had been too frightened to mention them previously. The patient's view of her own illness became clear during this discussion and her view of any illness in other family members was also explored.

As well as obtaining a detailed account of physical and psychological symptoms during this initial interview the patient was encouraged to discuss her feelings. This included feelings about various doctors — in particular previous gastroenterologists, most of whom were perceived as being unable to help, and her feelings about being seen by a psychiatrist. There was usually some ambivalence about the latter which could be overcome in the majority of cases provided it was explored openly. Feelings about the abdominal pain and bowel symptoms were also explored in depth. The patient was asked to describe the symptoms in as many ways as possible, and the frustration, fear, anger, guilt or suffering that became apparent was discussed in relation to the patient's life in general as well as in relation to the pain and bowel symptoms.

*The psychotherapy*   The psychotherapy is based on the model of Hobson (1985) which assumes the patient's presenting problems arise from a disturbance of significant personal relationships. If a healthy therapeutic relationship can be established then links can be made with other relationships in the patient's life and useful insights and new solutions to interpersonal problems can be found.

During the long initial interview the patient and therapist get to know each other, establish a therapeutic relationship and begin to work at the transference relationship. Within this setting the therapist focuses on the patient's physical symptoms and emotional feelings and attempts to draw parallels between the two. The bowel symptoms are viewed as a metaphor of distress and the therapist deliberately uses the patient's phrases such as 'loss of control', 'something being twisted inside', 'a constant nagging that never leaves me alone' to highlight the distress. In this way the patient is encouraged to understand how she really feels about herself and any bad feelings that have not previously been disclosed. This can lead to a discussion of how feelings intrude in personal relationships, the aim being that the experiences and learning that occur during the therapeutic relationship can be generalized to other relationships in the patient's life.

Finally, two further aspects of treatment are used. The patient keeps a detailed daily record of her bowel symptoms so that any exacerbations or improvements are noted. Simultaneously the record can include any comments about the situations and mood states that accompany such changes. This makes the patient more aware of the link between stressful situations (personally meaningful ones, rather than the classic 'overwork' etc.) and exacerbation of bowel symptoms, and allows discussion with the therapist of the situations which induce distress. The chart also allows a

record of symptom severity which may demonstrate over time the improvement in symptoms (or lack of it).

The patient is also given a relaxation tape to use regularly at home. This is
often the first time that the patient recognizes how tense she has been, and
may provide another opportunity to experience the link between emotional
state and bowel symptoms — when the patient relaxes the pain is relieved.

This approach has been successful with approximately two-thirds of
patients, as the following vignette demonstrates. (Full results are to be
published elsewhere (Guthrie *et al.*, 1990).)

> A 45-year-old builder had been off work for 4 years with IBS. He opened
> his bowels up to 10 times a day and experienced considerable
> abdominal pain. Although he had suffered from a 'nervous tummy' for
> many years, his symptoms had only become disabling a short while
> after his second marriage. He had been investigated at two hospitals;
> no organic cause was found for his bowel disturbance but he remained
> convinced that it resulted from an industrial accident 10 years
> previously. The usual treatment had not improved his symptoms, and
> although he was very sceptical about psychological treatment he was
> prepared to 'try anything' that might help.
>
> His bowel symptoms improved after psychotherapy and relaxation
> so that he only had to open his bowels frequently for an hour or so each
> morning; thereafter he was able to go out and work. When asked at the
> final interview why the treatment had helped he mentioned three
> factors: being able to disclose personal matters in confidence to the
> doctor (he felt this at the second or third interview); coming to accept
> that his bowel disturbance was unrelated to the accident and was
> related to stress; and sharing his feelings of inadequacy in relation to
> his young wife. He was not a psychologically minded person and had
> certainly never previously entertained the idea of seeing a psychiatrist
> — he was pleasantly surprised that it had helped.

Although the majority of patients treated in this way demonstrated
overall improvement, some patients did not improve or got worse. The
principal features of the disorder in those who were not helped were the
presence of constant pain (as opposed to that which fluctuated over time),
very long standing symptoms, and absence of clinical anxiety or depression.
Those patients who did poorly demonstrated a number of abnormal illness
behaviours in order to indicate the severity of their pain to the doctor; they
also had great difficulty in describing their complaints in anything but very
concrete terms so they could not adjust to the use of metaphor or develop a
meaningful therapeutic relationship.

Finally, it is essential to put this treatment in perspective. Most patients with IBS do not reach the gastroenterologist (Sandler *et al.*, 1984; Drossman *et al.*, 1988), and 85% of those who do will be helped by the first line of treatment and can be discharged within 6 months (Harvey *et al.*, 1987). Two-thirds of the remainder respond to psychiatric treatment (a satisfactory treatment has yet to be found for those with constant abdominal pain). For those whose symptoms did not respond there are two possibilities; either they have disturbed bowel function that is unrelated to stress or they strongly resist a psychological exploration because they would be unable to cope with the problems with which they would then be faced. The former group would previously have included those with lactase deficiency, and further organic causes may yet come to light. Patients in the latter category are seen by all of us.

## Conclusion

This chapter has reviewed physical and psychological aspects of functional abdominal pain and outlined a treatment approach which addresses both aspects of the disorder. It was the close co-operation of physician and psychiatrist that led to the successful inclusion of many IBS patients in psychological treatment, and which helped some in whom physical treatment had failed. It is likely that in the future concurrent study of physical and psychological factors will increase our understanding of the causes and treatment of functional abdominal pain.

## References

Almy, T.P., Kern, F. & Tulin, M. (1949). Alterations in function in man under stress. II. Experimental production of sigmoid spasm in patients with spastic constipation, *Gastroenterology*, **12**, 437–449.

Barsky, A.J. (1987). Investigating the psychological aspects of irritable bowel syndrome, *Gastroenterology*, **93**, 902–904.

Bennett, P. & Wilkinson, S. (1985). A comparison of psychological and medical treatment of the irritable bowel syndrome, *British Journal of Clinical Psychiatry*, **24**, 215–216.

Blanchard, E.B., Schwarz, S.P., Neff, D.F. & Gerardi, M.A. (1988). Prediction of outcome from the self-regulatory treatment of irritable bowel syndrome, *Behavioural Research Therapy*, **26**, 187–190.

Bond, P.R. (1987). Abdominal symptoms in general practice. A case control study, *Bristol Medico-Chirurgical Journal*, **102**, 33–34.

Bordie, A.K. (1972). Functional disorders of the colon, *Journal of the Indian Medical Association*, **58**, 451–456.

Bouchier, I.A.D. & Mason, C.M. (1979). A study of patients with abdominal symptoms of undefined cause, *Scottish Medical Journal*, **24**, 199–205.

Brown, G.W. & Harris, T. (1978). *Social Origins of Depression*, Tavistock, London.

Calloway, S.P. & Fonagy, P. (1985). Aerophagia and irritable bowel syndrome, *Lancet*, **ii**, 1368.

Cann, P.A. & Read, N.W. (1985). A disease of the whole gut? in *Irritable Bowel Syndrome* (Ed. Read, N.W.), pp. 53–63, Grune & Stratton, New York.

Canton, G., Santonastaso, P. & Fraccon, I.G. (1984). Life events, abnormal illness behaviour and appendectomy, *General Hospital Psychiatry*, **6**, 191–195.

Chaudhary, N.A. & Truelove, S.C. (1961). Human colonic motility: a comparative study of normal subjects, patients with ulcerative colitis, and patients with the irritable colon syndrome, *Gastroenterology*, **40**, 27–36.

Chaudhary, N.A. & Truelove, S.C. (1962). Irritable colon syndrome. A study of the clinical features, predisposing causes, and prognosis in 130 cases, *Quarterly Journal of Medicine*, **31**, 307–322.

Colgan, S., Creed, F.H. & Klass, H. (1988). Symptom complaints, psychiatric disorder and abnormal illness behaviour in patients with upper abdominal pain, *Psychological Medicine*, **18**, 887–892.

Cook, I.J., van Eeden, A. & Collins, S.M. (1987). Patients with irritable bowel syndrome have greater pain tolerance than normal subjects, *Gastroenterology*, **93**, 727–733.

Craig, T.K.J. & Brown, G.W. (1984). Goal frustration and life events in the aetiology of painful gastrointestinal disorder, *Journal of Psychosomatic Research*, **28**, 411–421.

Crean, G.P. (1985). Towards a positive diagnosis of irritable bowel syndrome, in *Irritable Bowel Syndrome* (Ed. Read, N.W.), pp. 29–41, Grune & Stratton, New York.

Creed, F.H. (1981). Life events and apendicectomy, *Lancet*, **i**, 1381–1385.

Creed, F.H., Craig, T.K.J. & Farmer, R. (1988). Functional abdominal pain, psychiatric illness, and life events, *Gut*, **29**, 235–242.

Creed, F.H. & Guthrie, E. (1987). Psychological factors in the irritable bowel, *Gut*, **28**, 1307–1318.

Creed, F.H. & Lennard-Jones, J.E. (1982). Gastrointestinal symptoms, in *Medicine and Psychiatry* (Eds. Creed, F.H. and Pfeffer, J.M.), pp. 329–337, Pitman, London.

Cumming, W. (1849). *London Medical Gazetteer*, 3rd Series, **9**, 969.

Dotevall, G. & Groll, E. (1974). Controlled clinical trial of mepiprazole in irritable bowel syndrome, *British Medical Journal*, **4**, 16–18.

Drossman, D.A., McKee, D.C., Sandler, R.S. *et al.* (1988). Psychosocial factors in irritable bowel syndrome. A multi-variate study of patients and non-patients with I.B.S., *Gastroenterology*, **91**, 701–708.

Drossman, D.A., Sandler, R.S., McKee, D.C. & Lovitz, A.J. (1982). Bowel patterns among subjects not seeking health care. Use of a questionnaire to identify a population with bowel dysfunction. *Gastroenterology*, **83**, 529–534.

Esler, M.D. & Goulston, K.J. (1973). Levels of anxiety in colonic disorders, *New England Journal of Medicine*, **288**, 16–20.

Farmer, R. & Creed, F.H. (1989). Life events, hostility and deliberate self-harm, *British Journal of Psychiatry*, (in press).

Feinmann, C. (1985). Pain relief by antidepressants: possible modes of action, *Pain*, **23**, 1–8.

Ferguson, A., Sircus, W. & Eastwood, M.A. (1977). Frequency of 'functional' gastrointestinal disorders, *Lancet*, 613.

Ford, M.J., Miller, P.McC., Eastwood, J. & Eastwood, M.A. (1987). Life events, psychiatric illness and the irritable bowel syndrome, *Gut*, **28**, 160–165.

Greenbaum, D., Abitz, L., VanEgeren, L., Mayle, J. & Greenbaum, R. (1983). Irritable bowel symptom prevalence, rectosigmoid motility and psychometrics in symptomatic subjects not seeing physicians, *Gastroenterology*, **84**, 1174.

Greenbaum, D., Mayle, J.E., Vanegeran, L.E. *et al.* (1987). Effects of desipramine on irritable bowel syndrome compared with atropine and placebo, *Digestive Diseases and Sciences*, **32**, 257–266.

Guthrie, E., Creed, F.H., Dawson, D. & Thomenson, B. (1990). A controlled trial of psychological treatment for the irritable bowel syndrome, *Gastroenterology* (in press).

Guthrie, E., Creed, F.H. & Whorwell, P.J. (1987). Severe sexual dysfunction in women with irritable bowel syndrome: comparison with inflammatory bowel disease and duodenal ulceration, *British Medical Journal*, **295**, 577–578.

Harvey, R.F., Mauad, E.C. & Brown, A.M. (1987). Prognosis in the irritable bowel syndrome: a 5-year prospective study, *Lancet*, **i**, 963–965.

Harvey, R.F., Salih, S.Y. & Read, A.E. (1983). Organic and functional disorders in 2000 gastroenterology outpatients, *Lancet*, **i**, 632–634.

Hawkins, C.F. & Cockel, R. (1971). The prognosis and risk of missing malignant disease in patients with unexplained and functional diarrhoea, *Gut*, **12**, 208–211.

Heefner, J.D., Wilder, R.M. & Wilson, I.E. (1978). Irritable colon and depression, *Psychosomatics*, 540–547.

Hislop, I.G. (1980). Effect of very brief psychotherapy on the irritable bowel syndrome, *Medical Journal of Australia*, **2**, 620–623.

Hobson, R.F. (1985). *Forms of Feeling*, Tavistock, London.

Holdsworth, C.D. (1985). Drug treatment of irritable bowel syndrome, in *Irritable Bowel Syndrome* (Ed. Read, N.W.), pp. 223–232, Grune & Stratton, New York.

Holmes, K.M. & Salter, R.H. (1982). Irritable bowel syndrome — a safe diagnosis? *British Journal*, **285**, 1533–1534.

Ingram, P.W., Evans, G. & Oppenheim, A.N. (1965). Right iliac fossa pain in young women, *British Medical Journal*, **ii**, 149–151.

I.B.S. Working Team Report (1988). *Handbook of International Congress of Gastroenterology*, Rome.

Johnsen, R., Jacobsen, B.K. & Forde, O.H. (1986). Association between symptoms of irritable colon and psychological and social conditions and lifestyle, *British Medical Journal*, **292**, 1633–1635.

Joyce, P.R., Bushnell, J.A., Walshe, J.W.B. & Morton, J.B. (1986). Abnormal illness behaviour and anxiety in acute non-organic abdominal pain, *British Journal of Psychology*, **149**, 57–62.

Kapoor, K.K., Nigam, P., Rastogi, C.K., Kumar, A. & Gupta, A.K. (1985). Clinical profile of irritable bowel syndrome, *Indian Journal of Gastroenterology*, **4**, 15–16.

Keeling, P.W.N. & Fielding, J.F. (1975). The irritable bowel syndrome: a review of 50 consecutive cases, *Journal of Irish College of Physicians and Surgeons*, **4**, 91–94.

Kingham, J.G.C. & Dawson, A.M. (1985). Origin of chronic right upper quadrant pain, *Gut*, **26**, 783–788.

Klein, K.B. (1988). Controlled treatment trials in the irritable bowel syndrome: a critique, *Gastroenterology*, **95**, 232–241.

Kumar, D. & Wingate, D.L. (1985). The irritable bowel syndrome: a paroxysmal motor disorder, *Lancet*, **ii**, 973–977.

Lancaster-Smith, M.J., Prout, B.J., Pinto, T., Anderson, J.A. & Schiff, A.A. (1982). Influence of drug treatment on the irritable bowel syndrome and its interaction with psychoneurotic morbidity, *Acta Psychiatrica Scandinavica*, **66**, 33–41.

Lane, D. (1973). The irritable colon and right iliac fossa pain, *Medical Journal of Australia*, **1**, 66–67.

Lasser, R.B., Bond, J.H. & Levitt, M.D. (1975). The role of intestinal gas in functional abdominal pain, *New England Journal of Medicine*, **293**, 524–526.

Latimer, P., Sarna, S., Campbell, D. *et al.* (1981). Colonic motor and myoelectrical activity: a comparative study of normal subjects, psychoneurotic patients, and patients with irritable bowel syndrome. *Gastroenterology*, **80**, 893–901.

Liss, J.L., Alpers, D.H. & Woodruff, R.A. (1976). The irritable colon syndrome and psychiatric illness, *Diseases of the Nervous System*, **34**, 151–157.

Lydeard, S. & Jones, R. (1988). *A Study of Factors Associated With Consultation for Dyspepsia*. Paper presented at Primary Care Society for Gastroenterology Annual Conference, University of Warwick, June 11th 1988.

McCloy, R. & McCloy, E. (1988). *The Irritable Bowel: Clinical Perspectives*, Meditext, London.

McDonald, A.J. & Bouchier, P.A.D. (1980). Non-organic gastrointestinal illness: a medical and psychiatric study, *British Journal of Psychiatry*, **136**, 276–283.

MacEwan, W. (1904). The function of the caecum and appendix, *Lancet*, **ii**, 996–1000.

Manning, A.P., Long, T.T. & Tyor, M.P. (1980). Analysis of patients referred to a gastroenterologist practicing in a community hospital, *Gastroenterology*, **79**, 566–570.

Mitchell, C.M. & Drossman, D.A. (1987). Survey of the AGA membership relating to patients with functional gastrointestinal disorders, *Gastroenterology*, **92**, 1282–1284.

Office of Population Censuses and Surveys (1974). *Morbidity Statistics from General Practice. Second National Study 1970–71*, H.M.S.O., London.

Palmer, R.L., Stonehill, E., Crisp, A.H., Waller, S.L. & Misiewicz, J.J. (1974). Psychological characteristics of patients with the irritable bowel syndrome, *Postgraduate Medical Journal*, **50**, 416–419.

Piloswky, I. & Spence, N.D. (1981). *Manual for the Illness Behaviour Questionnaire (IBQ)*, University of Adelaide, Adelaide.

Pimparkar, B.D. (1970). Irritable colon syndrome, *Journal of the Indian Medical Association*, **54**, 95–105.

Rang, E.H., Fairbairn, A.S. & Acheson, E.D. (1970). An enquiry into the incidence and prognosis of undiagnosed abdominal pain treated in hospital, *British Journal of Preventative & Social Medicine*, **24**, 47–51.

Ritchie, J.A. (1973). Pain from distension of the pelvic colon by inflating a balloon in the irritable colon syndrome, *Gut*, **6**, 105–112.

Ritchie, J.A. (1985). Mechanisms of pain in the irritable bowel syndrome, in *Irritable Bowel Syndrome* (Ed. Read, N.W.), pp. 163–171, Grune & Stratton, New York.

Ritchie, J.A. & Truelove, S.C. (1979). Treatment of irritable bowel syndrome with lorazepam, hyoscine butylbromide, and ispaghula husk, *British Medical Journal*, **1**, 376–378.

Royal College of Physicians (1984). The need for an increased number of consultant physicians with specialist training in gastroenterology, *Gut*, **25**, 99–102.

Sandler, R.S., Drossman, D.A., Nathan, H.P. & McKee, D.C. (1984). Symptom complaints and health care seeking behaviour in subjects with bowel dysfunction, *Gastroenterology*, **87**, 314–318.

Schonecke, O.W. & Schuffel, W. (1975). Evaluation of combined pharmacological and psychotherapeutic treatment in patients with functional abdominal disorders, *Psychotherapeutics and Psychosomatics*, **26**, 86–92.

Snape, W.J., Carlson, G.M., Matarazzo, S.A. & Cohen, S. (1977). Evidence that abnormal myoelectric activity produces colinic motor dysfunction in the irritable bowel syndrome, *Gastroenterology*, **72**, 383–387.

Sullivan, S.N. (1983). Management of the irritable bowel syndrome: a personal view, *Journal of Clinical Gastroenterology*, **5**, 499–502.

Svedlund, J., Sjodin, I., Olloson, J.O. *et al.* (1983). Controlled study of psychotherapy in irritable bowel syndrome, *Lancet*, **ii**, 589–592.

Svedsen, J.H., Munck, L.K. & Anderson, J.R. (1985). Irritable bowel syndrome — prognosis and diagnostic safety. A 5-year follow-up study, *Scandinavian Journal of Gastroenterology*, **20**, 415–418.

Swarbrick, E.T., Hegarty, J.E., Bat, L., Williams, C.B. & Dawson, A.M. (1980). Site of pain from the irritable bowel, *Lancet*, **ii**, 443–446.

Switz, D.M. (1976). What the gastroenterologist does all day, *Gastroenterology*, **70**, 1048–1050.

Taylor, I. (1985). Colonic motility and the irritable colon syndrome, in *Irritable Bowel Syndrome* (Ed. Read, N.W.), pp. 89–103, Grune & Stratton, New York.

Thompson, W.G. (1984). The irritable bowel, *Gut*, **25**, 305–320.

Thompson, W.G. & Heaton, K.W. (1980). Functional bowel disorders in apparently healthy people, *Gastroenterology*, **79**, 283–288.

Waller, S.L. & Misiewicz, J.J. (1969). Prognosis in the irritable bowel syndrome, *Lancet*, **ii**, 753–756.

Welche, G.W., Hillman, L.C. & Pomare, E.W. (1975). Psychoneurotic symptomatology in the irritable bowel syndrome: a study of reporters and non-reporters, *British Medical Journal*, **291**, 1381–1384.

White, H. (1905). A study of 60 cases of membranous colitis, *Lancet*, **ii**, 1229–1235.

Whitehead, W.E., Bosmajian, L., Zonderman, A., Costa, P. & Schuster, M.M. (1988). Symptoms of psychological distress associated with irritable bowel syndrome: comparison of community and clinic samples, *Gastroenterology*, **92**, 709–714.

Whitehead, W.E., Winget, C., Fedoravicius, A.S., Wooley, S. & Blackwell, B. (1982). Learned illness behaviour in patients with irritable bowel syndrome and peptic ulcer, *Digestive Diseases and Sciences*, **27**, 202–208.

Whorwell, P.J., Clouter, C. & Smith, C.L. (1981). Oesophageal motility in the irritable bowel syndrome, *British Medical Journal*, **282**, 1101–1102.

Whorwell, P.J., Lupton, E.W., Erduran, D. & Wilson, K. (1986a). Bladder smooth muscle dysfunction in patients with irritable bowel syndrome, *Gut*, **27**, 1014–1017.

Whorwell, P.J., McCallum, M., Creed, F.H. & Roberts, C.T. (1986b). Non-colonic features of irritable bowel syndrome, *Gut*, **27**, 37–40.

Whorwell, P.J., Prior, A. & Colgan, S.M. (1987). Hypnotherapy in severe irritable bowel syndrome: further experience, *Gut*, **28**, 423–425.

Whorwell, P.J., Prior, A. & Faragher, E.B. (1984). Controlled trial of hypnotherapy in the treatment of severe refractory irritable bowel syndrome, *Lancet*, **ii**, 1232–1234.

Wise, T.N., Cooper, J.N. & Ahmed, S. (1982). The efficacy of group therapy for patients with irritable bowel syndrome, *Psychosomatics*, **23**, 465–469.

Young, S.J., Alpers, D.H., Norland, C.C. & Woodruff, R.A. (1976). Psychiatric illness and irritable bowel syndrome: practical implications for the primary physician, *Gastroenterology*, **70**, 162–166.

# 7

# Functional Cardiorespiratory Syndromes

C.M. BASS

## Introduction

Previous descriptions of patients with cardiovascular manifestations of psychiatric disorder have always emphasized cardiac symptoms, but in clinical practice cardiovascular and respiratory symptoms often coexist. These functional cardiorespiratory disorders, which so frequently mimic ischaemic heart disease, are the subject of this chapter.

### Historical note

One of the earliest clinical descriptions of patients with these disorders was by Hartshorne (1864), but probably the best known historical account was by an American physician called Da Costa (1871). He described 300 patients who became ill during the American Civil War with a combination of cardio-respiratory and neurotic symptoms. Da Costa called this 'irritable heart', and his belief in a physical aetiology influenced subsequent investigators for 70 years. The disorder was particularly common among military personnel during wartime, and led to numerous publications on the subject between 1914 and 1950 (see Skerritt, 1983 for review).

The importance of hyperventilation in this disorder has been recognized for at least 50 years (Baker, 1934), but its exact contribution is uncertain. To some it is merely one of a number of diverse symptoms (Wood, 1941), whereas to others it is the causal mechanism responsible for the disorder (Soley & Shock, 1938; Hardonk & Beumer, 1979). This issue will be discussed later.

Numerous synonyms have been used to describe patients without cardiac disease but with a combination of cardiorespiratory and psychiatric symptoms (Table 7.1). The protean nature of the symptoms ensures that patients are referred to a variety of specialists, who have used descriptive terms for the disorder that reflects their clinical bias. For example, to a chest physician it is hyperventilation (Lum, 1976); to a cardiologist hyperdynamic beta-adrenergic circulatory state (Frohlich *et al.*, 1962); and to a psychiatrist cardiovascular neurosis (Caughey, 1937). Perhaps the most accurate description is an anxiety disorder with cardiorespiratory manifestations, but panic disorder (DSM-III-R) would include most (but not all) cases.

**Table 7.1.**   Synonyms for patients with cardiorespiratory and psychiatric symptoms (FCSs): 1860–1980

| Year | Description | Author |
|---|---|---|
| 1864 | Muscular exhaustion of heart | Hartshorne |
| 1869 | Neurasthenia | Beard |
| 1871 | Irritable heart | Da Costa |
| 1873 | Cerebro-cardiac neuropathia | Krishaber |
| 1895 | Anxiety neurosis | Freud |
| 1901 | Cardiac neurosis | Herrick |
| 1914–1918 | Soldier's heart | Medical Research |
|  | Disordered action of the heart (DAH) | Committee (UK) |
| 1918 | Effort syndrome | Lewis |
| 1918 | Neurocirculatory asthenia | Oppenheimer *et al.* |
| 1937 | Hyperventilation syndrome | Kerr *et al.* |
| 1939 | Cardiovascular neurosis | Caughey |
| 1941 | Da Costa's syndrome | Wood |
| 1952 | Somatization psychogenic cardiovascular reaction | DSM-I |
| 1952 | Somatization psychogenic asthenic reaction | DSM-I |
| 1957 | Vasoregulatory asthenia | Holmgren *et al.* |
| 1962 | Hyperkinetic heart syndrome | Gorlin |
| 1966 | Hyperdynamic beta-adrenergic circulatory state | Frohlich |
| 1968 | Psychophysiologic cardiovascular disorder | DSM-II |
| 1968 | Nervous heart complaint | Nordenfelt *et al.* |
| 1980 | Psychogenic cardiac non-disease | Lipowski |
| 1980 | Panic disorder | DSM-III |

## Epidemiology

Chest pain is commonly reported in all surveys of general populations and primary care attenders (Shepherd *et al.*, 1966). It is also a common symptom of anxiety disorders in the general population (Weissman & Merikangas, 1986). In one survey Hannay (1978) asked a random sample of 1344 patients drawn from the practice lists of a health centre about symptoms they had experienced in the previous 2 weeks. Fifty-one (3.8%) complained of ill-defined pain or discomfort in the chest. This compares with 26 (1.9%) with angina and 18 (1.3%) with symptoms attributable to coronary thrombosis.

In a recent questionnaire survey of adult enrolees of a large health maintenance organization, von Korff *et al.* (1988) asked whether 5 different types of pain had been present in the previous 6 months. Respondents were asked to report only pain problems that had lasted a whole day or more or that had occurred several times in a year. The prevalence of pain in the 6 month period was 12% for chest pain (compared with 41% for back pain; 26% for headaches; 17% for abdominal pain; and 12% for facial pain). Chest pain (like back pain) showed no relationship to either age or sex, but a higher proportion of chest pain patients had sought treatment in the previous 6 months (35%). These findings suggest that although pain in the chest is less common than pains affecting other major organs, it is associated with higher utilization of health care.

Studies of the prevalence of functional cardiovascular syndromes (FCSs) in cardiac clinics have been sparse. This is in stark contrast to studies of functional bowel complaints (see Chapter 6, p. 143). One of the earliest studies was carried out over 50 years ago by White (1937), who reported that 14% of consecutive referrals to his clinic had functional complaints. But his sample was comprised largely of private patients.

Using the 60-item General Health Questionnaire (GHQ), Vazquez-Barquero *et al.* (1985) found that 44% of a consecutive series of 194 patients attending a cardiac clinic had evidence of psychiatric morbidity. Although there was no estimate of the proportion of these patients without ascertainable organic disease, the authors noted that rates of psychiatric morbidity were highest in patients with atypical chest pain.

In a recent study of consecutive referrals to a cardiac clinic for chest pain or palpitations just over half the patients were diagnosed as not having ischaemic heart disease or any other significant physical disorder. Only one-third of patients were given a definite diagnosis of IHD (Mayou *et al.*, 1990). In another study of 113 patients with chest pain undergoing routine exercise testing only 19% had abnormal tests (Bass *et al.*, 1988). This low rate is probably a consequence of the inclusion criteria (i.e. patients whose pain has 'atypical' characteristics are more likely to be referred for an exercise test than those with more 'typical' pains). By contrast, an even greater proportion (21%) had evidence of hyperventilation, which is often associated with anxiety and panic. Interestingly, a large number of patients (50–60%) in this study had neither cardiac disease nor demonstrable psychiatric morbidity.

Patients with non-cardiac chest pain also attend gastrointestinal clinics (Dart *et al.*, 1983), emergency departments (Roll & Theorell, 1987), and coronary care units (Wilcox *et al.*, 1981).

**Diagnostic dilemmas in patients with cardiorespiratory symptoms**

Heart attacks are a common cause of sudden death in Western society, and so chest pain complaints often alert doctors (and patients) to the possibility of cardiac ischaemia. This is understandable, because cardiac ischaemia is treatable, and misdiagnosis may result in sudden death. But it is not always easy to diagnose IHD on the basis of symptoms, signs and non-invasive tests, and there are pitfalls in establishing the diagnosis. These can be grouped as follows:

**1** It is not easy to predict the results of investigations designed to establish the extent of IHD. For example, there is a poor correlation between reports of the frequency and severity of clinical symptoms and objective evidence of coronary artery disease (Quyyumi *et al.*, 1985). Moreover, there is a *negative* correlation between the extent of coronary atherosclerosis and measures of psychiatric symptomatology and somatic complaints (Elias *et al.*, 1982; Bass & Wade, 1984). This suggests that patients who undergo coronary angiography are either severely ill or they are insistent and persuasive complainers (Costa *et al.*, 1985).

**2** Non-invasive tests also have shortcomings: although treadmill exercise testing is a safe investigation which is non-invasive and cheap, there is a high incidence of false positive tests (specially in women) (Cumming *et al.*, 1973; Petch, 1987). This reduced specificity may lead to further diagnostic difficulties.

**3** Ischaemic heart disease and cardiorespiratory symptoms attributable to psychiatric illness frequently coexist (Bass & Wade, 1984; Bass *et al.*, 1988).

Not surprisingly, these diagnostic difficulties have led to increased reliance on high technology procedures as *diagnostic aids*. For example, an invasive test such as a coronary angiogram may be performed when a doctor cannot decide whether a patient's pain is due to IHD or non-cardiac causes. Todd (1983) has argued that the angiogram *cannot* answer this question because coronary stenoses may be coincidental rather than causal. Moreover, the injudicious use of high technology medicine to investigate patients with chest pain, especially when accompanied by ambiguous advice and inappropriate prescribing, may result in functional disability and invalidism. For these reasons the patient with chest pain is at risk of undergoing numerous investigations, some of which have limited diagnostic power. This risk may be increased if the pain is 'atypical', i.e. not induced by exertion or relieved by rest.

One way to prevent unnecessary investigations in these patients is to enquire routinely about positive evidence of psychiatric illness and to examine each patient for signs of a non-cardiac disorder (see later). Concurrent measurement of end-tidal $PCO_2$ also provides objective evidence of hyperventilation and has diagnostic utility. Early and appropriate intervention is also important.

## Clinical features

### Physical symptoms

Cardiorespiratory syndromes are never monosymptomatic. The finding of characteristic *multiple* symptoms is the most important diagnostic aid (Lipowski, 1980). The symptoms are probably a consequence of both increased autonomic activity secondary to anxiety and heightened awareness of bodily sensations. The symptoms can be brought on by effort (hence the outmoded term 'effort syndrome') as well as by emotional distress. The cardinal symptoms are breathlessness, palpitations, fatigue, left inframammary pain, and dizziness (Table 7.2).

There have been numerous clinical descriptions of these patients since Da Costa's seminal investigation, and most are remarkably consistent. For example, Da Costa described a typical patient as follows:

> He complained much of shortness of breath, and is still troubled with palpitations; sometimes they occur when he is quiet, and he is

**Table 7.2.** Cardinal symptoms reported by patients with functional cardiovascular syndromes. Figures are % of total number of patients with each symptom

| Symptom | Friedlander & Freyhof (1918) (n=50) | Craig & White (1934) (n=50) | Wood (1941) (n=200) | Wheeler et al. (1950) (n=60) | Bass et al. (1983) (n=46) |
|---|---|---|---|---|---|
| Breathlessness | 80 | 77 | 93 | 90 | 65 |
| Palpitations | 74 | 80 | 89 | 97 | 54 |
| Fatigue | 44 | 68 | 88 | 95 | 65* |
| Sweating | 54 | 20 | 80 | 45 | 57 |
| Chest pain | 88 | 64 | 78 | 85 | 100 |
| Faintness, giddiness | 54 | 36 | 79 | 78 | 59 |
| Paraesthesiae | | | 56 | 58 | 57 |
| Syncope | 10 | 20 | 35 | 37 | 26 |
| Sighs | | 35 | 62 | 79 | 50 |
| Nervousness | 44 | | 79 | 88 | 61† |

Patients in column 5 have no significant cardiac disease.

* Feelings of fatigue that either caused considerable distress or caused the patient to modify his/her activities.

† 61% of patients in this study were designated psychiatric 'cases' using a standardized psychiatric interview.

perfectly unable to undergo any great exertion; the cardiac pain,
however, left some years ago. He grew worse after leaving the army,
and while attempting to work actively at his trade as a baker he
became much weaker, and has frequent smothering sensations (1871,
p. 32, Case 73).

The cardinal symptoms will now be discussed in more detail. *Breathless-*
*ness* may occur at rest, when the patient will report being unable to obtain a
satisfactory breath or 'to get air into the lungs'. This sensation, which may
amount to smothering or suffocation, is called 'air hunger' and is often
accompanied by objective evidence of frequent audible and visible sighs (see
later). Occasionally nocturnal attacks may wake the patient from sleep, mimicking bronchial asthma or pulmonary oedema. The following case illustrates
the problems that occur:

> This 50-year-old solicitor was referred from a chest physician whose
> letter began as follows: 'This man has been through the well trodden
> route of cardiologist, coronary angiogram, and respiratory physician!'
> The patient gave a 4-year history of cardiorespiratory complaints
> which had a characteristic pattern and had led to repeated admissions
> to hospital for investigation of angina. The symptoms began with
> dizziness, and progressed to paraesthesiae in the left face and arm,
> chest tightness, gasping for breath, profuse sweating, a feeling of
> detachment and occasionally collapse. An ambulance had been called
> to his aid on at least 10 occasions in 4 years, and two angiograms
> performed 9 months apart had failed to establish a cardiac cause for his
> symptoms. He had given up his law practice 12 months previously and
> had been advised not to drive. He had stopped smoking 30 cigarettes
> per day, but treatment of his mild airflow obstruction with inhaled
> steroids and salbutamol failed to relieve his symptoms.
>
> On further enquiry it was evident that he had been overextending
> himself before the illness began, sleeping only 4 hours a night and
> failing to delegate work. He was also addicted to tranquillizers, and
> his third marriage was failing. At interview he was tense and affable
> although evasive on matters relating to his family or personal life. He
> acknowledged that his symptoms may have had a psychological basis.
> On examination his chest was grossly over-expanded and his breathing
> was punctuated by audible and visible sighs. Measurement of end-tidal
> $PCO_2$ confirmed resting hypocapnia (27 mmHg) in the presence of mild
> airflow obstruction, and forced overbreathing for 2 minutes reproduced
> all of his symptoms except depersonalization. He was admitted to a
> ward in the general hospital for further assessment and treatment
> of his anxiety disorder, hyperventilation-related symptoms and

tranquillizer abuse but absconded after 2 days, ostensibly because of a pressing business engagement. The following week his family doctor reported that although he had improved and benefited from our advice, he felt unable to continue with 'psychological' treatment.

A subgroup of patients, like the one above but most often those with habitual sighing and chronic diurnal hypocapnia (Bass & Gardner, 1985; Gardner & Bass, 1989), often experience an exacerbation of dyspnoea (and other symptoms) within 30 seconds of lying flat.

A proportion of patients will have situational breathlessness, when there is a subjective sensation of dyspnoea in specific situations such as crowds, public transport, or enclosed spaces. Patients report an inability to breathe, chest tightness and dizziness, usually accompanied by frightening thoughts or an urge to escape before they are overcome by an imagined catastrophe. Subsequent avoidance of these situations may occur. The presence of situational breathlessness discriminates between patients with and without significant IHD (Bass, 1984) and is more likely to be associated with psychiatric than cardiac disease.

*Palpitations* are often associated with sinus tachycardia or benign ventricular premature beats, both of which occur in anxiety. Patients may also develop an enhanced awareness of their own heartbeat (Tyrer *et al.*, 1980). *Fatigue* is a common but illunderstood symptom which may fluctuate in intensity throughout the day or be expressed as overwhelming lassitude after exertion. Earlier this century a clinical syndrome characterized by excessive fatigue and functional cardiorespiratory symptoms was called neurocirculatory asthenia (see Chapter 5, p. 112).

*Chest pain* in FCSs may be situated in any part of the thorax. It is commonly reported in the left inframammary region but may be pectoral or more central. Occasionally it is constricting and cramplike, and in these cases it may be difficult to distinguish from angina. Pains that are described as sharp and stabbing in quality are more likely to be non-cardiac. The pain may occur during anxiety or effort or, more likely, after exercise, when it may coexist with breathlessness. Many patients with FCSs have multiple pains with differing location, quality and duration. This variability is characteristic of a psychiatric rather than an ischaemic aetiology.

In a study which compared 46 patients with haemodynamically insignificant IHD with a group of 53 with significant disease, Bass (1984) found that the following were reported significantly more often by the 'non-ischaemic' group: Pain in the left submammary and left axillary region, or pain in more than one site; pain described as sharp or stabbing, aching or of mixed quality; pain occurring at rest or inconsistently related to physical exertion. By contrast, chest pain brought on by cold or relieved by GTN within 5 minutes was more likely to be associated with ischaemic heart disease. Chest pain (and other) characteristics that suggest a non-cardiac source are shown in Table 7.3.

## Physical signs

There are important and conspicuous signs of FCSs, which are summarized in Table 7.4. Regrettably, they are probably the most underdiagnosed and infrequently documented signs in medicine. The alert physician also has the potential to provoke symptoms and signs if he/she adopts certain bedside procedures.

Resting tachycardia and cold extremities are common, but the most useful physical sign is sighing or 'suspirious' respiration. Breathing may be interrupted by visible and audible gasping, which may involve the accessory muscles of the neck. These large breaths are an attempt by the patient to overcome the sensation of not being able to breathe satisfactorily (Fig. 7.1). Conspicuous sighing (with or without chest tightness) may be provoked by

**Table 7.3.** Chest pain (and other) characteristics that suggest a non-cardiac source

| | |
|---|---|
| Location | Chest wall tenderness |
|   Left inframammary | |
|   Left pectoral | Association of pain with other symptoms |
|   More than one site |   Sighing |
|   Right sided |   Dizziness |
| | |
| Quality | Behavioural measures |
|   Sharp, stabbing |   Anxiety |
|   Mixed quality |   Depression |
| |   Extreme concern with somatic complaints |

NB Non-cardiac chest pain is suggested by a *combination* of current physical and psychological factors, which should be considered together with relevant past history (especially response to adverse life stress).

**Table 7.4.** Important physical signs in non-cardiac chest pain

1 Obvious sighs and gasping respirations (involves accessory muscles of neck)
2 Respiratory 'tics', e.g. throat clearing
*3 Inability to lie flat without bringing on gasping and chest tightness
†4 Short breath-holding time (less than 20 seconds at peak inspiration)
5 Localized (one-finger) or diffuse areas of chest wall tenderness

* This sign has important diagnostic power, provided that the patient does *not* have obvious pulmonary oedema.
† The effect of breath-holding may provoke extreme breathlessness and, sometimes, the patient's usual non-cardiac pain.

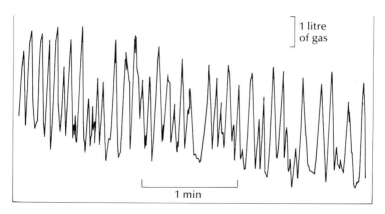

**Fig. 7.1.** Spirogram trace of a patient with gross sighing and gasping respirations and non-cardiac chest tightness (tidal volume of 3 litres).

asking the patient to lie flat. This sign has important diagnostic power provided, of course, that the patient does not have pulmonary oedema.

The respiratory rate may be increased to more than 20 breaths per minute (normal range 12–16 breaths per minute) and the rate may be irregular.

Breath-holding capacity may also be reduced. Patients with FCSs are more likely to have shorter breath-holding times (less than 20 seconds at total lung capacity or peak inspiration; Friedman, 1947; Wood, 1968; Chambers *et al.,* 1988). Occasionally the effort of breath-holding provokes extreme breathlessness and, sometimes, the patient's usual chest pain(s) (Fig. 2.2). Other patients may be required to walk up a flight of stairs before the breathlessness and chest pains are reproduced.

The chest wall should always be examined for localized or diffuse areas of tenderness. These are most common in the left inframammary region, but can also occur in any area of the chest wall, especially over the sternum and left pectoral region. Areas of tenderness should be noted on a chart.

**Psychiatric disorders associated with cardiorespiratory symptoms**

Cardiorespiratory symptoms can occur in a wide variety of psychiatric disorders (Table 7.5). Anxiety neurosis (ICD-10, WHO) or panic disorder (DSM-III-R) are the most common psychiatric diagnoses that subsume the diverse somatic and psychic symptoms. When cardiovascular symptoms such as chest pain and palpitations occur as part of the panic episode, this makes secondary handicaps more likely to develop. These include anticipatory anxiety and ultimately agoraphobia. Breier *et al.* (1986) have suggested that this sequence of events is more likely to occur when the somatic accompani-

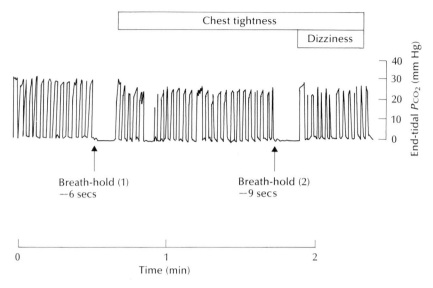

**Fig. 7.2.** This patient has a resting end-tidal $P_{CO_2}$ of 32 mmHg (4.3 kPa) and experienced non-cardiac chest pain during an exercise treadmill test. During the first breath-hold (6 seconds only) she experienced her usual stabbing chest pain which was associated with tachypnoea and continuous chest tightness. This led to more severe hypocapnia. The second breath-hold (9 seconds) was followed by dizziness. The most likely sequence of events was as follows: breath-hold → increased tension in intercostal muscles → chest pain → increased anxiety → hyperventilation (hypocapnia) → further symptoms of hypocapnia such as dizziness and further anxiety. This sequence is shown schematically in Fig. 7.3.

ments of panic are attributed to a *physical* as oppposed to a *psychological* cause, i.e. a 'heart attack' rather than 'nervous tension'. The somatic symptoms in these patients may be so persistent and preoccupying that psychiatric disorder is often overlooked and referral to a psychiatrist occurs relatively late in the course of the illness. Sheehan *et al.* (1980) provided evidence for this delay when they found that 70% of patients with agoraphobia and panic attacks had visited at least 10 different physicians with somatic complaints before the correct diagnosis was established. Patients also tend to report more somatic complaints when their panic anxiety is associated with phobic avoidance than when it is not (Beitman *et al.*, 1987a).

   Pain is a common symptom in depressed patients, and atypical chest pain may occur as part of a depressive illness. Kreitman *et al.* (1965) found that subjective complaints of depression were as common in patients with persistent somatic symptoms who were referred from a general hospital outpatient department as in a control group of depressed patients attending a psychiatric clinic. It is important to recall that depressive and anxiety symptoms frequently coexist. Among a group of patients with atypical or

**Table 7.5.** Main psychiatric syndromes associated with cardiorespiratory symptoms

| ICD-10 (April 1988 draft) | | DSM-III-R (1987) | |
|---|---|---|---|
| F40.0 | Agoraphobia | 300.21 | Panic disorder with agoraphobia |
| | | 300.22 | Agoraphobia without history of panic disorder |
| F41.0 | Panic disorder (episodic paroxysmal anxiety) | 300.01 | Panic disorder without agoraphobia |
| F41.1 | Generalized anxiety disorder | 300.02 | Generalized anxiety disorder |
| F41.2 | Mixed anxiety and depressive disorder | 296.2 | Major depression |
| F45.0 | Multiple somatization disorder | 300.81 | Somatization disorder |
| F45.1 | Undifferentiated somatoform disorder | 300.70 | Undifferentiated somatoform disorder |
| F45.2 | Hypochondriacal syndrome (hypochondriasis, hypochondriacal neurosis) | 300.70 | Hypochondriasis |
| F45.3 | Psychogenic autonomic dysfunction: cardiovascular system, respiratory system | | |
| F45.4 | Pain syndromes without specific organic cause | 307.80 | Somatoform pain disorder |
| F48.0 | Neurasthenia | | |
| | | 301.51 | Factitious disorder with physical symptoms |

non-cardiac chest pain, those with panic disorder (PD) *and* coexisting major depression have a more severe affective disturbance (as measured on self-report questionnaires) than those with PD and past major depression or PD alone (Beitman *et al.*, 1987b).

Cardiorespiratory symptoms can also occur as part of somatization disorder, which is historically linked to Briquet's syndrome (see Chapter 12, p. 301). Regrettably, this diagnosis is usually established in the 4th or 5th decade, by which time the condition may be untreatable and the patient is invariably in receipt of disability benefits. In a recent study of 41 patients satisfying research criteria for somatization disorder, Smith *et al.* (1986) found that cardiovascular symptoms (chest pain, breathlessness, and palpitations) were among the most frequently reported. Previous episodes of panic,

claustrophobia and phobic avoidance can often be elicited in patients diagnosed as having somatization disorder (see Chapter 12, p. 312). Hyperventilation may be one (of many) important pathophysiological mechanisms in
these latter cases (see below).

Atypical chest pain may also occur as part of a hypochondriacal illness,
when the complaint may be accompanied by the belief that the heart is in
some way irreparably damaged. Although not deluded, the patient may be
thoroughly convinced that he is ill. This form of hypochondriasis is aligned
phenomenologically and aetiologically to the overvalued idea, i.e. a non-
delusional, non-obsessional belief to which the sufferer's whole life becomes
subordinated (McKenna, 1984). Hypochondriacal complaints, especially
exaggerated fears about heart disease, are not uncommon in patients with SD,
and in our experience SD and hypochondriasis (as defined in DSM-III-R) are
not mutually exclusive.

It is very rare for chest pain to occur as part of a delusional disorder
(somatic type) as defined in DSM-III-R, although the following patient presented diagnostic problems in the cardiac clinic with his bizarre symptoms:

> This 62-year-old park keeper was referred from the cardiac outpatient
> clinic where his behaviour was noted to be 'bizarre and uncontrol-
> lable'. He had presented to hospital 6 months previously complaining
> of palpitations, and subsequently developed an episode of ventricular
> tachycardia during an exercise treadmill test. A subsequent coronary
> angiogram revealed a dyskinetic left ventricle but normal coronary
> arteries and he had been treated with amiodarone. For the next 6
> months he paid repeated visits to his GP, the Accident and Emergency
> Department, cardiology and the neurology services. His complaints
> were expressed with delusional intensity as follows: 'My chest has
> gone, my lips are curling in, my jaw protrudes, my legs have gone
> bony'. He was restless and agitated, talked incessantly and was
> impossible to interrupt. He was distressed that his delusional beliefs
> (of his body changing shape and his chest being transparent) were not
> being taken seriously by doctors. At various times in his past he had
> sought plastic surgery for imagined blemishes on his lips and face,
> although he had never visited a psychiatrist. A diagnosis of delusional
> disorder (somatic type) was made and treatment was commenced with
> stelazine. He became much less aroused and preoccupied with his
> symptoms during the next month but defaulted from outpatient
> follow-up.

Chest pain(s) are not commonly encountered as part of a factitious illness,
although a variant of Munchausen's syndrome with predominantly cardiac
symptoms has been described by Dickinson and Evans (1987). These authors

described 36 admissions over a 10-year period at a London teaching hospital (one man was admitted 6 times and one woman twice under different names). All but two admissions were male patients, most walked into the Emergency Department, and only two had referral letters — neither from their general practitioner. The most common presentation was simulated myocardial infarction with or without factitious complications.

## Prognosis

Prognosis in patients with functional cardiorespiratory complaints depends on many factors. Among these are the nature and duration of psychopathology, the personality, social factors, and the setting in which the patient is seen. Reported prognosis also depends on the measures used to assess outcome.

**Table 7.6.** Prognosis in patients with functional cardiovascular syndromes (FCSs)

| Outcome | Grant (1925) No. (%) | Wheeler *et al.* (1950) No. (%) |
|---|---|---|
| Recover completely | 92 (15.3) | 7 (11.7) |
| Improved | 107 (17.8) | 21 (35)* |
| Remain stationary | 338 (56.2) | 23 (38.3)** |
| Worse | 19  (3.2) | 9 (15) |

In the study by Wheeler *et al.* (1950), two-thirds remained symptomatic, one-third with mild** and another third without* disability.

The most impressive outcome studies in this field were published many years ago. They will be described in some detail because rigorous efforts were made to trace the patients. In the first study Grant (1925) attempted to contact 665 patients with a diagnosis of effort syndrome who passed through Hampstead and Colchester Military Hospitals during the years 1916–18. Five years later 601 cases (90.4%) had been traced, and only 14 (2.3%) had died. The results are shown in Table 7.6. In the second study Wheeler *et al.* (1950) followed up 173 patients with FCSs after a period of 20 years. It is clear that agoraphobics were included in this sample and, since agoraphobia is more common in women, this may have overemphasized the female prevalence. In addition, all patients had been seen at a cardiology clinic and recruited from private practice, so the sample cannot be regarded as unselected. The findings were very similar to those of Grant: approximately 1 in 6 recovered completely and one-half remained symptomatic, with varying degrees of disability (Table 7.6).

The results of these two studies suggest that the long term prognosis in FCSs is not favourable: at least half remain symptomatic. But both studies were published before the introduction of 'modern' pharmacological and psychological treatments, and it is important to establish whether such an unfavourable outcome would befall a contemporary sample of patients.

### Patients with chest pain and normal coronary arteries (NCA)

One group of patients that attend cardiac clinics and have high rates of psychiatric morbidity are those with normal coronary arteries (NCA). Among these patients, who comprise about 20% (range 6–31%) of those undergoing angiography (Chambers & Bass, 1990), almost two-thirds (61%) have psychiatric illness — most commonly an anxiety disorder, compared with 23% of those with significant IHD (Bass *et al.*, 1983). Similar findings were reported in an American sample by Katon *et al.* (1988) who found that 70% of patients with chest pain and a normal coronary angiogram had either panic disorder, major depression or both illnesses compared with about 9% of those with marked IHD.

Patients with NCA have a low long term cardiac morbidity and mortality but continuing high rates of functional disability. Three-quarters continue to visit a physician, one-half become unemployed and one-half regard their life as significantly disabled (Chambers & Bass, 1990). About three-quarters report residual pain at follow-up and one-third continue to visit accident and emergency departments. Only about one-third to one-half appear reassured that they do not have serious heart disease. Bass *et al.* (1983) found that those patients assessed initially as having higher levels of psychiatric morbidity and raised neuroticism scores were more likely to complain of chest pain 1 year after angiography. Patients with persistent pain also had significantly higher levels of psychiatric and social morbidity at 1 year than those whose chest pain had lessened during the follow-up period.

The high rates of psychiatric morbidity and functional disability in this patient group are startling. The interactions between physical symptoms and psychological factors are complex but there are opportunities for intervention which have not yet been exploited. There is a need for controlled intervention studies beginning immediately after the diagnosis of NCA is established (Chambers & Bass, 1990).

## Aetiological factors

The pathophysiological mechanisms responsible for the cardiorespiratory symptoms in this disorder have attracted considerable interest but little consensus. That there is activation of the sympathetic branch of the autonomic nervous system (ANS) in FCSs is not disputed, but it is becoming increasingly evident that psychosocial factors are also involved. This was demonstrated by Starkman *et al.* (1985), who found that none of the 17 patients with catecholamine-secreting phaeochromocytomas (cited in text books as a cause of anxiety with cardiovascular symptoms) met clinical criteria for panic disorder.

## Predisposing and precipitating factors

As with most other functional disorders, a consideration of predisposing and precipitating factors is important in any discussion of aetiology. *Predisposing* factors usually include enduring personality attributes such as neuroticism, which is known to be correlated with somatic complaints (Costa & McCrea, 1985); previous *personal* experience of illness — especially lung or heart disease; and previous exposure to cardiorespiratory illness in a close family member or friend. *Precipitating* factors nearly always involve life events which carry a major threat to the individual.

Studies of life events before the onset of FCSs are sparse, but there is some evidence that patients under the age of 40 who attend the emergency room with acute non-cardiac chest pain have experienced significantly more stressful life events during the previous year than randomly sampled matched controls (Roll & Theorell, 1987). These events, in particular uncontrollable ones, appear to interact with the personality trait of neuroticism, resulting in somatic symptoms in the form of chest pain. The authors suggested that enhanced tension in the thoracic muscles could cause chest pain.

Burns and Nicholls (1972) hypothesized that certain kinds of personal life event render some patients more preoccupied with specific bodily functions than others. They compared depressed patients with chest pain with a matched group of depressed controls without localized somatic symptoms. The chest pain group comprised patients with anxiety and hypochondriacal symptoms: all experienced non-exertional breathlessness, 82% had recurrent attacks of hyperventilation, and 88% feared death from heart or chest disease. Their hypothesis was supported by finding that the following factors were reported significantly more often by the chest pain group: a previous and current organic respiratory disease; a pre-existing excessive health-conscious obsessional personality; a family history of severe lower respiratory tract disease, including recollection of prolonged breathlessness in a parent; and recent bereavement, including witnessing the death with associated gross emotional impact. They concluded that somatic symptoms tend to occur in the area of a patient's body which is considered to be the most vital part. The importance of life events in the onset of a functional cardiovascular disorder are illustrated below:

> A highly strung 45-year-old shop manager with no previous history of psychiatric illness reported severe dizziness, headaches and chest pains one week after two distressing life events. Both events concerned her two sons aged 21 and 22 respectively. One week after her younger son disclosed his homosexuality her older son was seriously injured in a road traffic accident. The symptoms began soon after visiting her older son in hospital, who was in a coma and on a life support machine.
>
> She was a devout Catholic and attempted to protect her husband from the knowledge of their younger son's homosexuality. She began to experience episodes of dizziness, headaches and lightheadedness which were associated with fears of a brain tumour. Her anxiety would escalate to the point of panic, and during this extreme anxiety she panted and reported crushing chest pain. She was admitted to the Accident and Emergency Department on three separate occasions before finally being admitted to a medical ward for investigations. All tests, including coronary angiography, ventilation/perfusion scan and lung function tests were within normal limits. A diagnosis of severe panic attacks with pseudoangina was made. After referral to the psychiatric service the patient was able to understand her attacks as being 'anxiety attacks with chest pain', and stated that she had understood this from the beginning. Despite this she found it difficult to make any links between the two major events in her life and the onset of the chest pain complaints.

The somatic symptoms in such patients may sometimes be a consequence of increased activation of the sympathetic branch of the autonomic nervous system (ANS); a rapid fall in $P\text{CO}_2$; or a generalized or localized increase in muscle tension. But bodily symptoms are only one component of the disorder; the patient's reaction to these sensations is equally important. Ehlers *et al.* (1988) proposed a positive feedback loop between bodily symptoms of anxiety (mediated by the ANS) and the person's reaction to and appraisal of those symptoms (Fig. 7.3). In support of this, there is evidence that patients with cardiorespiratory symptoms (CRSs) may be more aware of their physiological functions than normal controls. In self-reports, panic patients describe high awareness of their heartbeat and other visceral functions (King *et al.*, 1986), and patients with normal coronary arteries have greater bodily awareness than those with angina (Frasure-Smith, 1987). Tyrer *et al.* (1980) also demonstrated that in anxious and hypochondriacal patients with predominantly cardiac symptoms, much of the patient's somatic preoccupation was explained by *heightened levels of cardiac awareness*. These

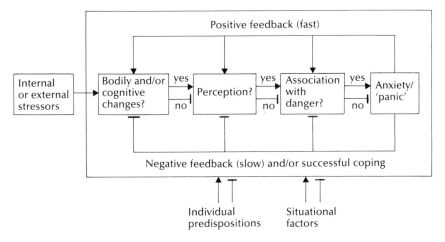

**Fig. 7.3.**   Schematic presentation of the psychophysiological model of panic attacks. Black arrows indicate panicogenic effects, small black rectangles indicate inhibitory effects. (Reproduced with permission from Ehlers *et al.*, 1988.)

patients were troubled by symptoms from essentially normal physiological activity, and the reason for this enhanced awareness of bodily function was in turn probably related to personality and *attributional* factors (the pain may be maintained and aggravated by the belief that it arises in the heart).

**Maintaining factors**

*Maintaining factors* in FCSs also need to be considered, especially as many patients will be referred for a psychiatric opinion after they have experienced symptoms for a considerable time. Personality traits such as 'anxiousness' and excessive health-consciousness (hypochondriacal personality traits) are clearly important, but in the author's experience *iatrogenic factors* are also contributory. In particular, injudicious prescribing of antianginal medication in patients without conspicuous heart disease is particularly difficult to justify, and the impact of repeated cardiac examinations and investigations should not be underestimated, as the following vignette illustrates:

> A woman was admitted to hospital for investigation of chest pain at the age of 38. Her first coronary angiogram revealed normal coronary arteries, but because of a slight irregularity in the proximal right coronary artery further tests were ordered. A thallium scan and myocardial biopsy were normal. Despite this she continued to report frequent and severe chest pain, and because medical treatment had failed and the ECG showed transient infero-lateral T wave inversion,

coronary angiography was repeated 1 month later. An ergometrine study revealed spasm of the left coronary artery (50%), reversed by isosorbide. However, 2 weeks later she had a cold blue foot and an emergency femoral artery thrombectomy was performed. In the next 12 months she visited numerous other hospitals with chest pain and on one occasion was admitted to a psychiatric unit with suicidal ideas and family problems. Eventually a third angiogram was performed (14 months after the first), and following confirmation of normal coronary artery anatomy she was referred to the pain clinic. Bilateral thoracic sympathectomies were complicated in turn by bilateral pneumothoraces, which were treated conservatively. Despite this her chest pain continued but by this time a new symptom had emerged: intermittent claudication in the right calf. This led to a translumbar arteriogram which revealed a complete block of the external iliac artery, which required further surgery with an ileo-femoral bypass graft.

The emergence of a new set of complaints in the ensuing 6 months (sweating, nausea and vomiting after meals) aroused the suspicions of the physicians and surgeons, whose combined efforts to alleviate her chest pain had only partly succeeded, but at a price: her iatrogenic illness now led to difficulty walking. She complained of loss of power and sensation in her legs, and in the next 4 years she underwent numerous investigations by the neurologists and other physicians for a paraparesis. None of these established an organic cause. She soon acquired a wheelchair and multiple benefits, including the installation of a lift into her house at the cost of £25,000. She continued to exasperate the doctors who were investigating her sweating, and the authenticity of this complaint was doubted when a relative informed the medical staff that it only occurred in hospital!

In the space of 4 years this woman had experienced an alarming array of iatrogenic disorders, some of which required surgical intervention. This in turn led to complaints which she used to considerable advantage. Thus overinvestigation of her non-cardiac pain led her to seek refuge in a wheelchair in her early 40s. Could this have been avoided? The patient's notes contained evidence of psychosocial problems, documented by one of the cardiologists, and further exploration by the psychiatrist revealed important information which might have predicted such a disastrous outcome. She had been treated for anxiety and depression during her 20s and 30s and her delinquent daughter had been placed in care because of the patient's bout drinking. Furthermore, there was a long history of somatization *before* the onset of the left-sided chest pain: numerous visits to gynaecology outpatients, gastrointestinal clinics and ENT clinics had failed to establish an organic cause for her multiple and diverse complaints. Interestingly, her long-suffering husband had distanced himself from her medical odyssey, but wryly commented that his wheelchair-bound wife *always* got her own way with *everyone*.

## The influence of exercise

Earlier this century it was noted that patients with functional cardiorespiratory syndromes could not tolerate hard work, as it induced their symptoms (hence the term 'effort syndrome'). During exercise on a treadmill and stepping up and down certain abnormalities appeared — a reduced oxygen intake, a higher rise in pulse rate, blood lactate, and pulmonary ventilation, and earlier fatigue than in normal controls (Cohen *et al.*, 1947; Jones & Scarisbrick, 1941; Jones, 1948).

These observations led some investigators to suggest that HV was an important cause of the chest-localized sensations in these patients. Perhaps the best known study of this causal factor was conducted by Friedman (1947), who demonstrated that the chest pain in these patients was of musculoskeletal origin. He conducted an experiment in which neurotic patients with chest pain had their upper chest walls immobilized with tight strapping for 6 days. After 2 days the chest pain was abolished in all patients, but reappeared when the adhesive tape was removed. Friedman also demonstrated that healthy volunteers developed considerable tachypnoea and dyspnoea during exercise when they were forced to breathe almost exclusively from the upper third of the chest (by immobilizing the lower third of the chest and upper abdomen with tight strapping). Nine of these ten subjects subsequently developed precordial pain after exercise, which disappeared after the adhesive tape restraints were removed. This suggests that mechanical or musculoskeletal factors are important in the aetiology of chest pain.

We have used exercise as a 'physiological stressor' in an attempt to understand the pathophysiological mechanisms; in particular the association between chest pain complaints, reports of subjective anxiety and hyperventilation (measured objectively as hypocapnia). In a previous study we found that hypocapnia during or after exercise occurs commonly in patients suspected of HV-related symptoms (70%) and chest pain of unknown cause (40%) but only rarely in patients with cardiac ischaemia (14%; Chambers *et al.*, 1988). These findings suggested that HV might be one (of possibly many) important mechanisms involved in the production of non-cardiac chest pain. We therefore requested patients with chest pain undergoing diagnostic tread-

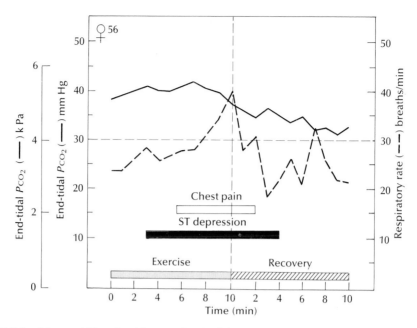

**Fig. 7.4(a).** 56-year-old female with normal end-tidal $P_{CO_2}$ response to exercise and chest pain with ischaemic ST segment changes.

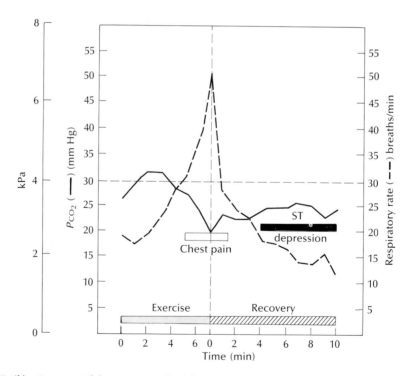

**Fig. 7.4(b).** Patient with low resting end-tidal $P_{CO_2}$ who develops a rapid rise in respiratory rate and pronounced hypocapnia after exercise. This is accompanied by chest pain which extends into the recovery period when pseudo-ischaemic ST segment depression occurs.

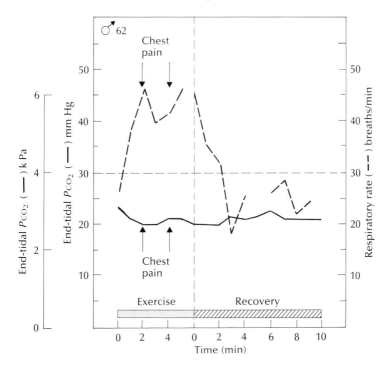

**Fig. 7.4(c).** 62-year-old female with resting end-tidal $P_{CO_2}$ 24 mmHg (3.2 kPa) in whom $P_{CO_2}$ fails to rise on exercise. Two separate epsiodes of stabbing chest pain occur in association with rapid increases in respiratory rates, and there are no ST segment changes on the ECG.

mill exercise testing to report whether their pain(s) occurred during either the exercise procedure or a 10 minute recovery phase. End-tidal $P_{CO_2}$ and respiratory rate were measured throughout. Chest pain was reported by 37 of 92 patients and there was an association between reports of chest pain *during exercise* and rapid rise in respiratory rate, whereas during the *recovery period* the more marked associations were between rates of fall of $P_{CO_2}$ and chest pain complaints. The respiratory responses to exercise in a patient with ischaemic heart disease and two with functional cardiovascular symptoms are shown in Fig. 7.4a, b & c.

We have identified a subgroup of patients who hyperventilate in response to exercise (Bass *et al.*, 1988). In this group $P_{CO_2}$ fails to rise during the first minute of exercise (in normal subjects $P_{CO_2}$ rises by about 5 mmHg in the first minute of exercise). These 'fail to rise' patients reported previous episodes of chest pain that occurred significantly more often on exercise or with emotion than those with normal rises (Fig. 7.5). Possibly either the anticipation of exercise or anxiety caused by the treadmill made them hyperventilate at the start of exercise. These findings suggest that an abnormal response of

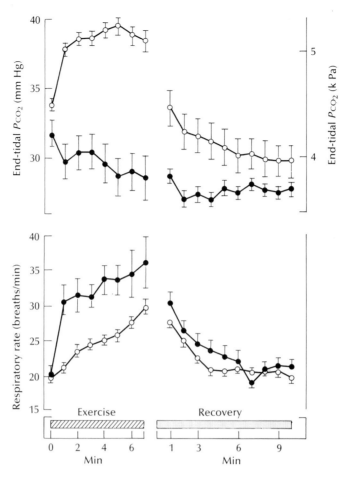

**Fig. 7.5.** Response of end-tidal $P_{CO_2}$ and respiratory rate to exercise in patients with initial hyperventilation (closed circles; $n = 24$) and those with normal rise in $P_{CO_2}$ (open circles; $n = 89$). (Reproduced with permission from Bass *et al.*, 1988.)

$P_{CO_2}$ to exercise provides objective data (hypocapnia) to support a clinical suspicion of chest pain associated with hyperventilation.

### Hyperventilation provocation tests and chest pain

It has often been suggested that hyperventilation is aetiologically relevant in this disorder (Evans & Lum, 1977; Channer *et al.*, 1985). Regrettably, these claims are rarely supported by objective data. Hyperventilation occurs commonly in the general population (Health and Lifestyle Survey, 1987) and is not always accompanied by chest pain. Moreover, some of the possible causes of chest pain in patients with HV (Table 7.7) can be associated but not necessarily causally related to the physiological changes induced by over-breathing. If, however, voluntary overbreathing at rest (the Hyperventilation

**Table 7.7.** Possible causes of chest pain in patients who hyperventilate

| | |
|---|---|
| Cardiac | Coronary artery spasm/vasoconstriction |
| Oesophageal | Spasm<br>Reflux<br>?Aerophagy |
| Chest wall | Localized tetany<br>Intercostal muscle fatigue |
| Psychological | Anxiety leads to enhanced awareness of and selective attention to bodily sensations |

**Table 7.8.** Hyperventilation provocation test

1 The patient should be asked to breathe at a rate of 30–40 breaths/minute for 3 minutes and then told to 'stop overbreathing'
2 After about 1 minute ask how many symptoms were produced during and/or after overbreathing
3 If the patient recognizes the bodily sensations induced by HV as similar to those experienced during naturally occurring symptoms, this observation is used as the basis for a discussion in which the doctor tries to help the patient reattribute the sensations and to suggest that he or she is suffering from stress-induced hyperventilation
4 In a positive test dizziness and digital paraesthesiae may occur before chest pain
5 Hyperventilation may continue (with chest pain complaints) for 5–10 minutes *after* the test has ended
6 If coexisting ischaemic heart disease is suspected in patients with angina-like chest pain, the test should be performed along with ECG monitoring

Provocation Test or HPT — Table 7.8) can reproduce a patient's usual chest pain, this suggests that HV-related changes rather than other factors, e.g. aerophagy, skeletal muscle spasm, are causal.

We therefore subjected 44 patients with a negative exercise treadmill test and non-cardiac chest pain to a 3 minute HPT, all of whom had been reassured about the absence of significant IHD (Bass *et al.*, 1990). Chest pain was reproduced during or after this procedure in 39% of patients (positive test), and this group had shorter breath-holding times, lower mean resting $PCO_2$ and higher mean respiratory rates than those with negative tests. There were no significant differences between those with positive and negative tests with regard to resting pulse rate or blood pressure, which suggests that there is no simple difference in physiological arousal between the two groups.

Retrospective examination of the treadmill exercise response in patients with positive provocation tests also revealed that, during the early stages of exercise their $P_{CO_2}$ fell significantly lower and respiratory rates rose higher than in those with negative tests (Fig. 7.6). Thus during the HPT and exercise test the patients with positive tests displayed evidence of excessively reactive respiratory responses, reflected in rapid increases in respiratory rate and falls in end-tidal $P_{CO_2}$. These patients also had significantly higher phobic avoidance scores for agoraphobia, which may predispose them to become breathless (and develop cardiorespiratory complaints) in phobic situations such as crowds and public transport.

Only 10 of the 17 patients who reported chest pain during the exercise treadmill also experienced pain during the HPT, however. This suggests that treadmill exercise (performed standing) and voluntary overbreathing (performed in a semirecumbant position) are qualitatively different stressors. One possible explanation for these differential responses to provocations is that the HPT was performed *after* each patient with a negative exercise test had been reassured about the absence of significant IHD. This would be expected to reduce levels of anxiety and preoccupation about heart disease.

These findings suggest that chest pain in patients with non-cardiac pain is associated with physiological arousal involving the respiratory system, i.e. an increased drive to breathe, which is evident at the time of assessment. Other disorders such as oesophageal spasm may also have a causal role, either independently of or in concert with HV (hypocapnia has been reported to induce disorders of oesophageal motility) (Rasmussen *et al.*, 1986).

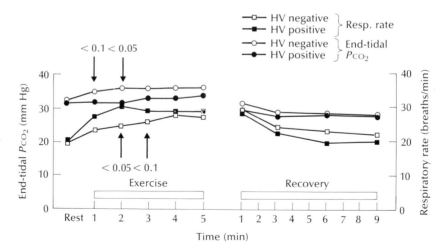

**Fig. 7.6.** End-tidal $P_{CO_2}$ and respiratory rates during exercise and recovery in patients with positive $(n = 17)$ and negative $(n = 27)$ hyperventilation provocation tests (HPTs). See text for further explanation.

That hyperventilation occurs commonly in patients with FCSs is not disputed. It is possible however that hyperventilation is an epiphenomenon, i.e. that it is secondary to anxiety, and that the main objective in the treatment of a patient with such a disorder should be to reduce anxiety rather than to cure the HV. It is also worth repeating that non-cardiac chest pain is a heterogeneous disorder and is unlikely to be caused by a single aetiological factor. In some patients more than one aetiological factor may be implicated. The complex interrelation between psychological and pathophysiological factors is shown in Figure 7.7.

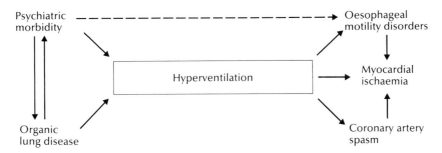

**Fig. 7.7.** Complex relation between hyperventilation and other physical and psychological factors. The probability that HV coexists with other *physical* mechanisms should not be overlooked.

## Summary

To conclude, no single factor has been implicated in the pathophysiology of this heterogeneous disorder. It is difficult to be precise about causal mechanisms, which are likely to be multifactorial. In many cases there is an interaction between (i) *physical* factors (characterized by an increased drive to breathe, manifest as tachypnoea and exercise-induced hyperventilation. This may lead to increased tension in the intercostal muscles and poor exercise tolerance); (ii) *psychological* factors (enhanced awareness of and selective attention to bodily sensations, possibly allied to a 'cognitive vulnerability', whereby bodily symptoms or even normal sensations such as rapid heart beating are misattributed to catastrophic causes, e.g. heart attacks); and (iii) *environmental* factors, such as previous exposure to cardiorespiratory disease in first degree relatives or significant others, and the experience of a major life event such as bereavement. These three contributory factors are not, of course, mutually exclusive. It is also important to disentangle initiating from maintaining factors. Possible initiating factors have already been described, but maintaining factors are more complex to investigate. Many of the cardio-vascular symptoms, most notably chest pain, are exaggerated and perpetuated by the belief that they arise in the heart.

## Assessment and management

### The referral process

It is not uncommon for patients with cardiovascular symptoms who have already consulted one or more specialists in internal medicine to balk at the suggestion of a psychiatric referral. For this reason it is important to ask a patient about the referral process. In particular, how was the referral made, what was the patient told about the reason for referral, and what was the patient's response to the request for psychiatric assessment? The replies to these enquiries yield useful information about the patient's attitudes and should be recorded in the notes. Members of the cardiology staff may need to be informed of the most appropriate ways of 'preparing' a patient for psychiatric referral.

### Psychiatric assessment

This should always include a comprehensive illness history (see Chapter 3, p. 42). Mental state assessment should include enquiry about a variety of neurotic phenomena, including irritability, poor concentration, insomnia, fatigue, depersonalization, depressed mood and intrusive thoughts about illness. The relation of somatic symptoms to certain situations should also be elicited, as should any phobic avoidance.

It is important to elicit the patient's attitudes and beliefs about the symptoms, because these may have a bearing not only on the natural history of the disorder but also, possibly, on response to treatment. It is mandatory to interview a relative of the patient or someone who knows him/her well, and to record the impact of the complaints on the patient's life. For example, has the patient restricted his/her social and recreational life? Is he/she absent from work and in receipt of disability benefits?

### Assessment for evidence of hyperventilation

This should be attempted in all patients with FCSs because HV-related disorders are common and treatable. Symptoms such as 'air hunger' and sensations of suffocation, together with signs of audible and visible gasping or sighing respirations suggest HV. The resting respiratory rate should be noted, and breath-holding time should be measured three times, 1 minute apart. The patient should be asked to breath-hold (at total lung capacity) for as long as possible and the time measured with a stopwatch (Fig. 7.2).

Next, an HV provocation test should be performed, ideally in an outpatient room or laboratory with a facility for measurement of end-tidal $P_{CO_2}$. This procedure should be standardized, so that each patient is requested to complete a symptom checklist which includes symptoms related to HV as well as dummy symptoms (to prevent response bias). This is followed by 3 minutes of HPT and a further 3 minute recovery period (Table 7.9). After this each patient is requested to complete the symptom checklist (for symptoms experienced during the HPT) as well as a 'similarities questionnaire', which enquires about the similarity of the experience to the usual complaints. If the patient rates the experience as very similar or identical to his/her usual complaints then this suggests that HV is a *possible* provoking factor. The test is useful but has many shortcomings. For example, some patients are unable to complete the test, others report that some, but not all of their usual symptoms were produced, and still others may feel so reassured by the presence of the doctor that they report nothing whatsoever except mild discomfort (even when the clinical history is very suggestive of HV and/or there is objective hypocapnia). However, the test is always worth performing and the results should be documented.

Because of the possibility of *lung disease*, lung function testing should be undertaken, e.g. $FEV_1$, vital capacity, and peak respiratory flow rate before and after bronchodilator. A histamine challenge test and ventilation–perfusion scan should be performed in certain patients. For example, those with HV of sudden onset or in whom the symptoms appear to be unrelated to life events or psychiatric disorder; patients with risk factors for deep vein thrombosis, e.g. after recent abdominal or gynaecological surgery; and those in whom there is a strong clinical suspicion of asthma, e.g. wheeze, atopic diathesis, or a positive family history of asthma. These tests may help to establish a diagnosis of asthma and pulmonary embolus, both of which can cause hyperventilation (Gardner & Bass, 1989). Continuous monitoring of $CO_2$ during sleep may occasionally be necessary to differentiate between organic and psychogenic causes of hyperventilation (Gardner *et al.*, 1986).

## Treatment

### Reassurance

In patients with unexplained chest pain it is important to establish a causal role for psychosocial factors or, at least, a plausible explanation for the pain.

This may be expressed to the patient as 'an overstretching or tension of the chest wall muscles' or 'a tension headache in the chest wall' etc. The explanation should be congruent with the patient's sociocultural background. This approach offers new and relevant information, and is more likely to be effective than bland reassurance that 'the tests are normal so there's nothing to worry about'. The limitations of this latter approach were recently revealed by Channer *et al.* (1987), who examined a group of patients with atypical chest pain 1 month after a normal treadmill exercise test. All patients had been reassured by the cardiologist that there was no significant IHD. Despite this reassurance two-thirds of these patients continued to complain of cardiorespiratory symptoms. Not surprisingly, those with continued pain had higher scores on anxiety and depression scales when assessed 1 month previously. These findings reveal the shortcomings of reassurance. Nevertheless, one-third of the patients in this study improved, and it is important to know why. Future studies should concentrate on those factors that predict failure to respond to reassurance.

### Withdrawing cardiac medication

If the patient with a FCS has been in receipt of antianginal medication before referral to the psychiatrist or psychologist, then this should be withdrawn gradually. This phase of management requires skilful handling, especially if the patient had been prescribed nitrates or calcium-channel blockers for months (or years) before referral. In effect the therapist is inviting the patient to negotiate the transition from a 'sick' to a 'healthy' mode of living. Each patient's response to the suggestion should be carefully noted, as it usually has an important bearing on prognosis. It is essential that the therapist not only gains the patient's trust but also is satisfied that there is an alternative explanation for the genesis of the complaints *before* this topic is broached. Prolonged unemployment and being in receipt of disability payments increases the likelihood of the patient remaining in the sick role.

### Psychological treatments

There is a paucity of controlled intervention studies in patients with unexplained cardiovascular symptoms. This is probably a consequence of both the heterogeneous nature of the disorder and the difficulty of engaging patients with essentially physical complaints in psychologically based treatments. It has to be remembered that a proportion of these patients neither perceive their illness as having a psychological component nor wish to see a psychiatrist. However, many patients can be engaged in treatment and there is increasing evidence to suggest that cognitive–behavioural approaches offer promise.

### Cognitive–behavioural treatments (CBT)

It is not only for diagnostic purposes that attempts are made to establish whether HV occurs in this disorder. There are important implications for treatment if HV is demonstrated to be of aetiological significance; it may be possible for the patient to reproduce the symptoms voluntarily, and this offers the potential for cognitive change, with the patient attributing the chest pain to chest wall discomfort rather than to serious heart disease. CBT involves three basic processes:

1  Attempting to *replicate* the symptoms using a variety of provocation techniques, e.g. chest pain by asking the patient to pant rapidly after fully expanding the chest; palpitations by asking the patient to run on the spot or up some stairs; breathlessness by forced hyperventilation. Occasionally, simply asking the patient to breath-hold as long as possible is sufficient to provoke chest pain. The aim of these procedures is to:

2  help the patients to *reattribute* their somatic sensations and to correct erroneous assumptions or 'symptom equations' (Beck & Greenberg, 1988). This can often be accomplished in writing, so that patients can remind themselves, during an attack, of the factual explanation of symptoms. For example, if the initial equation reads, 'Unable to breathe = death from suffocation' the new equation might read 'Unable to breathe = normal, harmless reaction of the body to chest wall sensations and anxiety, related to hyperventilation'. A self-instruction may follow: 'slow your breathing, remember symptoms do not last long' (see below). This process of symptom reattribution is crucial to cognitive treatment because it reduces the fear associated with the catastrophic and distorted thoughts that are central to anxiety (Clark & Beck, 1988).

3  *coping strategies* for the symptoms. These may involve positive self-talk, e.g. 'these symptoms are not in the least harmful or dangerous, just unpleasant. Nothing worse will happen'. Another commonly employed strategy is breathing exercises (respiratory control). These exercises are aimed at converting the patient from a predominantly thoracic pattern of breathing to one characterized by slow (8–12 breaths per minute) regular diaphragmatic breathing. It is not clear whether it is the cognitive (reattribution, reassurance) or behavioural component (respiratory control) that is most efficacious in this technique (Clark *et al.*, 1985; Bass & Lelliott, 1989).

However, evidence from a recent study of panic patients by Hibbert and Chan (1989) suggests that respiratory retraining in pure form adds only modestly to the effects of conventional treatment. Moreover, these authors found that training in controlled breathing was *not* of specific benefit for patients with panic attacks identified as 'hyperventilators' by the provocation test. It may have a non-specific effect in the treatment of patients with panic.

Klimes *et al.* (1990) used a cognitive–behavioural treatment in a sample of 38 patients with persistent (greater than 3 months) atypical chest pain. After baseline assessment they randomized the patients to either ten sessions of treatment or a waiting list. The essential components of treatment included stress management, home practice and diary keeping. Specific attention was given to ruminations, seeking reassurance, pulse taking and other checking habits. Most of those who completed treatment reported improvements in mental state and reduction in chest pain complaints. Four were unchanged and in nine symptoms persisted but were less frequent and less distressing. Most improvements were maintained at 3 months follow-up. Those patients randomly allocated to the waiting list were unchanged at reassessment.

A proportion of patients with chest pain and fear of heart disease make repeated visits to the emergency room. It is important that these patients are identified early and referred for psychological treatment. Successful management of such a case with re-education, relaxation training and biofeedback has been described by Schwartz *et al.* (1984).

## Drug treatments

### Tricyclic antidepressants (TCAs)

These drugs should be reserved for patients in whom the cardiorespiratory symptoms are accompanied by either depressed mood or panic attacks. There is evidence from a recent multinational study that imipramine is of benefit in patients with panic episodes that are accompanied by predominantly cardiorespiratory symptoms (Briggs, 1989).

Because these patients may be exquisitely sensitive to the side effects of TCAs it is usually advisable to start with small dosage, e.g. Dothiepin 25 mg on, gradually increasing to 50 mg/day by the end of the first week. Thereafter the dose should be increased by 25 mg increments every 3 days up to 150–200 mg/day. If depression fails to improve after 2–3 weeks at this dose then blood levels should be checked. Panics should also be 'blocked' at this dosage, but if the patient continues to panic then the dose should be increased to 250 mg or even 300 mg/day if necessary.

## Monoamine oxidase inhibitors (MAOIs)

Because cardiovascular symptoms are very common in patients with panic episodes, drugs which block panics have enormous potential in the treatment of these disorders. The most widely used is phenelzine, particularly useful when symptoms of panic avoidance, anergia, irritability and mild depression accompany the cardiorespiratory complaints (Bass & Kerwin, 1989). The method of prescribing these drugs is described in Chapter 3 (p. 61).

There have been no placebo controlled studies of MAOIs in patients with FCSs. In spite of this there is considerable evidence to suggest that patients with anxiety (with or without panic) and somatic symptoms (the most common of which are cardiorespiratory) show good therapeutic response to phenelzine compared with placebo (Liebowitz *et al.*, 1988). The efficacy of these drugs in patients with anxiety and predominantly cardiorespiratory symptoms is illustrated in the case report described in Chapter 3 (pp. 62–63).

## Benzodiazepines

The risks of dependence and withdrawal symptoms limit the use of these drugs in the treatment of FCSs. In spite of this, Beitman *et al.* (1988) have recently shown in an open trial of alprazolam that 7 of 8 chest pain patients without IHD and with PD experienced a 50% or greater reduction in panic frequency as well as decreases in anxiety and depression. Clearly, placebo controlled trials need to be carried out before claims are made about the efficacy of this drug, which, like the older benzodiazepines, carries the risk of dependence and withdrawal symptoms (Tyrer, 1989).

## Betablockers

Sympathetically mediated symptoms such as palpitations, trembling and sweating (but no other autonomic symptoms) may well respond to beta-blockers (Tyrer, 1976). Although the drugs only act peripherally on specific symptoms, they may reduce subjective anxiety indirectly because of the interaction betwen physiological and cognitive components of anxiety (Ehlers *et al.*, 1988). Patients with tachycardia in excess of 90 per minute may also benefit from betablockade, the dose of which should be titrated against the pulse rate, e.g. metoprolol 50–100 mg bd.

# Conclusions

Although precise figures are lacking, FCSs account for approximately 10–20% of all patients seen in a cardiac clinic. As many as a third of patients with established IHD also have concurrent psychiatric morbidity. The diagnosis of this disorder can be established on the basis of positive evidence of psychiatric symptomatology as well as characteristic somatic symptoms and physical signs. In some patients there is evidence of coexisting hyperventilation (hypocapnia), which is usually a consequence of anxiety.

Assessment should involve a search for predisposing, precipitating and maintaining factors, as well as evidence of hyperventilation, which is useful both as an aid to diagnosis and (when used as the hyperventilation provocation test) as a provocative agent in treatment. Management is aimed at treating the underlying psychiatric illness, most often an anxiety disorder with or without panic. Cognitive–behavioural treatments are probably as effective as psychotropic drugs in the short term. Over half the patients recover from the acute episode, but a proportion (particularly those with a phobic diathesis) may develop chronic illnesses, with relapses and remissions. Concurrent measurement of end-tidal $P_{CO_2}$ during exercise testing offers the cardiologist one method of establishing positive evidence of hyperventilation at an early stage in the evolution of the disorder. Because syndromes such as chest pain with normal coronary anatomy are associated with severe functional impairment, early and appropriate treatment of psychiatric disorder is essential in patients who present with cardiovascular symptoms.

# Acknowledgement

I thank Dr J.B. Chambers and Dr W.N. Gardner for stimulating discussions, and helpful comments on the manuscript.

# References

American Psychiatric Association (1987). *Diagnostic and Statistical Manual of Mental Disorders* (DSM-III-R) (3rd edn., revised), Washington D.C.

Baker, D. (1934). Sighing respiration as a symptom, *Lancet*, **i**, 174–177.

Bass, C. (1984). *Unexplained Chest Pain: psychosocial studies in presumptive angina*, University of London (MD Thesis), London.

Bass, C., Cawley, R.H., Wade, C. *et al.* (1983). Unexplained breathlessness and psychiatric morbidity in patients with normal and abnormal coronary arteries, *Lancet*, **i**, 606–609.

Bass, C., Chambers, J.B. & Gardner, W.N. (1990). Hyperventilation provocation in patients with chest pain and negative treadmill exercise test, *Journal of Psychosomatic Research* (in press).

Bass, C., Chambers, J.B., Kiff, P., Cooper, D. & Gardner, W.N. (1988). Panic anxiety and hyperventilation in patients with chest pain, *Quarterly Journal of Medicine*, **69**, 949–959.

Bass, C. & Gardner, W.N. (1985). Respiratory and psychiatric abnormalities in chronic symptomatic hyperventilation, *British Medical Journal*, **290**, 1387–1390.

Bass, C. & Kerwin, R. (1989). Rediscovering monoamine oxidase inhibitors, *British Medical Journal*, **298**, 345–346.

Bass, C. & Lelliott, P. (1989). Hyperventilation in the aetiology and treatment of anxiety disorders, in *Fresh Perspectives on Anxiety Disorders* (Eds. Emmelkamp, P.M.G. *et al.*), Swets & Zeitlinger, Lisse.

Bass, C. & Wade, C. (1984). Chest pain with normal coronary arteries: a comparative study of psychiatric and social morbidity, *Psychological Medicine*, **14**, 51–61.

Beard, G.M. (1869). Neurasthenia, or nervous exhaustion, *Boston Medical and Surgical Journal*, **3**, 217–221.

Beck, A.T. & Greenberg, R.L. (1988). Cognitive therapy of panic disorder, in *Review of Psychiatry* Vol. 7 (Eds. Frances, A.J. and Hales, R.E.), American Psychiatric Press, Washington, D.C.

Beitman, B.D., Basha, I.M., Flaker, G., De Rosear, L., Mukerji, V. & Lamberti, J.W. (1987a). Non-fearful panic disorder: panic attacks without fear, *Behaviour Research and Therapy*, **25**, 487–492.

Beitman, B.D., Basha, I.M., Flaker, G., De Rosear, L., Mukerji, V. & Lamberti, J.W. (1987b). Major depression in cardiology chest pain patients without coronary artery disease and with panic disorder, *Journal of Affective Disorders*, **13**, 51–59.

Beitman, B.D., Basha, I.M., Trombka, L.H., Jayaratna, M.A., Russell, B.D. & Tarr, S.K. (1988). Alprazolam in the treatment of cardiology patients with atypical chest pain and panic disorder, *Journal of Clinical Psychopharmacology*, **8**, 127–130.

Breier, A., Charney, D.S. & Heninger, G.R. (1986). Agoraphobia with panic attacks, *Archives of General Psychiatry*, **43**, 1029–1036.

Briggs, A.C. (1989). *Subtyping Panic Disorder by Symptom Clusters*, presented at the Royal College of Psychiatrists Quarterly Meeting, Leeds, England, April 4–5.

Burns, B.H. & Nicholls, M.A. (1972). Factors related to the localisation of symptoms to the chest in depression, *British Journal of Psychiatry*, **121**, 405–409.

Caughey, J.L. (1939). Cardiovascular neurosis — a review, *Psychosomatic Medicine*, **1**, 311–324.

Chambers, J.B. & Bass, C. (1990). Chest pain with normal coronary anatomy. A review of natural history and possible aetiological factors, *Progress in Cardiovascular Diseases* (in press).

Chambers, J.B., Kiff, P.J., Gardner, W.N., Jackson, G. & Bass, C. (1988). Value of measuring end-tidal partial pressure of carbon dioxide as an adjunct to treadmill exercise testing, *British Medical Journal*, **296**, 1282–1285.

Channer, K.S., James, M.A., Papouchado, M. & Rees, J.R. (1987). Failure of a negative exercise test to reassure patients with chest pain, *Quarterly Journal of Medicine*, **63**, 315–322.

Channer, K.S., Papouchado, M., James, M.A. & Rees, J.R. (1985). Anxiety and depression in patients with chest pain referred for exercise testing, *Lancet*, **i**, 820–823.

Clark, D.M. & Beck, A.T. (1988). Cognitive approaches, in *Handbook of Anxiety Disorders* (Eds. Last, C.G. and Hersen, M.), Pergamon, New York.

Clark, D.M., Salkovskis, P.M., Chalkley, A.J. (1985). Respiratory control as a treatment for panic attacks, *Journal of Behaviour Therapy and Experimental Psychiatry*, **16**, 23–30.

Cohen, M.D., Consolzaio, R.D. & Johnson, R.E. (1947). Blood lactate response during moderate exercise in neurocirculatory asthenia, anxiety neurosis or effort syndrome, *Journal of Clinical Investigation*, **26**, 339–347.

Costa, P.T. & McCrea, R.R. (1985). Hypochondriasis, neuroticism, and ageing. When are somatic complaints unfounded? *American Psychologist*, **40**, 19–28.

Costa, P.T., Zonderman, A.B., Engel, B.T., Baile, W.F., Brimlow, D.L. & Brinker, J. (1985). The relation of chest pain symptoms to angiographic findings of coronary stenosis and neuroticism, *Psychosomatic Medicine*, **47**, 285–293.

Craig, H.R. & White, P.D. (1934). Etiology and symptoms of neurocirculatory asthenia. Analysis of 100 cases, with comments on prognosis and treatment, *Archives of Internal Medicine*, **53**, 633–648.

Cumming, G.R., Dufresne, C., Kich, L. & Samm, J. (1973). Exercise electrocardiogram patterns in normal women, *British Heart Journal*, **35**, 1055–1061.

Da Costa, J.M. (1871). On irritable heart, a clinical study of a form of functional cardiac disorder and its consequences, *American Journal of Medical Sciences*, **61**, 17–52.

Dart, A.M., Alban-Davies, H., Griffith, T. & Henderson, A.H. (1983). Does it help to undiagnose angina? *European Heart Journal*, **4**, 461–462.

Dickinson, E.J. & Evans, T.R. (1987). Cardiac Munchausen's syndrome, *Journal of the Royal Society of Medicine*, **80**, 630–633.

Ehlers, A., Margraf, J. & Roth, W.T. (1988). Selective information processing, inerception and panic attacks, in *Panic and Phobias II* (Eds. Hand, I. and Wittchen, H.V.), Springer-Verlag, Berlin.

Elias, M.F., Robbins, M.A., Blow, F.C., Rice, A.P. & Edgecomb, J.L. (1982). Symptom reporting, anxiety and depression in arteriographically classified middle-aged chest pain patients, *Experimental Ageing Research*, **8**, 45–51.

Evans, D.W. & Lum, L.C. (1977). Hyperventilation: an important cause of pseudo-angina, *Lancet*, **i**, 155–157.

Frasure-Smith, N. (1987). Levels of somatic awareness in relation to angiographic findings, *Journal of Psychosomatic Research*, **31**, 545–554.

Freud, S. (1895). On the grounds of detaching a particular syndrome from neurasthenia under the description 'Anxiety neurosis', in *The Standard Edition of the Complete Psychological Works of Sigmund Freud* Vol. 3 (Ed. Strachey, J.), Hogarth Press, London (1962).

Friedlander, A. & Freyhof, W.L. (1918). Intensive study of neurocirculatory asthenia, *Archives of Internal Medicine*, **22**, 693–718.

Friedman, M. (1947). *Functional Cardiovascular Syndromes*, Williams & Wilkins, Baltimore.

Frohlich, E.D., Dunstan, H.P. & Page, I.H. (1966). Hyperdynamic beta-adrenergic circulatory state, *Archives of Internal Medicine*, **177**, 614–619.

Gardner, W.N. & Bass, C. (1989). Hyperventilation in clinical practice, *British Journal of Hospital Medicine*, **41**, 73–81.

Gardner, W.N., Meah, M. & Bass, C. (1986). Controlled study of respiratory responses during prolonged measurement in patients with chronic hyperventilation, *Lancet*, **ii**, 826–830.

Gorlin, R. (1962). The hyperkinetic heart syndrome, *Journal of the American Medical Association*, **182**, 823–829.

Grant, R.T. (1925). Observations on the after-histories of men suffering from the effort syndrome, *Heart*, **12**, 121–142.

Hannay, D.R. (1978). Symptom prevalence in the community, *Journal of the Royal College of General Practitioners*, **28**, 492–499.

Hardonk, H.J. & Beumer, H.M. (1979). Hyperventilation syndrome, in *Handbook of Neurology*, Vol. 38 (Eds. Vinken, P.J. and Brown, G.W.), N. Holland Biomedical Press, Amsterdam.

Hartshorne, H. (1864). On heart disease in the army, *American Journal of Medical Sciences*, **48**, 89–92.

Health and Lifestyle Survey (1987). Health Promotion Research Trust, London.

Herrick, J.B. (1901). The symptomatology of cardiac neuroses, *Chicago Medical Recorder*, Jan 30, 158–164.

Hibbert, G.A. & Chan, M. (1989). Respiratory control: its contribution to the treatment of panic attacks. A controlled study, *British Journal of Psychiatry*, **154**, 232–236.

Holmgren, A., Jonsson, B., Levander, M. *et al.* (1957). Physical training of patients with vaso-regulatory asthenia, *Acta Medica Scandinavica*, **158**, 437–446.

Jones, M. (1948). Physiological and psychological responses to stress in neurotic patients, *Journal of Mental Science*, **94**, 392–427.

Jones, M. & Scarisbrick, R. (1941). A comparison of the respiration in patients with effort syndrome and in normal subjects, *Proceedings of the Royal Society of Medicine*, **34**, 549–554.

Katon, W., Hall, M.L., Russo, J. *et al.* (1988). Chest pain: relationship of psychiatric illness to coronary angiographic results, *American Journal of Medicine*, **84**, 1–9.

Kerr, W.J., Dalton, J.W. & Gliebe, P.A. (1937). Some physical phenomena associated with anxiety states and their relationship to hyperventilation, *Annals of Internal Medicine*, **11**, 961–992.

King, R., Margraf, J., Ehlers, A. & Maddock, R. (1986). Panic disorder — overlap with symptoms of somatisation disorder, in *Panic and Phobias* (Eds. Hand, I. and Wittchen, H.V.), Springer-Verlag, Berlin.

Klimes, I., Mayou, R.A. & Pearce, M.J. (1990). Psychological treatment for atypical chest pain, *Psychological Medicine* (in press).

Kreitman, N., Sainsbury, P., Pearce, K. & Costain, W.R. (1965). Hypochondriasis and depression in out-patients at a general hospital, *British Journal of Psychiatry*, **123**, 607–615.

Krishaber, M. (1873). *De La Nevropathie Cerebro-cardiaque*, Masson, Paris.

Lewis, T. (1918). *The Soldier's Heart and the Effort Syndrome*, Shaw & Sons, London.

Liebowitz, M.R., Quitkin, F.M., Stewart, J.W. *et al.* (1988). Antidepressant specificity in atypical depression, *Archives of General Psychiatry*, **45**, 129–137.

Lipowski, Z.T. (1980). Cardiovascular disorders, in *Comprehensive Textbook of Psychiatry* (Eds. Freedman, A., Kaplan, S. and Sadock, S.), Williams & Wilkins, Baltimore.

Lum, L.C. (1976). The syndrome of chronic hyperventilation, in *Modern Trends in Psycho-somatic Medicine* Vol. 3 (Ed. Hill, O.), Butterworths, London.

McKenna, P.J. (1984). Disorders with over-valued ideas, *British Journal of Psychiatry*, **145**, 579–585.

Mayou, R. (1989). Atypical chest pain, *Journal of Psychosomatic Research*, **33**, 396–406.

Mayou, R., Bryant, B., Clark, D. & Forfar, C. (1990). Referrals to a cardiac clinic for chest pain or palpitations (submitted for publication).

Medical Research Committee (1918). *Report upon soldiers returned as cases of 'disordered action of the heart' (DAH) or 'Valvular Disease of the Heart' (VDH)*, HMSO, London.

Nordenfelt, I., Persson, S. & Redfors, A. (1968). Effect of a new adrenergic blocking agent H56/28 on nervous heart complaints, *Acta Medica Scandinavica*, **184**, 465–471.

Oppenheimer, B.S., Levine, S.A., Morrison, R.A., Rothschild, M.A., Lawrence, W. & Wilson, F.N. (1918). Report of neurocirculatory asthenia and its management, *Military Surgeon*, **42**, 711–719.

Petch, M.C. (1987). Misleading exercise electrocardiograms, *British Medical Journal*, **295**, 620–621.

Quyyumi, A.A., Wright, C.M., Mockus, L.J. & Fox, K.M. (1985). How important is a history of chest pain in determining the degree of ischaemia in patients with angina pectoris, *British Heart Journal*, **54**, 22–26.

Rasmussen, K., Ravnbaek, J., Funch-Jensen, P. & Bagger, J.P. (1986). Oesophageal spasm in patients with coronary artery spasm, *Lancet*, **i**, 174–176.

Roll, M. & Theorell, T. (1987). Acute chest pain without obvious organic cause before age 40 — personality and recent life events, *Journal of Psychosomatic Research*, **31**, 215–221.

Schwartz, D.P., Large, H.S., DeGood, D.E., Wegener, S.T. & Rowlingson, J.C. (1984). A chronic emergency room visitor with chest pain: successful treatment by stress management and biofeedback, *Pain*, **18**, 315–319.

Sheehan, D.V., Ballenger, J. & Jacobsen, G. (1980). Treatment of endogenous anxiety with phobic, hysterical and hypochondriacal symptoms, *Archives of General Psychiatry*, **37**, 51–59.

Shepherd, M., Cooper, B., Brown, A.C. & Kalton, G. (1966). *Psychiatric Illness in General Practice*, Oxford University Press, Oxford.

Skerritt, P.W. (1983). Anxiety and the heart — a historical review, *Psychological Medicine*, **13**, 17–25.

Smith, G.R., Monson, R.A. & Ray, D.C. (1986). Patients with multiple unexplained symptoms. Their characteristics, functional health, and health care utilisation, *Archives of Internal Medicine*, **146**, 69–72.

Soley, M.H. & Shock, N.W. (1938). The aetiology of effort syndrome, *American Journal of Medical Sciences*, **196**, 840–851.

Starkman, M.N., Zelnik, T.C., Nesse, R.M. & Cameron, O.G. (1985). Anxiety in patients with pheochromocytomas, *Archives of Internal Medicine*, **145**, 248–252.

Todd, J.W. (1983). Query cardiac pain, *Lancet*, **ii**, 330–332.

Tyrer, P. (1976). *The Role of Bodily Feelings in Anxiety*, Institute of Psychiatry Maudsley Monographs, Oxford University Press.

Tyrer, P. (1989). Treating panic, *British Medical Journal*, **298**, 201–202.

Tyrer, P., Lee, I. & Alexander, J. (1980). Awareness of cardiac function in anxious, phobic and hypochondriacal patients, *Psychological Medicine*, **10**, 171–174.

Vazquez-Barquero, J.L., Padierna Acero, J.A., Pena-Martin, C. & Ochoteco, A. (1985). The psychiatric correlates of coronary pathology: validity of the GHQ-60 as a screening instrument, *Psychological Medicine*, **15**, 589–596.

von Korff, M., Dworkin, S.F., Le Resche, L. & Kruger, A. (1988). An epidemiological comparison of pain complaints, *Pain*, **32**, 177–183.

Weissman, M.M., Merikangas, K.R. (1986). The epidemiology of anxiety and panic disorders: an update, *Journal of Clinical Psychiatry*, **47**, 11–17.

Wheeler, E.O., White, P.D., Reed, E.W. & Cohen, M.E. (1950). Neurocirculatory asthenia (anxiety, neurosis, effort syndrome, neurasthenia). A 20-year follow-up study of 173 patients. *Journal of the American Medical Association*, **142**, 878–889.

White, P.D. (1937). *Heart Disease*, Macmillan, New York.

Wilcox, R.G., Roland, J.M. & Hampton, J.R. (1981). Prognosis of patients with 'chest pain? cause', *British Medical Journal*, **282**, 431–433.

Wood, P. (1941). Da Costa's syndrome (or effort-syndrome), *British Medical Journal*, **i**, 767–772, 805–811, 845–851.

Wood, P. (1968). Cardiovascular disorders associated with psychiatric states, in *Diseases of the Heart and Circulation* (Ed. Wood, P.), Eyre and Spottiswoode.

# 8

# Disorders of Hysterical Conversion

B.K. TOONE

## Introduction

A distinction is often made between disorders of hysterical dissociation (disturbances of cognition and awareness) and hysterical conversion (sensorimotor disturbances) although the reasons for so doing are not always apparent. Terminology also remains a vexing issue. Hysteria is regarded by many as unduly pejorative (e.g., Hopkins & Clarke, 1987). The use of 'conversion' implies an acceptance of the validity of explanatory hypotheses (Freud, 1905) that few would consider proven (or indeed susceptible to proof). The International Classification of Diseases (World Health Organization, 1987) in its draft form, subsumes disorders of dissociation and conversion under one heading, dissociative disorders. This has much to recommend it. This chapter, however, is concerned primarily with disorders of hysterical conversion (although inevitably much of what follows will also apply to hysterical disorders as a whole) and so, as a matter of convenience, the present distinction will be retained.

## The development of the concept

Hysteria has a long history and there is room here only for a brief account (for a more detailed exposition, other authors (e.g., Merskey, 1979) are recommended). The ancients attributed a number of morbid states to displacement of the uterus, and a belief in the role of specific organ disease in the production of a wide array of somatic symptoms and emotional states persisted until relatively recent times.

Set alongside such mistaken assumptions, there developed a gradual understanding of the causal relationship between emotional stress and physical symptoms. Thus Whytt (1765) was able to ascribe 'the hypochondriac and hysteric affections' to '(i) A too great delicacy and sensibility of the whole nervous system', and '(ii) Uncommon weakness ... in some of the organs

207

of the body'. However, the variety of maladies subsumed within these two categories far exceed our present understanding, and the distinction between hypochondriasis and hysteria did not begin to take shape until the following century.

Popular thinking about hysteria continued to be influenced by ancient myths. Yet in 1853 Robert Brudenell Carter, a general practitioner, writing in his book on the pathology and treatment of hysteria, put forward views that would not be entirely out of place in a contemporary text book of psychiatry. Carter recognized that hysteria was due to the effects on the body of emotion, particularly 'sexual passion', working through the nervous system. It occurred in men, but was more common in women. He grasped the concept of secondary gain. He disregarded the role of uterine disease, the 'toxic hypothesis', and other theories that laid stress on the significance of disorders in vital organs.

By and large prominent medical thinking in the latter half of the century joined Carter in emphasizing the primacy of emotional stress acting through the central nervous system. Reynolds (1869) drew attention to the importance of a patient's idea about disease and how the manifestations of illness fulfil the patient's expectations. Single symptoms did not form a significant basis for a diagnosis of hysteria: multiple system involvement was necessary, a precondition which in recent years has been re-established as the central feature of one particular formulation of hysterical illness, Briquet's syndrome (see Chapter 12, p. 301). The school of Charcot is best remembered for its precise and detailed descriptions of hysterical fits, but other conversion syndrome phenomena, for example hemianaesthesiae and tubular vision, received careful attention and were interpreted in the light of signs elicited on physical examination and, in some cases, neuropathological examination. Charcot accepted the role of emotional and cognitive factors in the genesis of conversion but believed also in a constitutional diathesis, a susceptibility to develop conversion reactions in the presence of physical abnormalities within the territory of the syndrome, for example, vascular changes within the sensory distribution of an anaesthetic limb.

Later contributions came from Janet (1894) who, developing further the themes introduced by Reynolds, suggested that the conversion idea might form in the parent's mind 'below consciousness'. Janet laid more emphasis than did Freud on the personality characteristics of the hysteric, and in particular the capacity for dissociation. Freud's own contribution, primary gain, the use of conversion symptoms to resolve the unconscious forbidden oedipal wish, and the significance of symbolism, may now appear to be overly theoretical when seen through the eyes of a more pragmatic generation.

The first half of this century witnessed much discussion, but less clarification, of the distinction between so-called psychophysiological and conversion syndromes (Alexander, 1950); the experience of 'shell-shock' and the therapeutic efficacy of suggestion; and the rediscovery of one interpretaton of hysteria (Briquet's syndrome) and the introduction of another (illness behaviour). Each of these will be discussed in greater detail later in this chapter.

## Present definitions

The salient features of the hysterical conversion (HC) syndrome as it is presently understood have long been recognized and are not for the most part greatly disputed. The aetiology remains obscure at least in terms of neuropathological or neurophysiopathological change, and in that sense it has claim to syndrome rather than disease status. But as Lewis (1975) has noted the same could be said for other psychiatric entities. The relationship between hysterical personality and HC has been clarified considerably (see below), and the ever present possibility of underlying organic brain disease emphasizes the need for diagnostic vigilance, but does not challenge the nosological validity of the syndrome. Why then, more so perhaps than with any other psychiatric disorder, is that validity so frequently questioned? Slater (1965), to take one much quoted example, has concluded: 'the diagnosis of "hysteria" is a disguise for ignorance and a fertile source of clinical error. It is in fact not only a delusion but also a snare'. Others have confidently predicted a decline in prevalence (Steyerthal, 1908; Kranz, 1953) although this does not yet seem to have occurred (Trimble, 1982).

The reasons for this continuing state of dissatisfaction are not difficult to identify, but may have more to do with the state of mind of the physician than the patient. A diagnosis of HC is predicated on two sets of negatives: (i) signs and symptoms of physical ill health which the physician refuses to accept, and (ii) inferences (by the physician) of psychological disturbance which the patient (usually) rebuts. It is hardly surprising that many doctors find this state of affairs intolerable; but the unreliable evidence of physical disease is associated with disabilities and handicaps that are genuine and often incapacitating. The uncertain distinction between hysteria and malingering is also a source of disquiet. Faced with a mismatch between the complaints of the patient and the objective evidence of organic disease, many doctors incline to extreme positions: to give the patient the benefit of the doubt and to assume that all is organically determined, or to reject the patient out of hand as a malingerer. The third course, to accept the possibility that the patient may have a self-perception of bodily function that is genuine but at the same time quite incompatible with anatomical and physiological mechanisms as they are presently understood introduces a far more difficult concept. Finally, the very word has become a term of disapprobation. This has led to a search for fresh terminology, but adjectives such as 'simulated' and 'pretended' (Hopkins & Clarke, 1987) are no less judgemental.

Putting aside the personal reservations of individual clinicians, we may turn to present definitions of HC. DSM-III-R (1987) refers to a Conversion Disorder (or hysterical neurosis, conversion type) and lists a set of criteria for diagnosis (Table 8.1). These criteria incorporate the more important elements of the concept as it has evolved over the last century. The DSM-III-R definition avoids confusion with histrionic personality disorder which is defined elsewhere in the manual, and with Briquet's syndrome which also receives separate attention as Somatization Disorder. The accompanying text provides a useful descriptive summary and is in most respects an accurate reflection of consensual views on the subject. It is at its least explicit when it attempts to delimit the clinical area of the syndrome. Thus 'somatoform pain can be conceptualized as a conversion symptom' but is separately classified. Irritable colon is properly recognized as a physical disorder, albeit one in which psychological factors play a major part, and so is excluded; but psychogenic vomiting and pseudocyesis fall within the classification. The crucial distinction between a disturbance of function that, in the present state of knowledge, lacks any obvious physical explanation, and a disturbance of function that presents in a manner that is incompatible with our present knowledge of structure and function does not emerge. In practice this is not a distinction that is always easy to make, but recognition of it is fundamental to any classification of conversion syndrome.

In the draft version of ICD-10 (1987) all forms of either dissociation or conversion are subsumed within one category, Dissociative Disorders (F44),

**Table 8.1.**   Diagnostic criteria for conversion disorder

1  A loss of, or alteration in, physical functioning suggesting a physical disorder
2  Psychological factors are judged to be aetiologically related to the symptom because of a temporal relationship between a psychosocial stressor that is apparently related to a psychological conflict or need and initiation or exacerbation of the symptom
3  The person is not conscious of intentionally producing the symptom
4  The symptom is not a culturally sanctioned response pattern and cannot, after appropriate investigation, be explained by a known physical disorder
5  The symptom is not limited to pain or to a disturbance in sexual functioning

*Specify: single episode or recurrent*

and this further subdivided into disorders of memory awareness and identity, and disorders of movement and sensation. The diagnostic guidelines (Table 8.2) closely follow DSM-III-R but show a greater awareness of the difficulties in obtaining convincing evidence of psychogenesis. The disorders of dissociation are clearly delineated from Somatoform Disorders (F45), which are described in more detail in Chapter 2.

**Table 8.2.** Dissociative disorders (ICD-10, draft version, 1987)

*Dissociative disorders of memory awareness and identity*
Psychogenic amnesia
Psychogenic fugue
Psychogenic stupor
Trance and possession states
Multiple personality

*Dissociative disorders of movement and sensation*
Psychogenic disorder of voluntary movement
Psychogenic convulsions
Psychogenic anaesthesia and sensory loss
Other dissociative states
Unspecified dissociative or conversion disorder

A comparison of DSM-III-R and draft ICD-10 indicates close agreement concerning diagnostic criteria for a narrow definition of the conversion syndrome, but uncertainty about the classificatory position of some adjacent somatic syndromes, particularly 'psychogenic autonomic dysfunction' (draft ICD-10). In this respect the international classifications are a true reflection of the confusion evident in the literature. The exact relationship between conversion syndrome and other somatoform disorders merits further consideration.

## Somatization disorder

This disorder comprises a broad spectrum of somatic complaints in which HC may be but one component. Indeed the relationship between somatization disorder and HC may not be especially close. Woodruff *et al.* (1969) detected a history of conversion symptoms (somatic symptoms reported by the patient for which no medical explanation could be found) in 24 of an unselected series of 100 patients. They were encountered across a wide range of psychiatric diagnoses and were as common in patients with a primary diagnosis of alcoholism and of sociopathy as with the St Louis definition of hysteria. Somatization disorder and HC are therefore distinct and separate conditions which show some degree of overlap.

**Pain syndromes without specific organic cause**

Pain syndromes may contribute to the rich symptomatology of somatoform disorder. They may also coexist with HC and some earlier writers regarded them as one particular form of conversion (Walters, 1961). A contemporary view (DSM-III-R) is that pain syndromes of this type may be conceptualized as conversion symptoms but should, on account of differences in course and response to treatment, be classified separately. Where HC is concerned, such a distinction certainly serves the interests of diagnostic reliability; this in part depends on an opportunity to demonstrate an inconsistency between the subject's complaints and handicaps and objective evidence of dysfunction. The extremely varied nature of organic pain, much of which cannot be readily described in terms of neuro-anatomical distribution, makes this a difficult test to apply.

**Syndromes suggestive of autonomic dysfunction in the absence of any organic explanation**

This category, which finds a place in ICD-10 but not DSM-III-R, lacks adequate definition. It can probably best be understood as an interaction between generalized arousal and specific organ/system vulnerability. As such it is closer to anxiety disorder than to conversion (see also Chapter 2). Hyperventilation is of particular interest as it may give rise to atypical chest pain (Bass *et al.*, 1988) which may then become the source of hypochondriacal concerns. It may also result in altered states of consciousness, sensory disturbance and muscular spasm, circumstances in which suggestible subjects may come to believe that they are experiencing epileptic seizures. In some organ dysfunctional syndromes a disturbance of voluntary control may also be imputed, e.g. psychogenic vomiting, hysterical retention of urine. These conditions are then included under HC.

**Other conditions of uncertain aetiology**

There are a number of somatic syndromes in which the identification of a morbid state is almost entirely dependent upon the sufferer's own description of a recognizable constellation of symptoms. Laboratory tests and investigations that might provide confirmatory evidence do not exist and such physical signs as there are are of a kind that could be simulated by the patient. The majority of psychiatric disorders fall into this category and it is hardly surprising that psychogenic hypotheses have also been advanced to explain somatic symptoms of this type. But those who would seek to extend psychiatric boundaries need to proceed with caution. If attempts to find organic explanations for chronic fatigue syndromes (chronic brucellosis, neurasthenia, myalgic encephalomyelitis) have been largely unsuccessful (see Chapter 5, p. 110), diagnostic reassignation within the borderlines of psychiatry and neurology has been largely one way traffic. For example, a number of the less common movement disorders (spasmodic torticollis, dystonia, writer's cramp, stiff man syndrome) have followed epilepsy into the neurology camp. The case of dystonia is particularly germane to this discussion. Until quite recently most cases of dystonia were diagnosed by neurologists and psychiatrists alike as hysteria. The aetiology of primary dystonia remains uncertain, but identical syndromes develop in association with basal ganglia disease, Wilson's disease, encephalitis lethargica and exposure to neuroleptic drugs. In the only control study so far available, neither personality factors nor current stress appear to play a significant role in the development of the disorder (Cockburn, 1971).

**Malingering**

It is assumed that malingering patients have insight into the motives for their behaviour though they may rarely choose to confide these to the physician. This has led some to take a rather gloomy view of the distinction between malingering and dissociation. Hopkins and Clark (1987) quote Naish (1982) approvingly: 'There is no test to distinguish hysteria from malingering. Since differentiation is impossible, the decision of a doctor that a person is subconsciously deceiving and therefore ill is an entirely arbitrary one which depends more upon the doctor's prejudice than his reason'. The first statement is only partially true. Patient observation will not infrequently detect inconsistencies of behaviour that bring into question the possibility of deliberate simulation. However, the same authors go on to observe that 'the use of "malingering" and "hysteria" immediately polarises the issue with no acknowledgement that there may be, and are likely to be, intermediate positions'. It could well be that dissociation/malingering is better represented as a dimension than as distinct and separate categories and that individual patients may at different times, depending on their changing capacity for accurate introspection, occupy different positions on that dimension.

## Prevalence and incidence

Prevalence and incidence of HC are usually recorded indirectly (and often misleadingly) as rates of referral. These vary very considerably and in such a way as cannot be explained by cultural and geographical differences, important as these are undoubtedly are. For example, Guze *et al.* (1971) reported a history of one or more conversion symptoms in 24% of a series of 500 patients attending a university hospital. Stefansson *et al.* (1976), working in a similar setting, reported 4.5%. These discrepencies are almost certainly due to differing ascertainment procedures. The first author accepted a lifetime history of conversion symptoms in the absence of any objective evidence of the same; in the second study diagnosis was based on mental and physical state at the time of examination.

North European and American researchers who have adopted a similar approach have reported comparable figures. The most convincing estimates come from Scandinavian sources. Ljunberg (1957), on the basis of hospital referrals from a circumscribed regional population, calculated a community prevalence of 0.3%. Stefansson *et al.* (1976), in a comparative study of Icelandic and Monro County, USA cohorts, obtained considerably lower values. Other authors (Stephens & Kamp, 1962) found conversion features in between 1 and 3% of all outpatient referrals. Experience in specialist centres in similar; 1% of all diagnoses in postgraduate psychiatric (Reed, 1975) and neurological (Trimble, 1982) centres; 0.7% of all admissions to a group of neurosurgical units (Maurice-Williams & Marsh, 1985). The experience of developing countries is quite different. Hafeiz (1980) in Sudan and Pu *et al.* (1986) in Libya reported 10% and 8.25% of all new outpatient referrals respectively. Wig *et al.* (1982) found similarly in India.

Change in prevalence over time has received less attention. There is a view, more commonly expressed during the earlier part of the century (Steyerthal, 1908), that hysteria is a disorder on the wane and even that it may eventually disappear altogether. This may have seemed the case 50 years ago, but recent studies cast doubt on this assumption. Stephens and Kamp (1962) compared two cohorts (1913–20 and 1945–60) of patients attending the Henry Phipps Psychiatric Clinic in Baltimore. Hysterical syndromes comprised 2.14% of patients in the earlier series, 1.84% in the later. Stefansson *et al.* (1976) examined change over successive half decades (1960–70) and found a decline in prevalence (28 to 15 per 100000 population) in Monro County, but little change in Iceland. Trimble (1982) at the National Hospital, London found little substantial change during the period 1950–75 but Hare (1971) reported a decline from 4.0% of all admissions to the Maudsley Hospital in 1955–57 to 2.0% in 1967–69. Changing diagnostic concepts and criteria may make comparison difficult, particularly across large intervals, but the available evidence does suggest a modest decline over the past three to four decades, although less so than is often supposed.

It is also commonly held (e.g., Lazare, 1981) that HC is overrepresented 'in patients from rural areas or low socioeconomic classes ... and in certain immigrant populations.' There is some support for this view, but it is far from conclusive. Guze *et al.* (1971) found an excess of conversion symptoms in social classes 4 and 5, but Stephens and Kamp (1962), in an uncontrolled study, were unable to observe any relationship between the nature and severity of symptomatology and social class. The two major epidemiological studies also report differently: Stefansson *et al.* (1976) in Monro County found a disproportionate number of cases in non-whites and in classes 4 and 5. Ljunberg (1957) was unable to detect any social class effect, but found that for men, but not for women, urban dwellers were overrepresented.

Most studies are agreed that females outnumber males in a ratio that varies from 2:1 (Ljunberg, 1957; Stefansson *et al.*, (1976) to 10:1 (Raskin *et al.*, 1966). Ljunbeg has pointed out that the lower ratio differs little from neurosis in general.

# Clinical aspects

## Symptom pattern

A categorization according to symptom/syndrome choice for some of the more recently published studies is shown in Table 8.3. There is considerable variability. Amnesia, for example, is prominent in some studies, absent from others. Motor disorders (within which category are included not only paresis, but also tremor, incoordination and ataxia) form the largest single group in the majority of studies. The somatosensory and special senses are usually represented but account for a smaller proportion of cases.

## The signs of hysterical conversion

Consideration will be confined to sensorimotor syndromes.

Physical examination of the hysterical patient may provide incontestable evidence of the presence of a conversion syndrome. However, some caveats are in order. It is not enough that physical examination fails to provide confirmation of the organic nature of the patient's complaints; for a diagnosis of HC, an inconsistency between the patient's symptoms or observed disabilities and their state on physical examination must be demonstrated. For example, the patient who claims to be unable to move the left side of the body and yet, through various manoeuvres, is persuaded to demonstrate unacknowledged strength in the antagonist muscles in the presence of normal muscle tone and reflex responses. In such a case a diagnosis of conversion can be confidently made. Complaints of sensory loss or motor weakness are more amenable to this type of demonstration; periodic disorders, e.g. epilepsy, or conditions

**Table 8.3.** Frequency of conversion symptoms in 5 studies (1957–1986)

| Symptom | Ljungberg (1957)[1] (n=381) | Stefansson et al. (1976)[2] (n=64) | Roy (1980)[3] (n=50) | Hafeiz (1980)[4] (n=61) | Marsden (1986)[5] (n=34) |
|---|---|---|---|---|---|
| Gait disturbance | 62 | — | 4 | — | 18 |
| Fits (pseudo-seizures) | 36 | — | 64 | 10 | 33 |
| Tremor | 25 | — | — | 3 | — |
| Paralyses | 12 | 20 | 14 | 10 | 35 |
| Speech disturbances (incl. aphonia and mutism) | 4 | — | 6 | 23 | — |
| Sensory disturbances (incl. anaesthesia) | 13 | 28 | — | 3 | 15 |
| Pain | — | 69 | — | — | 15 |
| Visual field defects (incl. blindness) | 3 | 13 | 4 | 3 | 15 |
| Dyspnoea (breathlessness) | — | 28 | — | 20 | — |
| Vomiting | — | — | — | 16 | — |
| Syncope | — | 14 | — | — | — |
| Dizziness, faintness | — | 13 | — | — | — |
| Amnesia | 8 | — | 6 | — | 12 |
| Twilight states | 16 | — | — | — | — |
| Retention of urine | — | — | — | 3 | — |

Figures given are a % of the whole sample.
Patients in studies 1, 2 and 5 had more than one symptom:
1 Swedish case note study of 381 patients (1931–1945 data). Of this sample 233 (61%) were admitted to neurology and 148 (39%) to psychiatric clinics. Some patients had more than one symptom.
2 A retrospective psychiatric case register study (New York and Iceland) and consultation service survey (1960–1969 data). Of the 64 patients, 19 were 'probable' hysterical neurosis and 8 'misdiagnosed'. The mean number of conversion symptoms was 3.2.
3 A consecutive series of 50 patients (39 F, 11 M) seen in 10 London teaching hospitals between 1974 and 1977 (7 patients from specialist neurology hospital). Twenty patients (40%) had organic brain disease.
4 Study of 61 patients (56 F, 5M) referred to psychiatric clinic in Khartoum (Sudan) between 1975 and 1977. The high rate of dyspnoea and vomiting suggests that patients satisfied diagnostic criteria other than hysterical conversion.
5 Patients referred to a neurologist with an interest in movement disorders. Thirty-four cases (29 F, 5 M) among 3500 admissions (0.1%) over 5 years (1979–1984). Some patients had more than one symptom.

that lack readily objectifiable physical signs, e.g. dystonia, less so. In this context, the significance that may be attached to a physical sign is much influenced by the extent to which it is susceptible to simulation. This is largely determined by its physical parameters. Examination of the sensory system is generally less reliable, but disorders of gait are notoriously difficult to evaluate.

A thorough physical examination is of particular value in cases of paralysis. Hysterical weakness of the facial muscles and tongue seem not to occur and paralysis of the cervical and trunk muscles is extremely uncommon. Hysterical weakness therefore involves principally the extremities, and the legs more than the arms (Pincus, 1982). It is important to emphasize that a diagnosis of HC can be made with greater confidence if positive signs of hysteria can be adduced, rather than merely lack of evidence of organic disease. Thus, a demonstration of strength retained in the limbs is more important than the demonstration of preserved reflexes.

Hysterical paralysis is usually a paralysis of movement rather than a weakness of individual muscles. If the affected arm is held above the head, it may retain its position for a second or two before dropping. This indicates persisting strength in the antagonistic muscles. Discontinuous resistance, 'give way' weakness, is also typical of hysterical paresis. In the lower limbs leg raising provides a useful diagnostic test. In the supine position, the raising of one leg is naturally accompanied by a pushing down movement by the other leg. This may be tested by placing a hand below the stationary heel. This manoeuvre should be carried out on each leg in turn. Wasting, trophic changes, and contractures are said to be rare in HC but certainly do occur. Usually however they suggest the presence of organic disease (Merskey, 1979).

Hysterical gait disturbances are difficult to evaluate. To a considerable extent this is diagnosis by pattern recognition and patients who present with abnormalities of gait that do not fit any recognizable pattern, or are bizarre, are suspect. Inconsistency of gait disturbance is often put forward as a pointer to astasia abasia (hysterical gait), but anxiety may impair performance alike in organic and non-organic cases. The prevailing orthodoxy teaches that dystonia is always organic. This is undoubtedly true in the great majority of instances, but the writer has seen at least two cases in which this was not so. It is only in the last decade or so that torticollis has gradually come to be accepted as a neurological rather than a psychiatric condition. Many dystonics are still thought to be hysterics by neurologists and psychiatrists alike. The counterview, that dystonia is never hysterical, is an understandable reaction to this state of affairs but has to be resisted. Disturbances of sensation, anaesthesia or hyperaesthesia, are by their very nature less easy to substantiate or to refute. Again it is the presence of inconsistencies of function that may first arouse suspicion. For example, the patient who lays claim to a profound loss of position sense but can still perform complex tasks such as the knotting of a tie (Pincus, 1982). More precise tests may be unreliable. In organic hemisensory loss, due to midline dual innervation, the first 1–2 cm on either side of the midline are spared. Bone conduction ensures that a tuning fork placed asymmetrically on the skull or sternum will still be felt at either side, hemisensory loss notwithstanding. The hysterical subject, lacking this information, responds in accordance with his or her own concept of hemisensory loss. So unfortunately do some patients with organic sensory impairment and the tests lack discriminatory power.

# Aetiology

## Psychological factors

### *Personality*

The leading 19th century physicians were well aware of the significance of emotional factors in the development of hysteria, but it was not until the close of the century that Janet (1894) drew attention to that constellation of personality traits that taken together we now identify as the histrionic personality. Many of those who followed him failed to distinguish between personality abnormalities of this type and conversion symptoms, and saw them as different aspects of the same disorder. This important issue, which is relevant not only to HC but also to chronic somatization (somatization disorder), is discussed in more detail in Chapter 12, p. 315. Chodoff and Lyons (1958), collating information from the available literature, attempted an operational definition of the hysterical personality and showed that, in an admittedly small cohort, the relationship with HC was, to say the least, tenuous. Of 19 patients with HC only 3 were regarded as hysterical personalities. Passive dependent traits were twice as common.

Subsequent studies have largely confirmed these early findings. The data reported by Mersky and Trimble (1979) are particularly persuasive as a control sample was used. Hysterical personality was thought to be present in 21% of the conversion symptom group, but in none of the matched psychiatric patients who constituted the control group. However, the same proportions were noted for the passive-immature-dependent personality type. Personality was deemed to be normal in only 12% of the conversion patients. However, Wilson-Barnett and Trimble (1985) found no excess of hysterical personality types among HC subjects when compared with general psychiatric controls and significantly less than in neurological patients. Among other authors the proportion of HC patients with hysterical personality varies from 20% (Ljunberg, 1957) to 33% (Stefansson *et al.*, 1976) and to under 10% (Stephens & Kamp, 1962). Passive, dependent personalities (Stephens & Kamp, 1962) and dependency traits (Stefansson *et al.*, 1976) were observed more frequently. It seems therefore that there is a fair measure of concordance between the different studies. Hysterical personality may be seen, but only in a minority of conversion cases; other forms of personality disorder of immature dependent type are more usual. But the reliability of diagnosis of personality disorder remains unsatisfactory: 51% of HC cases in Monro County were thought to have character disorders; in Iceland it was only 4% (Stefansson *et al.*, 1976). These differences are likely to arise out of a lack of agreement between physicians from differing theoretical backgrounds rather than a true variation in prevalence. There is a particular need here for carefully conducted enquiries using matched control groups, standardized and objective instruments and appropriate statistical techniques. Regrettably, few studies have met these requirements. In one systematic study which compared HC patients with neurological patients and non-somatic psychiatric controls, Wilson-Barnet and Trimble (1985) used a battery of rating scales and questionnaires. The HC group admitted to more sexual difficulties but did not differ significantly from the other groups on the EPI or the Illness Behaviour Questionnaire (Pilowsky *et al.*, 1984). On the latter measure they did show a trend towards increased affective inhibition (defined as a difficulty in expressing personal and emotional feelings, especially negative ones, to others) and to denial of life's problems, and to diminished acknowledgement of anxiety and depression. In a cross correlative analysis these variables were found to correlate strongly with somatization. Response to mood scales did indicate levels of affective disturbance in the index group comparable to the psychiatric controls and greater than the neurological group. A familiar pattern thus emerges, with an emphasis on sexual difficulties, somatization, denial of problems, and affective symptomatology. But some group differences are less sharply defined than might be expected, and this underscores the possible limitations of self-report studies in a population of this kind.

### The role of stress in the development of conversion symptoms

It is the classical analytical view as originally expounded by Freud (1950) that HC represents an attempt to resolve a profound and deeply entrenched sexual conflict. Other authorities accept the central hypothesis of conflict resolution but believe that the causes may be more immediate and not necessarily of a sexual nature. The latter view has prevailed and has received ample confirmation both in published work and in general clinical experience. Raskin *et al.* (1966) and Stefansson *et al.* (1976) each found the presence of psychological precipitants among the more reliable criteria for diagnosis. Psychological problems could be identified in half of the cases at first assessment (Stephens & Kamp, 1962; Whitlock, 1967) and in all cases after further enquiry (Stephens & Kamp, 1962); but Whitlock has questioned whether these must always be regarded as aetiologically relevant rather than merely coincidental.

The role of stress will of course vary according to the population studied. In studies emanating from military psychiatry and reflecting wartime experience (e.g., Carter, 1972) severe stress is a constant factor. Once the stress is removed recovery is swift and complete in the majority of cases and some authorities (Slater, 1965; Meares & Horvath, 1972) have inclined towards the idea of an acute psychogenic subgroup with good personality and prognosis. The corollary that there may be an inverse relationship between certain types of abnormal personality traits and the degree of stress necessary to bring about a conversion episode is attractive but as yet insufficiently explored.

### Primary and secondary gain

The concept of gain is more complex. If as a consequence of illness a stressful situation is averted or ameliorated, primary gain may be said to have occurred. Admittedly this is to adapt a Freudian term to the needs of a more secular age, but the new meaning intended is clear enough. The benefits that accrue from the invalid role such as detention, sympathy, absolution from chores and responsibilities, are referred to as secondary gain. The first form of gain may merge imperceptibly into the second. Conversion symptoms that disrupt an unwanted engagement may then be permitted to resolve, but an adolescent illness that delays the taking up of adult responsibilities may harden into a lifetime of invalidism, in which case the distinction between primary and secondary gain becomes difficult to determine. The general principle of secondary gain, which is central to the concept of illness behaviour, has attracted interest (Pilowsky, 1969; Kendell, 1982; Marsden, 1986) but there are few detailed accounts of it in the HC literature. Raskin *et al.* (1966) judged it to be present in 26 of 32 patients with HC, but in only two of seven control patients with organic illness, and found it to be one of three observations which best discriminated between the two groups (the others were prior use of somatic symptoms as a psychological defence, and presence of precipitating stress — see above). Baker and Silver (1987), who also used an organic control group, also found the concept to have discriminatory value.

*Belle indifférence, modelling, and previous episodes of illness behaviour*

The same authors (Raskin *et al.*, 1966; Baker & Silver, 1987) have commented on the possible significance of other psychological factors. In one study (Raskin *et al.*, 1966) *belle indifférence*, a classical sign of HC, was judged to be present in just over half of both HC and control groups. Evidence for modelling, the hypothesis that conversion symptoms are literally a re-enactment of some earlier experience of illness, occurring in the patient or observed in others, was detected in one-third of Raskin *et al.*'s patients, but did not emerge in Baker and Silver's study. The prior occurrence of HC episodes has attracted surprisingly little attention. Raskin *et al.* (1966) found this a useful diagnostic criterion. Twenty-six of 32 patients admitted to such a history, and they fell into two groups: '19 patients responded to a variety of emotional stresses with multiple somatic symptoms involving various organ systems. The other 7 patients used conversion reactions as their only physical symptoms and developed these reactions in response to specific stresses.' Half of Baker and Silver's group described earlier episodes of functional disturbance of the central nervous system.

## Organic brain disease

The relationship between organic brain disease (OBD) and HC symptomatology is complex and continues to be the subject of much comment and disputation. Two principal themes emerge: the possibility that the presence of OBD may predispose to the development of HC; and the diagnostic difficulties in distinguishing between the clinical features OBD and HC, particularly when the two occur together.

The frequent occurrence of hysterical symptomatology in the presence of OBD has been remarked on for over one hundred years. A wide range of neurological disorders has been implicated (Merskey, 1979). Cohorts drawn from specialist neurological centres have reported particularly high prevalence rates (Merskey & Buhrich, 1975; Marsden, 1986). These may be a reflection of the particular type of problem referred to neurology clinics (Marsden, 1986). In some instances (e.g., the cohort reported by Slater & Glithero, 1965) a diagnosis of HC describes an elaboration of symptoms due to a recognized neurological disorder. The difficulty then lies less in diagnosis than in the accurate apportioning of disability to organic and non-organic causes. In other settings the presence of neurological disease is less remarkable. Among HC patients referred to psychiatrists, only 3% may have OBD (Roy, 1979). In a community survey Ljungberg (1957) was unable to find any increase in head injury among patients with HC compared with the general population.

Organic brain disease may operate on the probability of developing HC syndromes through a number of mechanisms (Merskey, 1979). Neurological disease may result in a state of handicap in which illness behaviour patterns may be encouraged; more speculatively, perhaps, it may disturb central functions in such a way as to permit the emergence of new forms of neurotic behaviour or exacerbations of pre-existing neurotic traits; and neurological disease in others may provide a symptom model. Modelling may determine symptom choice in suggestible subjects, in particular those who have had the opportunity to witness these symptoms in others, but this alone would not explain the pre-eminence of CNS symptomatology in the syndromology of factitious illness. Merskey (1975) compared the prevalence of hysterical symptoms in cerebral and peripheral physical illness. A substantial but statistically insignificant trend was found in the directon of the former. If disturbed cerebral function has a role to play, specific regional vulnerability may be sought. The possible association with right hemisphere dysfunction is discussed below. The aetiological significance of OBD would be enhanced if a close temporal relationship with HC syndromes could be demonstrated. Whitlock (1967) reported that among cases of hysterical conversion a substantially greater proportion had a history of organic brain disease than was the case for psychiatric controls. Moreover, he found that within the index group, all of those with a history of head injury (14 out of 56) developed conversion symptoms within one year of the cerebral insult, and 11 within one month. In the control group (10 out of 56) the average interval was 10.2 years.

The risks of overlooking organic pathology inherent in making a diagnosis of HC have attracted considerable attention (Lazare, 1981; Marsden, 1986). The studies of Slater and Glithero (1965) and Stefansson *et al.* (1976), who reported a rate of misdiagnosis of 30% and 12.5% respectively, are often cited. There seems little doubt that during the period to which these studies refer (1950–1970) errors of diagnosis were not uncommon. It is this author's impression (and there has been little recent work to confirm or to refute) that this is no longer the case. A diagnosis of HC is not lightly made, but it is no longer an excessively contentious issue. Often there is considerable doubt, and the provisional diagnosis is no more than a testable hypothesis; but in those cases in which the diagnosis is firmly made, revision is rarely necessary.

If this is so, what has changed? This is a matter only for speculation. Hysterical conversion disorders were common in wartime experience and inevitably received a great deal of attention. That may have led to overdiagnosis during the immediate post-war era. Criticism may have led to a reappraisal and a more rigorous approach to diagnosis. Neurological diagnostic precision has been greatly improved by technical advances, particularly in the field of neuroimaging. Psychiatric diagnosis has been refined (for example, pain syndromes, a source of considerable diagnostic confusion, have been excluded from the definition). The obverse, a reluctance even to consider the possibility of HC, the clinical evidence notwithstanding, accompanied by a single minded pursuit of increasingly unlikely organic aetiologies, may now represent the greater danger.

*Neurophysiological mechanisms*

If cerebral dysfunction does play a significant role in the genesis and evolution of HC symptoms (as is suggested by the concurrence of head injury and other forms of OBD), the means by which it does so remain obscure. HC symptoms are more commonly encountered on the left side of the body (Galin *et al.*, 1977) though this is also true of patients with psychogenic pain (Edmonds, 1947; Mersky & Spear, 1967), somatic symptoms due to hyperventilation (Tavel, 1964; Blau *et al.*, 1983) and hypochondriasis (Kenyon, 1964). Stern (1977) has shown that this is equally true of left and right handed subjects, disposing of the hypothesis that conversion symptoms occur on the left as a matter of convenience. The possible significance of the non-dominant hemisphere in the mediation of unconscious phenomena has long been a matter for conjecture (e.g., Ferenczi, 1926). Galin (1974), extrapolating from the findings of cerebral commissurotomy surgery, has speculated: 'in the human, the left hemisphere usually has preemptive control over the mainstream of body activity as well as of propositional speech. If repression in normal intact people is to some extent subserved by a functional disconnection of right hemisphere mental processes, we might expect to see the expression of un-conscious ideation through whatever output modes are not preempted by the left hemisphere'. Anosognosia, the denial of illness, is associated with parietal lobe disease of the non-dominant hemisphere. Direct objective evidence of neurophysiological dysfunction in HC remains inconclusive. Hernandez-Peon *et al.* (1963) investigated a patient with hysterical anaesthesia of one arm. Somatosensory Evoked Responses (ER) were absent from the afflicted arm, unremarkable from the normal side. Other studies e.g., Halliday (1968), fail to confirm these findings. These differences may be explained if attention is paid to stimulus parameters (Levy & Behrman, 1970). Impairment of ER to nerve stimulation may be demonstrated only if stimulus intensity is kept close to threshold level; stimuli applied directly to skin yield impaired ER on the affected side regardless of level of intensity.

Psychophysiological measures have also been used to attempt to clarify nosological distinctions both within HC and between HC and other psy-chiatric disorders. Meares and Horvath (1972) used electrodermal responsive-ness to demonstrate a greater degree of arousal in their chronic HC group. Lader and Sartorius (1968), using similar measures, compared groups of patients with HC and anxiety/phobic symptoms. The first group were more anxious according to their own self-ratings and confirmed by measures of electro-dermal activity, but not by observer ratings. That is to say, the HC patients *reported* more anxiety and were more aroused *physiologically*, but did not *appear* objectively anxious. This latter finding illustrates that *la belle in-différence* refers to only one facet of the disorder. Finally, the signs and symp-toms of HC are essentially the physical manifestations of a disease concept. The accuracy with which this mimics the features of a recognized physical disease will be a measure of the patient's informed understanding of that disease. This may derive from first hand experience. It is also influenced by the culture in which the patient moves. Hysterical conversion syndromes among primitive or medically unsophisticated peoples lack the biological verisimilitude found in better informed societies.

### The genetic inheritance

Early studies (Kraulis, 1931) are difficult to interpret as the concept of HC still lacks clarity. Ljungberg (1957) reported a modest excess (2.4% in male relatives; 6.4% in female relatives) of cases in the families of probands, which he considered to be consistent with a polygenic model of inheritance. How-ever, as Slater (1982) has pointed out, risk did not appear to be increased in either the families of the more severely effected probands nor of the male probands 'who, as the less frequently affected sex, might be expected to require more polygenes before becoming clinically manifest'. In Slater's own study (1971) of 12 MZ and 12 DZ twin pairs only one MZ pair was con-cordant for hysteria. Inouye (1972) has reported on the accumulated data from twin studies and case reports. There were at that time 9 concordant and 33 discordant MZ pairs, and no concordant but 43 discordant DZ pairs. The genetic contribution to risk of HC would appear on the basis of this admittedly very limited data to be inconsiderable; perhaps more surprisingly, DZ twin data do little to argue the case for the importance of early environ-mental influences of a psychosocial nature.

## Hysterical conversion syndrome and other psychiatric disorders

Some authors, Roy (1980) in particular, have been impressed by the frequency with which depressive symptoms are encountered among patients with HC. Others (McKegney, 1967) have obtained less conclusive results. Hysterical symptoms may also appear, perhaps less commonly, in depressed subjects.

Rarely conversion symptoms may presage the development of schizo-phrenia. Schizophrenic syndromes may also occasionally contain histrionic elements. These may reflect the underlying personality; or the syndrome may represent a conversion disorder in which schizophrenic rather than somatic features have been simulated (Hirsch & Hollender, 1969).

## Management

Much has been written about the concept of hysteria, its aetiology and its relationship to other physical and psychiatric disorders. By contrast, there has been very little interest in its treatment, particularly in recent years. Merskey, in perhaps the most authoritative single author account of the subject (1979), allows less than two pages in three hundred. Most studies refer to treatment only in passing; detailed accounts of new techniques or approaches are limited to single case reports or short series. A variety of physical and psychological methods may be used, alone and in combination, often in the same series. Suggestion often appears to play a central role (Carter, 1949; Hafeiz, 1980; Baker & Silver, 1987), unassisted or as part of other procedures, e.g. intravenous drugs, placebo or hypnosis. This may take the form of a physical examination, a reassuring statement, or exhortations to overcome the disability (Carter, 1949). Other authors, e.g. Hafeiz (1980) are less explicit. Abreactive techniques have been used in employing pentothol (Carter, 1949; Baker & Silver, 1987), sodium amylobarbitone (Hafeiz, 1980), methyl amphetamine (Hafeiz, 1980) and sterile water (Baker & Silver, 1987). Suggestion under faradic stimulation or electro-sleep (Hafeiz, 1980) and electrical stimulation applied directly to the paralysed limb (Pu, 1986) are also described. Behaviour therapy, principally operant conditioning and shaping, may be used in a ward or physiotherapy setting (Liebson, 1967; Dickes, 1974; Munford and Paz, 1978; Munford and Liberman, 1982).

It is not easy to evaluate the effectiveness of these various remedies. The methods are poorly described, case numbers are small and few studies used any form of controlled design. Dickes (1974) compared outcome for two groups of patients, one treated behaviourally, the other receiving 'traditional approaches.' The first achieved a 90% remission rate compared with 45% for the traditional group. Hafeiz (who did use adequate case numbers) found amylobarbitone sodium to be notably less effective than methyl amphetamine and soon abandoned the former.

### Management: a personal view

Recent published work, summarized above, has been mainly concerned with specific techniques. A brief account of the principles that govern general management would seem in order.

*The investigation of physical illness*

Most patients with HC symptoms are firmly wedded to the notion that their complaints have a physical basis and that eventually, if they show sufficient persistence, a doctor will be found who through a combination of patience and astuteness will make the correct diagnosis where others have failed. It follows from this that if the patient is to retain confidence in an investigatory process as it increasingly moves in an unwelcome direction towards diagnostic conclusions that the patient may find difficult to accept, then that process must be carried out with unusual thoroughness and the patient and relatives kept informed at every step. Physical examination should be thorough and the opinions of colleagues sought if there is any room for doubt. A final diagnostic formulation should be delayed until all investigations are complete and all lines of enquiry satisfied as far as they can be. The position should then be put to the patient. If an adequate explanation in physical terms for part or all of the patient's symptoms is lacking, this should be stated and any request for further physical examination firmly resisted. In discussing this with the patient and his/her family, the physician may not wish to appear unduly categorical, but should be firm. A finely weighed 'on the one hand . . . on the other hand' exposition may be intellectually satisfying, but will do little to help the patient in resolving his/her own feelings of ambivalence.

The response of the patient or the patient's family to this information is often highly instructive. Most people, on hearing that they do not have significant brain disease, possibly progressive or even mortal, react with pleasure and relief. Not so the individual with conversion symptoms. Dismay gives way to unconcealed disbelief and an array of evidence pointing to organicity is paraded before the bemused physician. Concern at the loss of a physical diagnosis rapidly gives way to angry suspicion that a re-evaluation of symptoms in psychological terms is underway, that the patient's probity is being questioned and so on. Of course not all patients react in this way but when they do the portents are ominous and indicative of a primary need to be ill or to be seen to be ill, the clinical evidence notwithstanding.

*The assessment of psychiatric illness*

HC symptomatology may occur in association with other psychiatric conditions, affective disorders in particular, but also panic disorder and, rarely, schizophrenia. These should be recognized and treated appropriately.

*The explanation to the patient*

Patients whose symptoms are thought to arise due to some dissociative process are apt to become extremely sensitive concerning their status as patients. They may angrily insist that they are not 'putting it on', are not 'mad' or 'psychiatric'. Friends and relatives are often eager to take up cudgels on behalf of the patient and to denounce unsympathetic staff attitudes, the carelessness or lack of interest of earlier medical advisors, and so forth.

In this emotional climate it is essential that the physician adopts a neutral, non-judgemental approach. It is better first to insist only that investigations have failed to uncover any disease process that could account for the patient's symptoms. Psychological explanations are best avoided until later. The aim at this stage is gently to detach the patient from an explanatory model based on organic disease while remaining on good terms. Stress-related somatic phenomena, for example muscular tension or hyperventilation, may play a significant part in the development of HC symptoms (see above) and patients who may not otherwise be ready to accept the relevance of emotional factors in their illness are often able to recognize the physical manifestations of anxiety and to consider how these may in various ways explain or contribute to their disability. This somewhat impersonal and mechanistic approach may seem to some an evasion, a collusion between clinician and patient to avoid confronting the true meaning of the symptoms, but in practice it is a useful method of effecting an introduction to the role of stress, motivation and other factors that the patient may not find easy to discuss.

*Involvement of other significant people in the patient's life*

The attitudes of friends and family to the patient's disability and to the explanations and advice offered by the medical team form possibly the most reliable guide to outcome. Outwardly reasonable and constructive, extended acquaintance may reveal attitudes that match the patient's own in their irrationality and deviancy. The family may seem to have a vested interest in the patient's continuing invalidism. The dynamics of family attitude and behaviour may be extremely complex and expert assistance may be required. In some cases a family interview involving the patient and key family members may prove fruitful, as the following case illustrates:

> A 23-year-old single woman (Jane) was referred from the neurology service with a 7 year history of multiple physical complaints, the most recent being a 'useless right arm' which was prone to intermittent shaking. These complaints began soon after two epileptic seizures, but

she had remained fit-free on carbamazepine 200 mg o.d. She had attended 6 different specialist departments in at least 2 London teaching hospitals, seeking an organic cause for her monoplegia. Three years before referral a neurologist had diagnosed a transient hysterical gait disorder. There was no other relevant past medical history.

Jane lived at home with both parents and her younger brother, an unemployed recluse. After leaving school at 15 she had worked briefly as a clerk before her first seizure at the age of 16. After her second seizure she began having 'attacks' at home accompanied by carpopedal spasm and digital paraesthesiae (probably panic episodes with hyper-ventilation) and she had not worked since. Premorbidly shy and timid, she had lived the life of an invalid since 16 and had no friends or social life. Her only hobby was embroidery but her disability prevented this.

Both parents were angered by the psychiatric referral, believing the symptoms to be a consequence of epilepsy. They had always discouraged independence in Jane and had become overinvolved in her health. Her father had instigated most of the referrals to specialists, but his demands for splints and disability benefits were not granted because the neurologists could not find an organic cause for her symptoms. The psychiatric diagnosis was hysterical monoplegia in an immature, dependent personality with a past history of epilepsy. The symptoms were thought to serve a function: they postponed any development in the psychological, sexual or work related spheres, principally because she lacked the resources to advance in these areas. The symptoms had prevented her from doing anything except to consult a succession of doctors and as a consequence she had become very socially isolated.

A family therapy approach was adopted and it became clear during the first 2 sessions that there was a 'model' in the family for not leaving home. Neither parent had separated from their own parents (Jane's mother had lived in her own mother's house since she was born, and Jane's father had also lived at home until his mid-thirties before moving in with his wife's parents). The central issue in this family concerned the children leaving home: Jane and her brother would be the first generation to do so. The family feared separation, perceived being alone as dangerous, and did all they could to postpone Jane's departure. They administered all her medicine, gave her physiotherapy and accompanied her to the lavatory 'just in case'.

At the third family therapy session Jane was presented with two options: the first was to stay at home and have her parents administer to all her needs, the second was to ask her parents to desist from acting as her therapist and to encourage Jane to initiate help from outside the family. She was asked to find a professional physiotherapist through her general practitioner and to visit a local youth club once a week. The family therapist acknowledged that Jane would find this difficult, but nevertheless encouraged her vigorously.

At the next session a remarkable transformation had occurred. Although Jane had not achieved the goals we had set, she had visited a local allergy clinic and 'discovered' that all her symptoms were caused by multiple food allergies. After dietary manipulation most of her symptoms had disappeared. Both parents were adamant that this had been the cause of Jane's symptoms from the beginning and they were very angry that the doctors had not considered this diagnosis. They brought books and pamphlets on food allergies to the session and Jane waved these gleefully (with her previously useless right hand) in the therapist's face.

Although taken aback by this display, the therapist decided to acquiesce with the family's new-found attribution of Jane's disorder. Jane was congratulated on initiating this consultation at the allergy clinic and we encouraged her to continue going to the clinic because it involved self-initiated activity, and unaccompanied travel on a bus, which were new departures for her. She had also made enquiries about employment, which we encouraged. No further family sessions occurred.

This case illustrates some crucial points about hysterical conversion in particular, and somatization in general. The function of the symptoms was evident from the family assessment, and the exhortations to Jane to initiate activity herself resulted in a pseudo-improvement. This led to a new (and increasingly fashionable) attribution of her symptoms which, although resulting in symptomatic recovery, effectively shifted the family's attention from their own problems to another pseudo-disorder (food allergies). Thus the blame-avoidance function of somatization was maintained and the family did not have to acknowledge their own difficulties involving separation and autonomy. The blame for Jane's paralysis was shifted to factors outside their control, but with less dangerous connotations than neurological disease. Jane's prognosis is uncertain, and we await further information from the family doctor with interest.

## Abreaction

This may be used diagnostically, particularly in regard to hysterical fugues and amnesias, or therapeutically, either as an adjunct to exploratory psychotherapy or as part of a cognitive approach to physical rehabilitation.

Dramatic responses to abreactive techniques are described in wartime psychiatry, but usually occurred in cases in which conversion symptoms had appeared in response to overwhelming physical threat and in which treatment had followed with little delay. Peacetime experience is rather different. Many patients are inclined to regard the technique used in this way with some suspicion and are reluctant to divulge information that may compromise their position. Abreaction may be used to particularly good effect in cases with motor conversion phenomena to demonstrate to the patient that they have greater powers of response than they would otherwise have believed. Intravenous sedation appears to produce a state of heightened suggestibility in which the patient may be successively encouraged to achieve and to sustain greater limb movements. It is essential that video recordings be made as the outcome of the session may subsequently be denied or genuinely forgotten. The recorded sessions may later be used in cognitive work to demonstrate to the patient (and sometimes to relatives) the potential for recovery.

## Prognosis

The outcome for HC syndromes is varied. In those cases in which conversion symptomatology has embellished or has been released by OBD, the prognosis will be determined by the course of the primary disorder. Likewise, if HC has been incorrectly diagnosed, the outcome is that of the neurological or psychiatric condition that has been overlooked. There remains a majority in whom the initial diagnosis was correctly reached and it is the outcome in this group that will be considered here.

Even within this restricted group, observations vary: some report a modestly encouraging outcome, but with a significant proportion who remain chronically handicapped; other studies record a brisk and gratifying response to treatment, but a tendency to relapse. These apparent differences may only reflect variability in time sampling.

Ljungberg again provides the most detailed and comprehensive long term study (1957). At 1 year 43% of males and 35% of females were symptomatic. At 5 years these figures were 25% and 22% respectively. At 10–15 years there had been little change. Of the females, 7.6% who had recovered at 1 year relapsed at 5 years with the same symptoms, 3.2% with different symptoms. For men the figures were 6% and 0%. Poor premorbid personality influenced outcome adversely; intelligence and age of onset were unimportant. Lewis (1975) retrospectively analysed a cohort of 98 patients who had been followed up for 5–7 years at the Maudsley Hospital. Fifty-four were well and working.

Poor outcome appeared to be related to personal inadequacies rather than to adverse circumstances or to untoward life events.

Results from a number of studies suggest that the prospects for immediate recovery are good, but that a significant number will quickly relapse. An acute onset related to highly stressful circumstances, e.g. wartime experiences, and prompt treatment are good outcome predictors. Eighty-three per cent of a cohort of 100 patients first seen between 1939 and 1943 were again working 4–6 years later (Carter, 1949). In a study of acute hysterical paraplegia (Baker & Silver, 1987) all of 23 patients had recovered within 8 days and 13 within 48 hours. A systematic follow-up was not attempted, but from information obtained it seems that five subsequently developed hysterical neurological syndromes (not all paraplegia) and four somatic syndromes of doubtful organic aetiology. Other studies of hysterical paraplegia (Maurice-Williams & Marsh, 1985) have stressed the importance of early diagnosis and treatment but some chronic conditions may still respond, particularly if there is an underlying organic lesion (Delargy *et al.*, 1986). If the incidence of HC is high in some developing countries, the response to treatment is prompt (Pu *et al.*, 1986) if not always sustained (Hafeiz, 1980). In the latter study one-fifth of a cohort of successively treated patients had relapsed within an interval of 1 year.

Prognosis may also be influenced by symptom pattern. Hysterical seizures have a poor outcome (Carter, 1949; Ljungberg, 1957; Hafeiz, 1980; Pu *et al.*, 1986) and cases presenting with tremor (Carter, 1949; Ljungberg, 1957) and amnesia (Carter, 1949) also faired badly. Hysterical blindness, aphonia (Carter, 1949), and motor disorders (Carter, 1949; Ljungberg, 1957; Hafeiz, 1980; Maurice-Williams & Marsh, 1985; Pu *et al.*, 1986) do better, though the rate of relapse in treated hysterical paraplegia is considerable (Baker & Silver, 1987).

It would seem therefore that outcome is determined by a diversity of factors which include acuteness of onset, the presence of major stress, the length of the interval before treatment is instituted, symptom pattern, personality type and the cultural setting in which the illness occurs. The majority of patients show a rapid response to treatment, but a significant proportion will relapse within a year of recovery.

# References

Alexander, F. (1950). *Psychosomatic Medicine*, Norton & Co., New York.

American Psychiatric Association (1987). *Diagnostic and Statistical Manual of Mental Disorders*, (DSM-III-R) 3rd edn revised, Washington, D.C.

Baker, J.H. & Silver, J.R. (1987). Hysterical paraplegia, *Journal of Neurology, Neurosurgery and Psychiatry*, **50**, 375–382.

Bass, C., Chambers, J.B., Kiff, P., Cooper, D. & Gardner, W.N. (1988). Panic anxiety and hyper-ventilation in patients with chest pain: a controlled study, *Quarterly Journal of Medicine*, **69**, 949–959.

Blau, J.N., Wiles, C.M. & Solomon, F.S. (1983). Unilateral somatic symptoms due to hyper-ventilation, *British Medical Journal*, **286**, 1108.

Carter, A.B. (1949). The prognosis of certain hysterical symptoms, *British Medical Journal*, **1**, 1076–1078.

Carter, A.B. (1972). A physician's view of hysteria, *Lancet*, **ii**, 1241–1243.

Carter, R.B. (1853). *On the Pathology and Treatment of Hysteria*, Churchill, London.

Chodoff, P. & Lyons, H. (1958). Hysteria, the hysterical personality, and hysterical conversion, *American Journal of Psychiatry*, **114**, 734–740.

Cockburn, J.J. (1971). Spasmodic torticollis: a psychogenic condition? *Journal of Psychosomatic Research*, **15**, 471–477.

Delargy, M.A., Peatfield, R.C. & Burt, A.A. (1986). Successful rehabilitation in conversion paralysis, *British Medical Journal*, **292**, 1730–1731.

Dickes, R.A. (1974). Brief therapy of conversion reactions: an in-hospital technique, *American Journal of Psychiatry*, **131**, 584–586.

Edmonds, E.B. (1947). Psychosomatic non-articular rheumatism, *Annals of Rheumatic Disease*, **6**, 36–49.

Ferenczi, S. (1926). *Further Contributions to the Theory and Technique of Psychoanalysis*, Hogarth Press, London.

Freud, S. (1905). Three essays on infantile sexuality, in *The Standard Edition of the Complete Psychological Works of Sigmund Freud* Vol. 7 (Ed. Strachey, J.), Hogarth Press, London (1960).

Galin, D. (1974). Implications for psychiatry of left and right cerebral specialisation, *Archives of General Psychiatry*, **31**, 572–583.

Galin, D., Diamond, R. & Braff, D. (1977). Lateralisation of conversion symptoms: more frequent on the left, *American Journal of Psychiatry*, **134(5)**, 578–580.

Guze, S.B. (1967). The diagnosis of hysteria: what are we trying to do? *American Journal of Psychiatry*, **124**, 491–498.

Guze, S.B., Woodruff, R.A. & Clayton, P.J. (1971). A study of conversion symptoms in psychiatric out-patients, *American Journal of Psychiatry*, **128(5)**, 643–646.

Hafeiz, H.B. (1980). Hysterical conversion: a prognostic study, *British Journal of Psychiatry*, **136**, 548–551.

Halliday, A.M. (1968). Computing techniques in neurological diagnosis, *British Medical Bulletin*, **24**, 253–259.

Hare, E.H. (1971). *Triennial Statistical Report*, Bethlem Royal Hospital and The Maudsley Hospital, London.

Hernandez-Peon, R., Chavez-Ibarra, G. & Aguilar-Figuroa, E. (1963). Somatic evoked potentials in one case of hysterical anaesthesia, *Electroencepholography and Clinical Neuro-physiology*, **15**, 889–892.

Hirsch, J.J. & Hollender, M.H. (1969). Hysterical psychosis. Clarification of the concept, *American Journal of Psychiatry*, **125**, 909–915.

Hopkins, A. & Clarke, C. (1987). Pretended paralysis requiring artificial ventilation, *British Medical Journal*, **294**, 861–862.

Inouye, E. (1972). Genetic aspects of neurosis, *International Journal of Mental Health*, **1**, 176–189.

Janet, P. (1894). *L'Etat Mental des Hysteriques*, Ruess, Paris.

Kendell, R.E. (1982). A new look at hysteria, in *Hysteria* (Ed. Roy, A.), pp. 27–36, John Wiley & Sons, London.

Kenyon, F.E. (1964). Hypochondriasis: a clinical study, *British Journal of Psychiatry*, **110**, 478–488.

Kranz, H. (1953). Die entwicklung des hysterie-begriffs, *Fortschritte der Neurologie und*

*Psychiatrie*, **21**, 223–238.

Kraulis, W. (1931). Zur vererbung der hysterischen reaktionsweise, *Zeitschrift fur die Pesamate Neurologie und Psychiatrie*, **136**, 174–258.

Lader, M. & Sartorius, N. (1968). Anxiety in patients with hysterical conversion symptoms, *Journal of Neurology, Neurosurgery and Psychiatry*, **31**, 990–995.

Lazare, A. (1981). Conversion symptoms, *New England Journal of Medicine*, **305**, 745–748.

Levy, R. & Behrman, J. (1970). Cortical evoked responses in hysterical hemianaesthesia, *Electroenkepholography and Clinical Neurophysiology*, **29**, 400–402.

Lewis, A. (1975). The survival of hysteria, *Psychological Medicine*, **5**, 9–12.

Liebson, I. (1967). Conversion reaction: a learning theory approach, *Behaviour Research and Therapy*, **7**, 217–218.

Ljungberg, L. (1957). Hysteria: a clinical, prognostic and genetic study, *Acta Psychiatrica et Neurologica Scandinavica*, **32** (Suppl. 112).

McKegney, F.P. (1967). The incidence and characteristics of patients with conversion reactions: I. A general hospital consultation service sample, *American Journal of Psychiatry*, **124**, 542–545.

Marsden, C.D. (1986). Hysteria — a neurologist's view, *Psychological Medicine*, **16**, 277–288.

Maurice-Williams, R.S. & Marsh, H. (1985). Simulated paraplegia: an occasional problem for the neurosurgeon, *Journal of Neurology, Neurosurgery and Psychiatry*, **48**, 826–831.

Meares, R. & Horvath, T. (1972). 'Acute' and 'chronic' hysteria, *British Journal of Psychiatry*, **121**, 653–657.

Merskey, H. (1975). The mode of action of organic lesions in promoting hysteria, *British Journal of Medical Psychology*, **48**, 373.

Merskey, H. (1979). *The Analysis of Hysteria*, Ballière-Tindall, London.

Merskey, H. & Buhrich, N.A. (1975). Hysteria and organic brain disease, *British Journal of Medical Psychology*, **48**, 359–366.

Merskey, H. & Spear, F.D. (1967). *Pain: Psychological and Psychiatric Aspects*, Ballière-Tindall, London.

Merskey, H. & Trimble, M.R. (1979). Personality, sexual adjustment, and brain lesions in patients with conversion symptoms, *American Journal of Psychiatry*, **136**, 179–182.

Mumford, P.R. & Liberman, R.P. (1978). Differential attention in the out-patient treatment of operant cough, *Journal of Behavioural Medicine*, **1**, 289–295.

Mumford, P.R. & Paz, G. (1978). Differential attention in the treatment of astasia-abasia, *Journal of Behavioural and Therapeutic Experimental Psychiatry*, **9**, 369–371.

Naish, J.M. (1982). A concept of hysteria, *Health Trends*, **14**, 15–17.

Perley, M.J. & Guze, S.B. (1962). Hysteria — the stability and usefulness of clinical criteria, *New England Journal of Medicine*, **266**, 421–426.

Pilowsky, I. (1967). Dimensions of hypochondriasis, *British Journal of Psychiatry*, **113**, 89–93.

Pilowsky, I. (1969). Abnormal illness behaviour, *British Journal of Medical Psychology*, **42**, 347–351.

Pilowsky, I., Spence, N., Cobb, J. & Katsikitis, M. (1984). The illness behaviour questionnaire as an aid to clinical assessment, *General Hospital Psychiatry*, **6**, 123–130.

Pincus, J. (1982). Hysteria presenting to the neurologist, in *Hysteria* (Ed. Roy, A.), pp. 131–144, John Wiley & Sons, London.

Pu, T., Mohamed, E., Iman, K. & El-Roey, A. (1986). One hundred cases of hysteria in Eastern Libya: a socio-demographic study, *British Journal of Psychiatry*, **148**, 606–609.

Purtell, J.J., Robins, E. & Cohen, M.E. (1951). Observations on clinical aspects of hysteria, *Journal of the American Medical Association*, **146**, 902–909.

Raskin, M., Talbott, J.A., Myerson, A.T. (1966). Diagnosis of conversion reactions: predictive value of psychiatric criteria, *Journal of the American Medical Association*, **197**, 530–534.

Reed, J.L. (1975). The diagnosis of hysteria, *Psychological Medicine*, **5**, 13–17.

Reynolds, J.R. (1869). Remarks on paralysis and other disorders of motions and sensations, dependent on idea, *British Medical Journal*, **2**, 3–5. Discussion, 378–379.

Roy, A. (1979). Hysteria: a case note study, *Canadian Journal of Psychiatry*, **24**, 157–160.

Roy, A. (1980). Hysteria, *Journal of Psychosomatic Research*, **24**, 53–56.

Slater, E. (1965). Diagnosis of 'hysteria', *British Medical Journal*, **1**, 1395–1399.

Slater, E. (1982). What is hysteria? in *Hysteria* (Ed. Roy, A.), pp. 37–40, John Wiley & Sons, London.

Slater, E. & Glithero, E. (1965). A follow-up of patients diagnosed of suffering from 'hysteria', *Journal of Psychosomatic Research*, **9**, 9–14.

Stefansson, J.D., Messina, J.A. & Meyerowitz, S. (1976). Hysterical neurosis, conversion type: clinical and epidemiological considerations, *Acta Psychiatrica Scandinavica*, **53**, 119–138.

Stephens, J.H. & Kamp, M. (1962). On some aspects of hysteria: a clinical study, *Journal of Nervous and Mental Disorders*, **134**, 302–315.

Stern, D. (1977). Handedness and the natural distribution of conversion reactions, *Journal of Nervous and Mental Diseases*, **164(2)**, 122–128.

Steyerthal, A. (1908). *Was ist Hysterie?* Halle a. S, Marhold.

Tavel, M.E. (1964). Hyperventilation syndrome with unilateral somatic symptoms, *Journal of the American Medical Association*, **187**, 301–303.

Trimble, M.R. (1982). Functional diseases, *British Medical Journal*, **2**, 1768–1770.

Walters, A. (1961). Psychogenic regional pain alias hysterical pain, *Brain*, **48(1)**, 1–18.

Whitlock, F.A. (1967). The aetiology of hysteria, *Acta Psychiatrica Scandinavica*, **43**, 144–162.

Whytt, R. (1765). *Observations on the Nature, Causes and Cure of those disorders which are commonly called Nervous, Hypochondriac, or Hysteric*, Becket & Du Hondt, Edinburgh.

Wig, N.N., Mangalwedhe, K., Herminder, B. & Murphy, R.S. (1982). A follow-up study of hysteria, *Indian Journal of Psychiatry*, **24**, 50–55.

Wilson-Barnett, J. & Trimble, M.R. (1985). An investigation of hysteria using the Illness Behaviour Questionnaire, *British Journal of Psychiatry*, **146**, 601–608.

Woodruff, R.A., Clayton, P.J. & Guze, S.B. (1969). Hysteria: an evaluation of specific diagnostic criteria by the study of randomly selected psychiatric clinic patients, *British Journal of Psychiatry*, **115**, 1243–1248.

World Health Organization (1987). Mental, behavioural and developmental disorders, in *International Classification of Diseases* (10th revision) Draft chapter V(F). Division of Mental Health, World Health Organization, Geneva (copyright reserved).

# 9

# Gynaecological Complaints

M. HUNTER

## Introduction

A woman's decision to seek gynaecological help is influenced by many factors unrelated to disease. These include not only personal factors such as health beliefs e.g. interpretation and attribution of symptoms and current mood state, but also social factors such as available social support and the nature and accessibility of medical services (see Mechanic, 1983; Rosenstock & Kirscht, 1979). Indeed, there is evidence to suggest that psychological and social factors (psychosocial stress and perception of one's own general health) are more likely to predict clinic attendance than organic factors (Tessler *et al.*, 1976; Mechanic, 1983).

## Explanatory models of distress in gynaecological patients

An understanding of the causes of distress in women has been hampered by polarized views and outdated assumptions. In Graeco-Roman times, emotional and health problems in women were attributed to the 'wandering womb'. Early psychological explanations, influenced by psychodynamic theory, emphasized the negative aspects of female reproductive events, such as menstruation and menopause. In addition, a woman's identity came to be seen as a function of her reproductive capacity. Biological explanations have tended to link high rates of distress with hormonal changes that occur during menstruation, the postpartum period and the menopause (Dalton, 1978). These views have led to various stereotyped beliefs which may be held to differing degrees by doctors and women seeking medical help.

More recently, psychological explanations of distress reported by women have emphasized the increased psychosocial stress associated with female roles as well as possible differences in expression of distress (Weissman & Klerman, 1981; Briscoe, 1982). It seems plausible that some women who

235

attend gynaecological clinics may express a latent need (Mechanic, 1983), using a particular somatic mode of complaint, about their lives and psychosocial state. However, the precise mechanisms underlying presentation of particular symptoms by distressed women are little understood.

Recent developments in psychology have emphasized the cognitive processes involved in perception, interpretation and explanations of physical sensations (Pennebaker, 1982; Leventhal *et al.*, 1980), attribution of symptoms and locus of control (Wallston *et al.*, 1987; Hewstone, 1983) and beliefs about health and illness (Becker & Maiman, 1983). Patients are seen as active in attempting to understand and explain their symptoms. They develop 'lay explanations' about their illness, its causes and possible outcome (see Chapter 4, p. 76).

A knowledge of cognitive processes is necessary to understand the determinants of somatization in gynaecology. For example, both the patient and the doctor will have causal attributions of the presenting symptoms, and an understanding of these is crucial to the outcome of the clinic visit and subsequent treatment.

Having highlighted the potential psychological needs of this client group let us consider gynaecological factors. Gynaecology emerged as a separate branch of medicine during the early part of this century. Before that general surgeons were responsible for major gynaecological problems. This may explain why gynaecology is still considered to be primarily a surgical specialty. Psychoanalytic and feminist writers have suggested that it is no accident that surgery has been used so extensively by physicians to remove female organs (Horney, 1932; Weideger, 1978).

There does appear to be a discrepancy between the needs of women attending gynaecological clinics and the treatment available to gynaecologists. Indeed, a leading gynaecologist has pointed out that: 'Gynaecologists see a large number of women with complaints that do not have their origin in recognised forms of pathology' (Beard, 1984).

For example, two of the most commonly reported presenting complaints, menorrhagia and pelvic pain, are frequently associated with distress but without known organic pathology. These conditions may lead to surgical intervention when a psychological approach might have been a more appropriate alternative (Pearce *et al.*, 1982; Greenberg, 1983).

This chapter is divided into three main sections. The first will deal with studies of the prevalence of psychiatric disorder and psychological distress in patients with gynaecological symptoms. Next, menstrual problems are discussed in detail with reference to possible mechanisms linking symptom experience and help-seeking behaviour. Examples from the author's own studies of menopausal women are included. Finally, treatment approaches are suggested which are aimed at alleviating distress and modifying help-seeking behaviour.

# Prevalence of psychiatric disorder and psychological distress in women with gynaecological complaints

## Community studies

A large *community survey* of gynaecological and psychological symptoms reported by middle-aged women was carried out in Oxford by Gath *et al.* (1987). The women in this sample were not reporting symptoms to their doctor but described internal bodily experiences which may or may not have been problematic. Five hundred and twenty one women aged 35–59 years completed the GHQ (Goldberg, 1972) and were interviewed using the Present State Examination (Wing *et al.*, 1974) and a structured gynaecological assessment. Overall rates of psychological illness were 17.3% and 9.6%, using the 60-item GHQ and PSE respectively. Current psychiatric state was significantly associated with reports of dysmenorrhoea and premenstrual symptoms but to a lesser extent with excessive menstruation (or menorrhagia).

Similar associations between menstrual problems and psychological distress have been reported in a community survey of dysmenorrhoea in Australia (Wood *et al.*, 1979) and in another study of premenstrual tension in women consulting their general practitioners in London (Clare, 1983).

## Gynaecological outpatient clinics

During the past decade several well-designed studies have been carried out examining the prevalence of psychological problems in general gynaecological outpatient clinics, as well as in groups of women presenting with specific gynaecological problems.

Byrne (1984) studied 230 consecutive new referrals, aged 18–65 years, to a gynaecological outpatient clinic at a London teaching hospital. The 60-item General Health Questionnaire (GHQ) (Goldberg, 1972), was used as a screening instrument to detect psychiatric disorder and a subsample of 35 women were also interviewed using the Present State Examination (PSE), (Wing *et al.*, 1974). There was a 92% response rate. Forty-six per cent of the sample scored as cases on the GHQ. PSE rates for affective illness were higher in the clinic sample (29%) than those found in a matched general population sample (17%).

High GHQ scorers and those rated as PSE cases tended to be younger and middle class, more likely to be divorced, separated or widowed and to present with pelvic pain (see Chapter 10, p. 259). In fact, 74% of women complaining of pelvic pain were GHQ cases. The majority of other problems such as menstrual symptoms, requests for sterilization and cervical smears were not particularly associated with psychiatric morbidity. Women who were asymptomatic according to the subsequent (blind) assessment by the gynaecologist were no less likely than those with symptoms to be rated as PSE cases.

The prevalence rates reported by Byrne (1984) are similar to those reported in an earlier Australian study by Worsley *et al.* (1977), who also used the 60-item GHQ and found that approximately 50% of the 97 clinic attenders reported psychological distress. These women were more likely to report having problems relating to their partners, children, and parents, as well as financial and other social problems. In this study those with high GHQ scores were more likely to present with menstrual disturbances — in particular menstrual irregularity, uterine bleeding and amenorrhoea. Unlike Byrne, Worsley *et al.* found that women complaining of pelvic pain were not overly distressed. There was no difference in the incidence of organic illness between high and low GHQ scorers. This implies that although a woman might be psychologically distressed as measured by the GHQ, she is just as likely to be suffering from organic illness as a non-psychologically distressed patient. Less than half the sample in this study were assigned a diagnosis of unambiguous organic disease, and in one-third it was 'unknown'.

Women with climacteric and postmenopausal symptoms who attend gynaecology clinics have been studied by Ballinger (1977) and Hunter (1988b). Ballinger used the 60-item GHQ in women aged 40–55 years and found that 53% were classified as psychiatric cases. Psychological distress was not significantly associated with reports of gynaecological status, such as being pre or postmenopausal. However, there was a tendency for menopausal women with abnormal menstrual bleeding to be more distressed. Women who had 3 or more children, were separated or divorced, and who had past emotional problems were more likely to suffer from current psychological distress. Similar levels of distress were reported by Hunter (1988b) in women attending a special menopause clinic, where 47% were estimated to be psychiatric cases. In this study divorce and separation were again associated with clinic attendance. The climacteric and postmenopause will be discussed in more detail in the next section.

To summarize, the prevalence rates of psychological distress reported by women attending gynaecological clinics are remarkably consistent. On average, 50% of this population are estimated to be psychiatric cases. This high level of distress is higher than that found in studies of other general hospital outpatient clinics (Mayou & Hawton, 1986) (Table 9.1).

**Table 9.1.** Rates of affective disorder in general hospital outpatient clinics

| Population | Reference | Number of patients | Cases (%) |
|---|---|---|---|
| Gynaecology | Byrne (1984)[1] | 230 | 46 |
| Cardiology | Vazquez-Barquero et al. (1985)[2] | 234 | 45 |
| Dermatology | Wessely & Lewis (1989)[3] | 133 | 40 |
| Neurology | Bridges & Goldberg (1984)[4] | 100 | 39 |
| Pain | Tyrer et al. (1986)[5] | 97 | 32 |
| Gastroenterology and general medicine | McDonald & Bouchier (1980)[6] | 100 | 26 |
| Venereal disease | Mayou (1975)[7] | 100 | 20 |

Adapted from Mayou & Hawton (1986).
[1] GHQ-60 (11/12); [2] CIS; [3] GHQ-12 and CIS; [4] GHQ-28 and CIS; [5] PSE; [6] GHQ-60 (9/10) and CIS; [7] CIS
CIS = Clinical Interview Schedule; GHQ = General Health Questionnaire; PSE = Present State Examination.

## Methodological shortcomings of these studies

In medical populations the sensitivity and specificity of an instrument such as the GHQ is low. The high proportion of false positive cases is usually attributed to items such as fatigue, insomnia and dizziness which are often endorsed by those with physical symptoms or disabilities. It is possible to improve specificity (reduce number of false positives) by raising the cut-off threshold, but this reduces sensitivity. Further discussion of the limitations of psychiatric screening methods in general hospital patients are described by Mayou and Hawton (1986). These authors concluded that although methods often overestimate the prevalence of affective disorder in the general hospital, disorders of moderate severity are considerably more common than in the general population, especially in younger women.

The 30-item GHQ is least dependent upon somatic symptoms, but false positives have been found using this form of the questionnaire in women with physical illness or social problems (Finlay-Jones & Murphy, 1979). Again, raising the cut-off threshold offers a partial solution. The Hospital

Anxiety and Depression scale (Zigmond & Snaith, 1983) was designed for use with patients suffering from physical illness and is an improvement on other self-assessment instruments since it avoids items such as insomnia and anorexia which are as likely to result from physical illness as from mood disorder (Snaith, 1988). Similarly, the scale developed by the author (Women's Health Questionnaire) to study menopausal women enables separation by factor analysis of depression, anxiety, sleep and somatic symptoms (Hunter *et al.*, 1986).

The results of studies of gynaecological samples outlined above suggest that women who have experienced divorce, separation or social problems may be more likely to suffer from psychological problems. While women who report menstrual problems and pelvic pain have been found to be particularly distressed, no clear relationship between psychological distress and signs of organic pathology has been demonstrated. In the next section the relationships between psychological distress and menstrual problems are presented in more detail.

## Specific gynaecological problems

In view of the association between psychological distress and menstrual problems in clinic attenders, this area will be discussed further under three headings: premenstrual tension; menorrhagia; and menopause. Pelvic pain will not be covered here since this topic is fully discussed in Chapter 10, p. 259. Other gynaecological problems such as dysmenorrhoea, cancer, and infertility are discussed elsewhere (Hunter, 1989).

### Studies of cyclical mood changes in women

This section will deal largely with the results of studies of clinic populations. However, it is important not to generalize from conclusions based on the results of such studies to members of the general population.

It is generally assumed that hormonal fluctuations underlie cyclic mood changes in women, but conclusive evidence of a specific physiological basis is lacking. There is some evidence of small changes in sensory acuity and sensitivity, and possibly small effects on motor activity across the cycle (Sommer, 1982). However, when higher cognitive processes, mood, and complex behaviours have been investigated, the evidence does not support a menstrual effect (Parlee, 1983). Environmental factors have generally been found to account for more of the variation in psychological measures than cycle phase (Wilcoxon *et al.*, 1976; Strauss & Appelt, 1983).

*Premenstrual tension or syndrome*

PMS refers to a wide range of symptoms, including tension, depression, irritability, abdominal bloating and breast tenderness. The concept is illdefined in terms of the nature and duration of symptoms. As a result prevalence rates vary from 25–90% (Coppen & Kessel, 1963; Reid & Yen, 1981). Evidence from recent factor analytic studies supports the existence of several clusters of symptoms (Warner & Bancroft, 1986). The existence of a severe form of debilitating PMS has been shown to be relatively rare (Halbreich & Endicott, 1982; Steiner *et al.*, 1980). Nevertheless, some consider that only those without psychiatric disorder and with clear relief of severe symptoms on menstruation are true PMS sufferers (Steiner *et al.*, 1980). Acceptance of this narrow definition would lead to a negative relationship between psychiatric disorder and PMS.

Clare (1983) carried out a large study to examine the relationship between psychiatric disorder and reports of menstrual, psychological and somatic symptoms. In a sample of 521 randomly selected women attending their General Practitioner's (GP) surgery, he found a consistent association between psychiatric disorder, assessed by the GHQ as well as interview, and reports of premenstrual symptoms, as assessed by a modified version of the Moos Menstrual Distress Questionnaire (MDQ) (Moos, 1968). The majority of women with psychological problems reported premenstrual symptoms. Seventy-five per cent of the sample were classified as being premenstrual complainers defined by retrospective reports of one or more symptoms at moderate level of intensity (MDQ score) during the premenstrual phase.

There is evidence that premenstrual symptoms are overreported in retrospective studies when patients are asked to complete symptom checklists during the premenstrual phase. By contrast, when women are ignorant of the purpose of the research and complete daily diaries, increases in negative affect during the premenstrual phase are generally not found (Wilcoxon *et al.*, 1976; Abplanalp *et al.*, 1979; Strauss & Appelt, 1983). The only symptoms that are consistently linked to the premenstrual phase in these studies have been pain and water retention.

Thus, there is a discrepancy between reports of symptoms in retrospective studies and symptoms reported in well controlled studies. Cognitive labelling and attribution theories help to explain this finding (Ruble & Brooks-Gunn, 1979; Sherif, 1980). In an elegant study Ruble (1977) found that women's descriptions of their bodily states, such as menstrual pain, were influenced by beliefs about their current menstrual phase. Using an attributional theory framework Koeske and Koeske (1975) found that when women performed actions that were evaluated in a negative way these tended to be attributed to the menstrual cycle, even when the actions could be accounted for by situational or other personal factors. Slade (1984) has provided evidence to suggest that the discrepancy between beliefs about the causes and diary ratings of symptoms may be explained by the random fluctuations in emotional state and differential patterns of attributions. For example, increased arousal in the context of good news may be interpreted as excitement, while the same level of arousal during family arguments may be perceived as irritability and attributed to the premenstrual phase (Schachter & Singer, 1962).

In a study of 60 women attending a family planning clinic Bains and Slade (1988) found that negative moods occurring premenstrually tended to be attributed to health factors while the mood states experienced intermenstrually were attributed to personality or environmental factors. Such attributions may result in premenstrual mood states being viewed as having unstable, internal and uncontrollable causes. As a result effective action may not be taken to solve situational or personal problems. If this attributional pattern is a general tendency then women who experience greater psychological and social problems may also be expected to be those who report PMS. Attribution theory may therefore explain the frequent coexistence of reports of PMT with general emotional problems in women attending medical services.

There have been few studies of help-seeking behaviour in women with menstrual problems. However, Coppen and Kessel (1963) noted that despite menstrual problems being very common they rarely result in consultations with general practitioners. In a recent community study Scambler and Scambler (1985) investigated menstrual symptoms, attitudes and consulting behaviour in 126 women aged 16–44 years. Using the Moos Menstrual Distress Questionnaire, modified by Clare (1983), they also found high rates of premenstrual symptoms (83%). However, only 28% of the total sample had consulted a doctor about these symptoms in the 6 months before the interview and a similar proportion had never sought help for menstrual problems. The major reason for not seeking help was disillusionment with the medical profession's attitude to menstrual problems. Other reasons included (i) symptoms not being sufficiently severe, and (ii) not construing menstruation as a health problem.

When women *do* consult doctors, careful analysis of the nature of the problem is essential. A daily diary used for a 2–3 month period should be used to clarify whether problems are chronic, associated with life stresses or with the menstrual cycle. The appropriateness or usefulness of certain attributions can be assessed using a problem solving approach. A small proportion of women do appear to have severe PMS.

Ms C presents an example of the function of a particular attribution of mood during the menstrual cycle. She was referred for help for PMS by a gynaecologist working in an outpatient clinic who could find no physical problems on examination. She was a 36-year-old single woman who had lived alone and not formed close relationships or a satisfactory occupation during her life. She described feeling rejected by her parents and clearly had anxiety and difficulties in meeting people and forming social relationships. She also became anxious and suffered from panic attacks in crowds or when travelling and was moderately depressed. During the initial interview she frequently returned to the subject of PMS when discussing the unhappy aspects of her life. It appeared that to attribute problems to PMS enabled her to maintain some level of self-esteem. Towards the end of the session she claimed that 'if it isn't PMS then it means that I'm a total failure'. However, by holding onto this explanation of her problem she had not sought solutions which might help her to overcome her general anxieties. Treatment continued by further discussion of explanations and her global assumptions about herself as a failure. Attempts were made to help her attain realistic goals that were within her reach. Daily diaries showed that her moods were variable and did *not* show a predictable relationship with her menstrual cycle. By monitoring her activities and achievements she was gradually able to learn that her moods were more under her own control than she had previously believed. Her anxiety and panic attacks also improved.

*Menorrhagia*

Menorrhagia or excessive menstrual bleeding is a common problem in women, specially those in their 30s and 40s. By comparison with other menstrual problems the psychological aspects of menorrhagia have been neglected. The specific causes of menorrhagia are not known. Diagnosis is usually based upon subjective reports which are only partially associated with blood loss as assessed by objective methods (Fraser *et al.*, 1984). The situation is further complicated by the fact that the number of sanitary towels and tampons used does not correspond with the amount of blood lost.

One of the few psychological studies of menorrhagia was carried out by Greenberg (1983). He demonstrated that 62% of women attending a gynaeco-logical clinic complaining of menorrhagia were also suffering from neurotic depression as assessed by the 60-item GHQ and clinical assessment. This represents a higher level than in gynaecology clinic attenders (see above). Intriguingly, the group of depressed women had significantly higher haemo-globin levels, less specific and less severe gynaecological symptoms and more social problems. They had also experienced more recent life stresses (as assessed by interview) than non-depressed women complaining of menorrhagia.

There are several possible interpretations of these results. Firstly, severe menstrual bleeding could lead to considerable psychological distress, with the added debilitating effects of anaemia. Secondly, depressed women could suffer from increased blood loss, possibly mediated by hormonal or central nervous system mechanisms. Thirdly, these women might be depressed but use the complaint of menorrhagia as a means of obtaining medical help. This need not be a conscious process. During depression bodily symptoms are more likely to be perceived in a negative light. In addition, gynaecological problems may be viewed as more acceptable complaints because there is less social stigma attached to them. Attention to physical rather than emotional problems is often reinforced by the medical system — so-called differential reinforcement (Goldberg *et al.*, 1987).

The first explanation appears less likely given the inverse relation between haemoglobin levels and GHQ caseness in Greenberg's study. Although the second explanation cannot be ruled out it is the third which appears most plausible, i.e. that some women adopt a particular pattern of illness behaviour in order to seek help for emotional and personal difficulties.

Greenberg provides a clue as to why they present with gynaecological problems. In his study women were asked about previous physical problems. Depressed women with menorrhagia were more likely than those without depression to have had a termination of pregnancy or miscarriage, as well as a family history in which there was a high prevalence of gynaecological disorder. While physical and genetic factors may be relevant, previous family and personal contact with medical services may have influenced help-seeking behaviour in these women.

Confirmation of these findings would have important implications. For example, intervention during the phase of initial consultation would be justified, and after this women could be referred for combined psychological and gynaecological help. Because a proportion of these women undergo subsequent hysterectomy (Gath *et al.*, 1982), the possibility of earlier intervention should be explored more fully. Hysterectomies are carried out twice as often in the USA as in the UK (Dennerstein & Ryan, 1982; van Keep *et al.*, 1983). In one study 57% of patients undergoing hysterectomy for reasons other than cancer were found to be psychiatrically ill, with one-quarter of these suffering from somatization disorder and one-fifth from depression (Martin *et al.*, 1977; Chapter 12, p. 317). Geographical differences in medical practice will obviously influence treatment decisions and the nature of the population who undergo hysterectomy. But it seems likely that some women with emotional problems may present with symptoms for which hysterectomy is seen as a possible treatment. In spite of this it is important to note that Gath and co-workers (Gath & Cooper, 1981; Gath *et al.*, 1982) found a *decrease* in psychiatric disorder (from 58% to 29%) after hysterectomy in a sample of women suffering from menorrhagia. This study is difficult to interpret, but it is possible that for some of these women preoperative distress was a reaction to menstrual symptoms.

The following case vignette illustrates how menorrhagia may be one of numerous somatic complaints that lead to surgical intervention:

> This 41-year-old woman was seen on many occasions in the gynaecological outpatient clinic during her teens with complaints of irregular periods. An episode of rheumatic fever at the age of 14 left her with mild mixed mitral and aortic disease but minimal cardiorespiratory symptoms. She was reared by a cold, rejecting mother and left home at the earliest opportunity (age 18) to marry. She disregarded advice to avoid pregnancy because of heart disease and gave birth to a child in her early twenties. One year later she took a drug overdose following a row with her husband, who was unwilling to engage in marital therapy. Marital problems continued but the couple were difficult to engage in marital therapy. During the next 5 years she developed functional cardiovascular and gastrointestinal symptoms requiring extensive investigations and one inpatient admission. At 27 she complained of lower abdominal pain, dyspareunia and menorrhagia, which led to repeated investigations by the gynaecologist (including examination under anaesthetic, dilatation and curettage and endometrial biopsy). All these investigations, performed on two separate occasions, were within normal limits. On her 30th birthday the following comment was made by the gynaecologist: 'In view of her long continued troubles, hysterectomy may ultimately be the answer, but I am not in a hurry to suggest it. Her domestic upheavals may be nearer the mark as a cause, and I have some misgivings about her mental state. She told me that she is so depressed she is almost suicidal, but as it seems to be her periods which are bringing her so low I think we should press on'. Six months later a hysterectomy was performed. During the next 10 years this woman complained of multiple somatic complaints involving other organ systems and acquired 3 extra files of notes. None of the investigations carried out during this time revealed an organic cause for her symptoms. Her husband eventually divorced her when she was 40, and after losing custody of her child she was admitted to a psychiatric hospital with depression. She satisfied diagnostic criteria for somatization disorder (see Chapter 12).

*The menopause*

This is primarily a physiological event, marked by cessation of the menstrual cycle, experienced by all women who have not undergone earlier disease or surgery. The menopause is generally defined by the following menstrual criteria: premenopausal women are regularly menstruating; perimenopausal women have experienced 2 or more irregular cycles but have menstruated during the past year; and finally, women who have not menstruated for at least a year are deemed postmenopausal.

Research in this area has been hampered by the numerous methodological problems encountered when assessing symptoms that are confounded by age and physiological change. There is general consensus that hot flushes, night sweats and vaginal dryness occur more frequently in postmenopausal women (McKinlay & McKinlay, 1973; Studd *et al.*, 1977). However, there is considerable confusion for women and their doctors about the emotional sequelae of the menopause and the causes of psychological distress during this phase of life. For example, symptoms could be attributed to age, hormonal changes, personal or social problems. There is evidence that treatment of such women in clinical settings may be idiosyncratic, depending upon the doctor's model of the menopause (as a disease process or natural event) and the woman's own explanations or needs (Lock, 1985). There is also some evidence that medical personnel hold views of the menopause that are more 'pathological' than those of menopausal women (Cowan *et al.*, 1985).

Studies of menopause in *non-clinic samples* carried out since 1980 in North America (McKinlay & McKinlay, 1986; Kaufert, 1984), Norway (Holte, 1987), and by the author in a sample of UK women (Hunter *et al.*, 1986) all suggest that for the majority the menopause is *not* a major stress. Previous depression, social factors such as stressful life events and attitudes and beliefs about the menopause appear to be more important than menopausal status (i.e. becoming peri or postmenopausal as defined by changes in menstrual cycle) in explaining distress in menopausal women (Holte, 1987; Hunter 1988b). For further discussion of psychological aspects of menopause, see Hunter (1988a).

Menopausal women are not particularly high users of the health care system (Kaufert, 1980), and peri and postmenopausal women are not more likely to consult doctors than premenopausal women (McKinlay & McKinlay, 1986; Hunter, 1988b). In the two studies carried out in North America (McKinlay & McKinlay, 1986; Kaufert, 1980) it was found that the women who had previously undergone surgical menopause were the highest users of medical services.

Comparisons of women who attend specialized menopause clinics with non-clinic samples have revealed important differences. For example, Ballinger (1985) found that the clinic sample were significantly more depressed, reported more life stress and general symptoms. She concluded that psychological symptoms were the main discriminators between clinic and non-clinic samples.

In a similar study the author compared 85 new attenders at the Menopause Clinic at King's College Hospital with a general sample of 474 women aged between 45 and 55 years (Hunter, 1988b). The general sample was drawn from a large pool of women attending an ovarian screening clinic at King's College Hospital and were found to be representative of women of this age band living in South East England with respect to social class, employment and marital status. They were not overly health conscious as assessed by the Whiteley Index (Noyes *et al.*, 1986). Comparisons between menopause clinic and general samples were made on a number of demographic, general health, psychological, somatic and attitudinal variables using the Woman's Health Questionnaire (WHQ — a questionnaire developed to assess general health, symptom reports and beliefs in menopausal women).

The results can be summarized as follows. The menopause clinic attenders were more likely to be divorced or separated and to describe their health as poor. They reported more hypochondriacal concerns as well as more symptoms in general. As expected, rates of psychiatric morbidity (estimated GHQ equivalent scores on the depression scale) were significantly higher in the clinic sample (47% compared with the non-clinic sample of 13%). The clinic attenders also were more likely to hold certain beliefs about the menopause. These are shown in Table 9.2. Thus they viewed the menopause as being not only personally uncontrollable but also associated with physical and emotional problems.

In order to summarize these findings a discriminant functional analysis was carried out to establish which combinations of variables best discriminated between clinic and non-clinic groups. Five variables correctly classified 74% of women into the appropriate groups and these are shown in Table 9.3.

**Table 9.2.** Beliefs about the menopause more often held by menopause clinic attenders than a non-clinic sample

The menopause:
1 Does not depend upon one's attitude of mind
2 Does not bring relief from menstruation
3 Is psychologically upsetting
4 Brings problems with physical health

From Hunter, 1988b.

**Table 9.3.**  Factors that predict menopause clinic attendance

| Variable | Wilks lambda | Discriminant function |
|---|---|---|
| Depressed mood | .81 | .33 |
| Vasomotor symptoms | .74 | .37 |
| Disease conviction | .71 | .29 |
| Difficulty coping with symptoms | .69 | .29 |
| Anxiety | .67 | .31 |

These 5 variables correctly classified 74% of women (clinic attendance vs. non-attendance) [discriminant function analysis].
From Hunter, 1988a.

These results suggest that decisions to seek medical help may occur when emotional distress occurs with vasomotor symptoms, and when these are experienced in the context of certain beliefs — in particular the belief that the symptoms are due to a current disease process. It seems possible that some women are attributing emotional distress to the menopause, which is seen as a disease process responsible for both psychological and physical problems. If these attributions are faulty then appropriate solutions to emotional problems may not be found and these women may continue to seek medical treatments with possible detrimental effects.

The following two examples illustrate the complex interactions between physical and psychological problems in menopausal women.

First, Mrs P, age 47 years, was referred to me from a hospital menopause clinic because her oestrogen levels were found to be within the premenopausal range. She had felt depressed for approximately 5 years and wondered if it was due to the menopause. It was clear that this was largely her husband's explanation. Following further discussion she revealed that her mother died 5 years previously and she had never felt able to grieve at home nor with her family. A joint session with the couple was arranged. Mr P's parents had died when he was in his teens as a result of a road traffic accident. He had discouraged discussion of death at home to protect himself and had unknowingly prevented his wife from overcoming her more recent bereavement. Treatment involved couple therapy focusing on grief and their reaction to loss.

The second patient — Mrs T, age 51 years, had experienced quite severe hot flushes. She had undergone psychiatric treatment in her 20s for panic attacks and depression and was very concerned that these symptoms were recurring. She had begun a course of oestrogen therapy which had reduced the severity of hot flushes. However, these symptoms continued to a lesser extent. In general her life was happy and she had not experienced major life changes in recent years. She kept a detailed diary of her anxiety symptoms and hot flushes. From this information and exploration of her cognitions it seemed that she was interpreting the palpitations, which are known to occur with hot flushes, as symptoms of anxiety. Using relaxation and cognitive reappraisal she was able to reconstrue these symptoms as being associated with hot flushes rather than as signs of a recurrence of her previous panic syndrome.

## Assessment

### The gynaecological consultaton

The gynaecological consultation may be particularly anxiety-provoking and beset by communication problems for several reasons. Firstly, all patients are women and most gynaecologists are men. In a recent survey Areskog-Wijma (1987) found that only 4% of women awaiting a gynaecological examination preferred a male doctor. Secondly, many experience embarrassment and anxiety when undergoing vaginal examination (Magee, 1975). If patients are overanxious then information imparted to them may not be retained and decisions may be made without adequate consideration. It is important that women are helped to feel at ease and allowed time to discuss their own explanations and theories about the gynaecological complaint as well as other general concerns.

Since consultations with gynaecologists often end with a definite decision being made, e.g. whether to be sterilized or to have a hysterectomy, it is essential that adequate and full details are provided both verbally and in written form. There is growing evidence to support the routine use of adequate psychological preparation for gynaecological operations and other interventions, as these have been shown to decrease reports of postoperative anxiety and pain (Wallace, 1984; Ridgeway & Matthews, 1982). In my opinion intervention should be provided in full, long before the patient enters hospital, at the decision-making stage. For example, women who are depressed and suffer from menorrhagia might benefit from the offer of psychological help *before* accepting advice to have a hysterectomy.

### Psychological assessment

Following thorough gynaecological assessment additional psychological assessment may be appropriate for those women considered by the gynaecologist or by screening questionnaire to suffer from emotional problems. Close working relationships are important so that the patient sees the gynae-cologist and psychologist as part of a team, thus reducing the split between physical and emotional problems. It is helpful if a possible interactive model can be presented to the patient by the gynaecologist which is reiterated by the psychologist. Fears of the term 'psychological' being equated with malinger-ing, imaginary problems or being insane often require acknowledgement and discussion.

A full psychological assessment should include the following:

**1** Exploration of the patient's views and explanations about her problem and its causes;

**2** Exploration of the strength of physical attributions of symptoms, e.g. 'do you think that your pain/tension could be made worse by your mood?'

**3** Assessment of illness-motivated behaviour, health beliefs and existing ways of coping with symptoms, e.g. distraction or asking for reassurance. Details of history of relationship with doctors (i.e. the *illness history* — see Chapter 3, p. 42) and current help-seeking network would also be of interest;

**4** Detailed discussion of relationships and past events which may influence attitudes to illness and illness behaviour;

**5** Examination of psychological and social factors occurring before and since the onset of symptoms. For example, bereavements and divorce/separation or chronic relationship problems;

**6** Daily diaries in which symptoms and mood are rated, together with brief notes of activities or stressful events. Key symptoms may be selected and rated on 5-point scales or as present or absent. These are valuable because they reinforce the link between subjective reports of somatic complaints and environmental events (see also Chapter 4, p. 95). In addition, diaries can clarify the relationships between menstrual cycle changes and psychological distress. An example of a typical diary is shown in Table 9.4.

Examination of these issues should help to provide an assessment of general distress, possible precipitating factors and factors which may be maintaining illness behaviour.

## Management

### Physical treatment

Apart from surgery, hormone treatments are the major physical treatments available for the types of problem described in the previous section. These will be outlined briefly here.

**Table 9.4.** Daily diary of menstrual cycle changes and psychological distress

*These questions are about the past 24 hours, that is, last night and the whole of today*

Date: ...............................................................................................

Has anything bothered or upset you today?
(please write down any worries, arguments, disappointments):

...............................................................................................

...............................................................................................

Has anything good or pleasant happened to you today?
(for example, good news, enjoyable activity):

...............................................................................................

...............................................................................................

Have you taken any tablets or medicines today?
(Please write their names and what you took them for):

...............................................................................................

...............................................................................................

...............................................................................................

...............................................................................................

Are you having a period today? ...... Yes  ...... No

*Please describe your experience of the following symptoms during the past 24 hours* (last night and the whole of today)

| | | | | |
|---|---|---|---|---|
| A gain in weight | none | slight | moderate | marked | severe |
| Tension | none | slight | moderate | marked | severe |
| Headache | none | slight | moderate | marked | severe |
| Stomach pains | none | slight | moderate | marked | severe |
| Anxiety/worry | none | slight | moderate | marked | severe |
| Backache | none | slight | moderate | marked | severe |
| Tiredness | none | slight | moderate | marked | severe |
| Feeling sick/vomiting | none | slight | moderate | marked | severe |
| Irritability | none | slight | moderate | marked | severe |
| Feeling swollen/bloated | none | slight | moderate | marked | severe |
| Depressed/feeling sad | none | slight | moderate | marked | severe |
| Painful/tender breasts | none | slight | moderate | marked | severe |
| Crying | none | slight | moderate | marked | severe |
| Sleeplessness | none | slight | moderate | marked | severe |
| Arguments/anger | none | slight | moderate | marked | severe |
| Increase in eating | none | slight | moderate | marked | severe |
| Increased clumsiness | none | slight | moderate | marked | severe |
| Any other symptoms | none | slight | moderate | marked | severe |

(Please specify & indicate severity)  ................................................

...............................................................................................

*Premenstrual syndrome*

A variety of physical treatments have been used in the treatment of PMS, including the contraceptive pill, oestradiol, progestins, progesterone, vitamins and diuretics. Controversy surrounds the use of hormone treatments, for example whether they serve only to disrupt the menstrual cycle or whether they have a specific therapeutic effect. Numerous methodological problems pervade this area of research, particularly with respect to the definition of PMS and selection of cases. Overall the results are negative or at best inconclusive. In a well known controlled trial, progesterone therapy was found to be no more effective than placebo treatment (Sampson, 1977). In a more recent study Sampson and her colleagues (1988) confirmed the earlier finding that progestin therapy was no more effective than placebo, again using a double-blind randomized design.

By contrast, Dalton (1984) claims success in the use of progesterone therapy. Limited support for her claims was reported by Dennerstein *et al.* (1985), who used a similar design to Sampson and showed that oral progesterone alleviated premenstrual complaints more effectively than placebo treatment. But there was a very small sample of women ($n=23$) in this study. Finally, the use of oestradiol implants and cyclical progestogens has been the subject of recent investigation. In one such prospective double-blind study, including 68 women with severe PMS, Magos *et al.* (1986) demonstrated significant improvements in premenstrual symptoms using a combination of oestradiol implants and cyclical progestogens.

*Menorrhagia*

Treatments of menorrhagia include progestogens, synthetic androgens and the contraceptive pill, but the results of treatments are variable and there are risks of side-effects.

*Menopausal symptoms*

Oestrogen therapy is advocated for the alleviation of hot flushes and in the prevention of osteoporosis in climacteric and postmenopausal women. Whilst this treatment is very effective for hot flushes there is little evidence that oestrogen therapy is effective for psychological symptoms over and above a placebo effect. As for PMS a strong placebo effect for psychological symptoms has been found (Campbell & Whitehead, 1977; Coope, 1981). Comparison of oestrogen and placebo treatments revealed improvements in minor psychological symptoms in some studies (Campbell & Whitehead, 1977; Durst & Maoz, 1979; Gerdes *et al.*, 1982) but not in others (Coope, 1981; Strickler *et al.*, 1977). But when such treatments have been compared using standardized psychological measures *no* differences were found between oestrogen therapy and placebo (using the Beck depression scale (Coope, 1981) or the GHQ (Campbell & Whitehead, 1977)). Minor improvements could be due to the secondary relief from troublesome vasomotor symptoms. Improvements in general well-being are often attributed to a biological effect of oestrogen or 'mental-tonic' effects. Further research is needed to demonstrate such an effect and its duration when using oestrogens. However, should an effect be demonstrated this does not mean that reduced levels of oestrogen actually caused emotional problems in menopausal women.

**Psychological treatment**

Women who present to gynaecological clinics with somatic symptoms or 'syndromes' such as PMS usually report a combination of emotional and physical symptoms. In many cases physical symptoms are not explained by organic pathology, and in these cases symptoms are maintained by a combination of somatic attribution of symptoms and somatized anxiety and/or depression.

I recommend a problem-solving approach to assess and explore these issues with the patient. Attributions of symptoms should be enquired about and alternative causal explanations explored. The use of relaxation during a session can help to demonstrate the relationship between tension and pain. Information about our current knowledge of gynaecological problems, e.g. premenstrual tension and the menopause, can help women to understand the most likely cause of their own distress. Single case studies can demonstrate the impact of interventions to both health professionals and patients alike. For patients with strongly held beliefs about disease processes and hypochondriacal concerns, cognitive therapy is recommended. In a single case study of a woman suffering from PMS, Morse *et al.* (1983) found that cognitive behavioural treatment was successful in countering maladaptive thought patterns. There is clearly a need for systematic intervention studies using cognitive–behavioural treatments or other psychological treatments in women suffering from severe premenstrual symptoms.

When the causes or correlates of emotional distress become evident then appropriate treatment can be offered. This may include grief therapy, marital therapy, or psychotherapy. Social support can be gained from self-help groups and voluntary organizations.

Finally, there are likely to be large individual differences in the causes of physical and emotional problems in women attending gynaecological clinics, and it is likely that for most complaints the causal factors are multiple.

## Conclusions

Approximately half the women who attend gynaecological clinics have psychiatric morbidity, often in association with marital and social problems. Retrospective studies with women with premenstrual symptoms (PMS) have found high rates of symptom-reporting in the premenstrual phase. By contrast, in women who rate symptoms and mood states prospectively such associations are not detected. These discrepancies may be due to *attributional* factors, i.e. the expectation that negative mood experienced premenstrually may be attributed to health factors rather than other personal/environmental factors.

Women who attend menopause clinics also have high rates of psychiatric morbidity and are more likely to view the menopause as a 'pathological' process than non-attenders. Careful assessment of patient's attributions is essential before commencing treatment in women who attend gynaecological clinics. There is no consensus about the efficacy of drug treatment in premenstrual syndrome. Psychologists need to educate both their patients and medical colleagues about the interactive processes that underlie complaint behaviour in women with somatic complaints who attend gynaecological clinics.

## References

Abplanalp, J.M., Rose, R.M., Donnelly, A.F. & Livingstone-Vaughn, L. (1979). Psychoendocrinology and the menstrual cycle: II the relationship between enjoyment of activities, moods and reproductive hormones, *Psychosomatic Medicine*, **14(8)**, 605–615.

Areskog-Wijma, B. (1987). The gynaecological examination — women's experiences and preferences and the role of the gynaecologist, *Journal of Psychosomatic Obstetrics and Gynaecology*, **6**, 59–69.

Bains, G.K. & Slade, P.C. (1988). Attributional patterns, moods and the menstrual cycle, *Psychosomatic Medicine*, **50**, 469–476.

Ballinger, C.B. (1977). Psychiatric morbidity and the menopause: survey of a gynaecological outpatient clinic, *British Journal of Psychiatry*, **131**, 83–89.

Ballinger, S. (1985). Psychological stress and symptoms of menopause: a comparative study of menopause clinic patients and non-patients, *Maturitas*, **7**, 315–327.

Beard, R.W. (1984). Preface to *Psychology and Gynaecological Problems* (Eds. Broome, A. and Wallace, L.), Tavistock, London.

Becker, M.H. & Maiman, L.A. (1983). Models of health related behaviour, in *Handbook of Health, Health Care and the Health Professions* (Ed. Mechanic, D.), Free Press, New York.

Briscoe, M. (1982). Sex differences in psychological well-being, *Psychological Medicine Monograph*, Supplement 1, 1–46.

Byrne, P. (1984). Psychiatric morbidity in a gynaecological clinic: An epidemiological study, *British Journal of Psychiatry*, **144**, 28–34.

Campbell, S. & Whitehead, M.I. (1977). Oestrogen therapy and the menopausal syndrome, *Clinics in Obstetrics and Gynaecology*, **4(1)**, 31–47.

Clare, A. (1983). Psychiatric and social aspects of premenstrual complaint, *Psychological Medicine Monograph*, Supplement 4.

Coope, J. (1981). Is oestrogen therapy effective in the treatment of menopausal depression? *Journal of Royal College of General Practitioners*, **31**, 134–140.

Coppen, A. & Kessel, N. (1963). Menstruation and personality, *British Journal of Psychiatry*, **109**, 711–721.

Cowan, G., Warren, L.W. & Young, J.L. (1985). Medical perceptions of menopausal symptoms, *Psychology and Women Quarterly*, **9(1)**, 3–14.

Dalton, K. (1978). *Once a month*, Fontana, Great Britain.

Dalton, K. (1984). *The premenstrual syndrome and progesterone therapy*, Heinemann, London.

Dennerstein, L. & Ryan, M. (1982). Psychosocial and emotional sequelae of hysterectomy, *Journal of Psychosomatic Obstetrics and Gynaecology*, **1–2**, 81–86.

Dennerstein, L., Spencer-Gardner, C., Gotts, G., Brown, J.B., Smith, M.A. & Burrows, G.D. (1985). Progesterone and the premenstrual syndrome: a double-blind crossover trial, *British Medical Journal*, **290**, 1617–1621.

Durst, N. & Maoz, B. (1979). Changes in psychological well-being during post-menopause as a result of oestrogen therapy, *Maturitas*, **11**, 301–315.

Finlay-Jones, R.A. & Burvill, P.W. (1977). The prevalence of minor psychiatric morbidity in the community, *Psychological Medicine*, **7**, 425–489.

Finlay-Jones, R.A. & Murphy, E. (1979). Severity of psychiatric disorder and the 30-item general health questionnaire, *British Journal of Psychiatry*, **134**, 604–616.

Fraser, I.S., McCarron, G. & Markham, R. (1984). A preliminary study of factors influencing perception of menstrual blood loss volume, *American Journal of Obstetrics and Gynaecology*, **149**, 788–793.

Gath, D. & Cooper, P.J. (1981). Psychiatric disorder after hysterectomy, *Journal of Psychiatric Research*, **25**, 347–355.

Gath, D., Cooper, P. & Day, A. (1982). Hysterectomy and psychiatric disorder 1. Levels of psychiatric morbidity before and after hysterectomy, *British Journal of Psychiatry*, **140**, 335–342.

Gath, D., Osborn, M., Bungay, G. *et al.* (1987). Psychiatric disorder and gynaecological symptoms in middle aged women; a community survey, *British Medical Journal*, **294**, 213–218.

Gerdes, L.C., Sonnendecker, E.W. & Polakow, E.S. (1982). Psychological changes effected by oestrogen-progestogen and clonidine treatment in climacteric women, *American Journal of Obstetrics and Gynaecology*, **142**, 98–104.

Goldberg, D. (1972). *The Detection of Psychiatric Illness by Questionnaire*, Maudsley Monograph, 21. Oxford University Press, London.

Goldberg, D., Benjamin, S. & Creed, F. (1987). *Psychiatry in Medical Practice*, Routledge, London.

Greenberg, M. (1983). The meaning of menorrhagia: an investigation into the association between the complaint of menorrhagia and depression, *Journal of Psychosomatic Research*, **27**, 209–214.

Halbreich, U. & Endicott, J. (1982). Classification of premenstrual syndromes, in *Behaviour and the Menstrual Cycle* (Ed. Freidman, R.), Marcel Dekker, New York.

Hewstone, M. (1983). Attribution theory and common sense explanations: an introductory review, in *Attribution Theory: Social and Functional Extensions* (Ed. Hewstone, M.), Basil Blackwell, Oxford.

Holte, A. (1987). *The Norwegian Menopausal Project*, paper presented at the 5th International Congress on the menopause — International Menopause Society, Sorrento, Italy.

Horney, K. (1932). The dread of women, *International Journal of Psychoanalysis*, **13**, 348–360.

Hunter, M. (1988a). Psychological aspects of the climacteric and post-menopause, in *The Menopause* (Eds. Studd, J. & Whitehead, M.I.), Blackwell, London.

Hunter, M. (1988b). *Determinants of symptom reporting and use of medical services by menopausal women*, paper presented at the 30th Annual Conference of the Society of Psychosomatic Research, London, November 1988.

Hunter, M. (1989). Gynaecology, in *Health Psychology* (Ed. Broome, A.), Chapman & Hall, London.

Hunter, M., Battersby, R. & Whitehead, M. (1986). Relationships between psychological symptoms, somatic complaints and menopausal status, *Maturitas*, **8**, 217–228.

Kaufert, P.A. (1980). The peri-menopausal woman and her use of the Health Services, *Maturitas*, **2**, 191–205.

Kaufert, P.A. (1984). Women and their health in the middle years: a Manitoba Project, *Social Science and Medicine*, **18**, 279–281.

Koeske, R.K. & Koeske, G.F. (1975). An attributional approach to moods and the menstrual cycle, *Journal of Personal and Society Psychology*, **31**, 474–478.

Leventhal, H., Meyer, D. & Nerenz, D. (1980). The commonsense representation of illness danger, in *Contributions of Medical Psychology* Vol. 2 (Ed. Rachman, S.), Pergamon Press, New York.

Lock, M. (1985). Models and practice in medicine: menopause as a syndrome or life transition? in *Physician of Modern Medicine* (Eds. Hahn, R.A. and Gaines, A.D.), D. Reidel Publishing Co., Boston.

McKinlay, S.M. (1987). *Overview of an ongoing investigation into psychosocial aspects of the menopause*, paper presented at the 5th International Congress on the Menopause, Sorrento, Italy.

McKinlay, S.M. & McKinlay, J.B. (1973). Selected studies of the menopause, *Journal of Biosocial Sciences*, **5**, 533–555.

McKinlay, S.M. & McKinlay, J.B. (1986). Health status and health care utilization by menopausal women, in *The Climacteric in Perspective*, Proceedings of the 4th International Congress on the Menopause, MTP Press Ltd., Lancaster.

Magee, J. (1975). The pelvic examination: a view from the other end of the table, *Annals of Internal Medicine*, **83**, 563–567.

Magos, A.L., Brincat, M. & Studd, J.W.W. (1986). Treatment of the premenstrual syndrome by subcutaneous oestradiol implants and cyclical oral norethisterone: a placebo controlled study, *British Medical Journal*, **i**, 1629–1633.

Martin, R.L., Roberts, W.V., Claydon, P.J. & Wetzel, R. (1977). Psychiatric illness and non-cancer hysterectomy, *Diseases of the Nervous System*, December, 974–980.

Mayou, R. & Hawton, K. (1986). Psychiatric disorder in the general hospital, *British Journal of Psychiatry*, **149**, 172–190.

Mechanic, D. (1980). The experience and reporting of common physical symptoms, *Journal of Health and Social Behaviour*, **21**, 146–155.

Mechanic, D. (1983). The experience and expression of distress: the study of illness behaviour and medical utilization, in *Handbook of Health, Health Care and the Health Professions* (Ed. Mechanic, D.), Free Press, New York.

Moos, R.H. (1968). The development of a menstrual distress questionnaire, *Psychosomatic Medicine*, **30**, 853–867.

Moos, R.H. (1977). *Menstrual Distress Questionnaire Manual*, Department of Psychiatry Standard University and Veterans Administration, Palo Alto, California.

Morse, C.A., Farrell, E. & Dennerstein, L. (1983). *A cognitive–behavioural treatment model for women with premenstrual syndrome*, paper presented at the 7th International Congress on Psychosomatic Obstetrics and Gynaecology, Dublin.

Noyes, R., Reich, J., Clancy, J. & O'Gorman, T.W. (1986). Reduction in hypochondriasis with treatment of panic disorder, *British Journal of Psychiatry*, **149**, 631–635.

Parlee, M.B.C. (1983). The psychology of the menstrual cycle: biological and psychological perspectives, in *Behaviour and the Menstrual Cycle* (Ed. Freidman, R.C.), Marcel Dekker, New York.

Pearce, S., Knight, C. & Beard, R.W. (1982). Pelvic pain — a common gynaecological problem, *Journal of Psychosomatic Obstetrics and Gynaecology*, **1**, 12–21.

Pennebaker, J.W. (1982). *The psychology of physical symptoms*, Springer-Verlag, New York.

Reid, R.L. & Yen, S.S.C. (1981). Premenstrual syndrome, *American Journal of Obstetrics and Gynaecology*, **139**, 85–104.

Ridgeway, V. & Matthews, A. (1982). Psychological preference for surgery: a comparison of methods, *British Journal of Clinical Psychology*, **21**, 271–280.

Rosenstock, I.M. & Kirscht, J.P. (1979). Why do people seek health care? in *Health Psychology: A Handbook* (Eds. Stone, G.C. and Adler, N.E.), Jossey Bass, San Francisco.

Ruble, D. (1977). Premenstrual symptoms: a re-interpretation, *Science*, **197**, 291–292.

Ruble, D.N. & Brooks-Gunn, J. (1979). Menstrual symptoms: a social cognition analysis, *Journal of Behavioural Medicine*, **2**, 171–191.

Sampson, G.A. (1977). Premenstrual syndrome: a double-blind controlled trial of progesterone and placebo, *British Journal of Psychiatry*, **135**, 209–215.

Sampson, G.A., Heathcote, P.R., Wordsworth, J., Prescott, P. & Hodgson, A. (1988). Premenstrual syndrome: a double-blind crossover study of treatment with dydrogesterone and placebo, *British Journal of Psychiatry*, **153**, 232–235.

Scambler, A. & Scambler, G. (1985). Menstrual symptoms, attitudes and consulting behaviour, *Social Science and Medicine*, **20**, 1065–1068.

Schachter, S. & Singer, J.E. (1962). Cognitive social and physiological determinants of emotional state, *Psychological Review*, **69**, 379–399.

Sherif, C.W. (1980). A social psychological perspective on the menstrual cycle, in *The Psychobiology of Sex Differences and Sex Role* (Ed. Parsons, J.E.), McGraw Hill, New York.

Slade, D. (1984). Premenstrual emotional changes in normal women: fact or fiction, *Journal of Psychosomatic Research*, **28(1)**, 1–7.

Snaith, P. (1988). Hospital Anxiety and Depression Scale, *British Journal of Psychiatry*, **152**, 424.

Sommer, B. (1973). The effects of menstruation on cognitive and perceptual motor behaviour: a review, *Psychosomatic Medicine*, **35**, 515–534.

Sommer, B. (1982). Cognitive–behaviour and the menstrual cycle, in *Behaviour and the Menstrual Cycle* (Ed. Friedmann, R.C.), Marcel Dekker, New York.

Steiner, M., Haskett, R.F. & Carroll, B.J. (1980). Premenstrual tension syndrome: the development of research, diagnostic criteria and new rating scales, *Acta Psychiatrica Scandinavica*, **62**, 177–190.

Strauss, B. & Appelt, H. (1983). Psychological concomitants of the menstrual cycle: a prospective longitudinal approach, *Journal of Psychosomatic Obstetrics and Gynaecology*, **2–4**, 215–219.

Strickler, R.C. (1977). The role of oestrogen replacement in the climacteric syndrome, *Psychological Medicine*, **7**, 631–637.

Studd, J.W.W., Chakravarti, S. & Oram, D.H. (1977). The climacteric, *Clinics in Obstetrics and Gynaecology*, **4**, 3–29.

Tessler, R., Mechanic, D. & Dimond, M. (1976). The effect of psychological distress on physician utilization: a prospective study, *Journal of Health and Social Behaviour*, **17**, 353–364.

van Keep, P.A., Wildemeerch, D. & Lehert, P. (1983). Hysterectomy in European countries, *Maturitas*, **5**, 69–77.

Vazquez-Barquero, J.L., Padierna Acero, J.A., Pena Martin, C. & Ochoteco, A. (1985). The psychiatric correlates of coronary pathology: validity of the GHQ-60 as a screening instrument, *Psychological Medicine*, **15**, 589–596.

Wallace, L. (1984). Psychological preparation of gynaecological surgery, in *Psychology and*

*Gynaecological Problems* (Eds. Broome, A. and Wallace, L.), Tavistock, London.

Wallston, K.A., Wallston, B.A., Smith, S. & Dobbins, C.J. (1987). Perceived control and health, *Current Psychology Research Reviews*, **6**, 1.

Warner, P. & Bancroft, J. (1986). *PMS Survey: one syndrome for 7000 respondents?* Paper presented at the annual conference of the Society of Reproductive and Infant Psychology, Bristol.

Weideger, P.C. (1975). *Female cycles*, The Women's Press, London.

Weissman, M.M. & Klerman, G.L. (1981). Sex differences and the epidemiology of depression, in *Women and Mental Health* (Eds. Howell, E. and Bayes, M.), Basic Books Inc., New York.

Wilcoxon, L.A., Schrader, S.L. & Sherif, C.W. (1976). Daily reports on activities, life events, moods, and somatic changes during the menstrual cycle, *Psychosomatic Medicine*, **38**, 399–417.

Wing, J.K., Cooper, J.E. & Sartorius, N. (1974). *The measurement and classification of psychiatric symptoms*, Cambridge University Press, London.

Wood, C., Larsen, L. & Williams, R. (1979). Menstrual characteristics of 2343 women attending the Shepherd Foundation, *Australian and New Zealand Journal of Obstetrics and Gynaecology*, **19**, 107–115.

Worsley, A., Walters, W.A.W. & Wood, C. (1977). Screening for psychological disturbance amongst gynaecological patients, *Australian and New Zealand Journal of Obstetrics and Gynaecology*, **17**, 214.

Zigmond, A.S. & Snaith, F.P. (1983). The hospital anxiety and depression scale, *Acta Psychiatrica Scandinavica*, **67**, 361–370.

# 10
# Chronic Pelvic Pain in Women

S. PEARCE AND R.W. BEARD

## Introduction

Pelvic pain is one of the most common presenting problems among women attending a gynaecological clinic (Henker, 1979; Morris & O'Neill, 1958). In this chapter we are concerned with chronic pelvic pain, by which we mean pain in the lower abdomen of at least 6 months' duration.

The condition has earned a range of descriptive diagnoses reflecting different theories of the cause of the pain. These diagnoses include pelvic congestion (Taylor, 1949), pelvic sympathetic syndrome (Theobald, 1951), pelipathia vegetativa (Prill, 1964, reported by Renaer, 1980), pelvic pain syndrome (Beard et al., 1977) and CPPWOP (chronic pelvic pain without obvious pathology) (Renaer, 1980). Despite sophisticated methods of investigation a large proportion of women with pelvic pain may have no obvious organic pathology. For example, Gillibrand (1981) reported that of 331 women presenting with pelvic pain only 31% had any identifiable pathology at laparoscopy. More recently studies by Beard et al. (1984) have shown, using techniques of pelvic venography and ultrasound scanning, that congestion in the pelvic veins is present in more than 80% of women experiencing chronic pelvic pain in the absence of obvious pathology.

It must be emphasized however that the identification of pathology does not mean that a *cause* of the pain has been found. Rapkin (1986) found that whereas 26% of a sample of pelvic pain patients had pelvic adhesions, among infertility patients who did not complain of pain the rate was 39%. The groups did not differ significantly in either the density or location of the adhesions. These findings suggest that pain is not closely related to pathology in the pelvis. It is possible that adhesions and other forms of pelvic pathology may provide a sensory input which is only labelled as painful under certain psychological conditions. Such a view is in line with recent biobehavioural models of other chronic pain conditions (Pearce & Erskine, 1989). A range of psychological factors have indeed been shown to influence the relationship between physical damage and subjective pain intensity in all pain conditions (Melzack, 1983). This concept of an interaction between physiological and psychological components of pain is central to recent progress in our understanding of chronic pain and a model of chronic pelvic pain based on these principles is presented below. Before presenting the model the background to its development is discussed.

## Psychogenic theories of chronic pelvic pain

A number of studies which claim to show psychological abnormalities of women with chronic pelvic pain have been reported. Typically, these compare patients with undiagnosed chronic pelvic pain with those without pain, using psychometric tests or psychiatric interviews. In an early example of such a study Gidro-Frank *et al.* (1960) found that 38 of 40 patients with chronic pelvic pain and 24 of 25 control (pregnant) patients had psychiatric abnormalities. The psychiatric disturbance in the pelvic pain group was classified as follows: schizophrenia (4) borderline psychosis (10), severe neurosis (20), moderate neurosis (3), mild neurosis (1). Remarkably, 8 of the 25 control subjects were classified as having a borderline psychosis and only one was categorized as normal. The high rates of psychiatric illness in this study were possibly a consequence of the low reliability and validity of the unstructured interviews. Furthermore, no mention was made of how ratings such as mild, moderate and severe were used to determine the severity of the neurotic disorder. A further problem is that American diagnostic labels at that time did not correspond exactly with the British use of the terms. It is therefore possible that the very high incidence of major psychotic disorders reported in this study is not typical of the patients with undiagnosed chronic pelvic pain presenting to British gynaecology clinics.

A number of other studies have similar shortcomings. Benson *et al.* (1959) described a series of 35 women presenting with unexplained pelvic pain who were interviewed by a psychiatrist. The last seven patients of their series were also assessed on formal psychological tests, including the Taylor Manifest Anxiety Scale and the Cornell Medical Index. All patients were diagnosed as psychiatrically ill, with six of the 35 diagnosed as schizophrenic and the remainder with neurotic disorders. The small subsample who were formally assessed had scores on the Cornell Medical Index which were significantly higher than the psychiatric outpatient norms.

Prill (1964, reported by Renaer, 1980) interviewed 163 patients with pelipathia vegetativa. He found 68 to be suffering from neurotic disorders, 34 from psychopathic or psychasthenic personality disorders and only 61 (38%) to have no evidence of psychopathology. This study is interesting in that it is the first to suggest that a proportion of these women may not show any psychiatric disorder. The authors also suggest that it is not possible to identify any specific underlying psychological conflicts or distress which characterize women with undiagnosed pelvic pain. Previous writers such as Benson *et al.* (1959) suggested that women with chronic pelvic pain had pathological relationships with their mothers that may have contributed to the development of their pain.

A later study which also questions the association between psychiatric disorders and undiagnosed chronic pelvic pain is by Castelnuovo-Tedesco and Krout (1970). Of 40 women with CPPWOP, 4 were diagnosed as schizophrenic, 33 as borderline disorders and only 3 as 'normal'. All 40 patients then underwent laparoscopy at which 25 were found to have organic pathology including endometriosis, ovarian cysts, pelvic congestion and inactive pelvic inflammatory disease. No relationship was found between pathology and psychiatric findings. That is to say, the incidence of psychiatric disorder was as high in the group with pathology as in those without. This finding does not support the view that psychological disorders play a causal role in the development of pelvic pain, but suggests instead that psychological disturbances may be a consequence of chronic pain, whatever its origin.

The problem of the direction of the relationship between chronic pain and psychopathology is one which has received considerable attention in other areas of pain research (Weisenberg, 1977). A number of studies investigating personality profiles of chronic pain patients have used the Minnesota Multiphasic Personality Inventory (MMPI). A commonly described MMPI profile for chronic pain patients is that which has become known as the 'conversion valley' (Sternbach, 1974). This term refers to the fact that for chronic pain patients, hysteria and hypochondriasis scores have been found to be higher than depression scores. Hence, their scoring profiles show peaks on the two scales, hypochondriasis and hysteria, but a trough or 'valley' on the intervening depression scale. This pattern became known as the 'conversion valley' from the psychoanalytic notion that feelings of depression or anxiety were not being acknowledged and were 'converted' into hypochondriacal complaints. Conversion valley findings have been reported for patients with undiagnosed chronic pelvic pain (Renaer *et al.*, 1979). They compared MMPI profiles of 28 patients with CPPWOP with those of 22 patients with known endometriosis. Whilst both groups were found to have elevated scores on the hypochondriasis, depression and hysteria scales, the undiagnosed pelvic pain group showed some evidence of the conversion valley profile whilst the endometriosis patients did not. However, these differences are not marked and Renaer acknowledges that the personality abnormalities may be consequences of the chronic pain condition.

Other studies attempting to isolate personality profiles of women with undiagnosed chronic pelvic pain have not resolved the problem. Beard *et al.* (1977) compared 18 women with pain in the absence of pathology detected at laparoscopy (laparoscopy negative), with 17 women for whom an organic basis to the pain had been identified (laparoscopy positive). The laparoscopy negative group obtained significantly higher neuroticism scores on the Eysenck Personality Inventory than the laparoscopy positive group. This supports the view that the high neuroticism may have been a causal factor in the development of chronic pelvic pain. However, although the two groups were carefully matched for social variables (e.g. age, parity), they were not matched for chronicity (duration of the pain). Hence it is possible that the laparoscopy negative groups may have endured the pain for longer and hence suffered more from its effects than those with demonstrable pathology. In a subsequent study Pearce (1988) confirmed this. After controlling for duration of pain, she failed to detect any difference on the neuroticism scale of the Eysenck Personality Questionnaire between women who were categorized as laparoscopy positive and laparoscopy negative.

In an attempt to identify abnormal psychological characteristics in women with undiagnosed chronic pelvic pain some investigators have explored sexual attitudes. The view that women with pelvic pain have sexual difficulties and are concerned about female identity probably developed as a consequence of the site of the pain and the frequent clinical observation that the pain is aggravated by sexual intercourse. Psychoanalytic writers, for example Gidro-Frank *et al.* (1960), make a clear distinction between 'organic' and 'psychogenic' pelvic pain and view the latter as a symptom of underlying conflicts about femininity. Although there are problems in making such a distinction, there are findings to support the view that women with un-diagnosed chronic pelvic pain may have anxieties about sex. Beard *et al.* (1977) used a semantic differential to assess sexual attitudes. They found that women with no obvious cause for pelvic pain rated themselves significantly less positively on a number of sex-related concepts than those with positive laparoscopic findings and a no pain control group.

Gross *et al.* (1980) have also suggested that sexual activities play a causal role in the development of undiagnosed chronic pelvic pain. They identified early traumatic sexual experiences (incest) in 9 out of 25 patients. They suggested that these early sexual experiences result in anxieties in adulthood which, unless resolved, will be manifested as pelvic pain. This view is supported by Harrop-Griffiths *et al.* (1988), who compared women under-going laparoscopy for chronic pelvic pain with those investigated for in-fertility. The pain patients showed more disturbance as reflected by greater depression, substance abuse and sexual dysfunction and they were more likely to be victims of childhood and adult sexual abuse. Not all studies, however, support the view that patients with undiagnosed chronic pelvic pain have anxieties about sex. Petrucco and Harris (1982) investigated 24 women with undiagnosed chronic pelvic pain. Seventy-two per cent of these were orgasmic and reported no sexual problems. Furthermore, their mean scores on a 20-item questionnaire measure of sexual pleasure were not indicative of sexual dysfunction. There is therefore disagreement about the extent of sexual problems or anxieties among these patients and more systematic investigation is required before concluding that sexual anxieties play a specific aetiological role in chronic pelvic pain.

Regrettably, very few studies have compared patients of equivalent chronicity in whom pathology has been categorized according to laparoscopic. findings rather than clinicians' judgement. In one study satisfying these criteria, Pearce (1988) found no evidence to support the view that women experiencing pelvic pain in the absence of observable pathology were more neurotic, more anxious, or more depressed than women with demonstrable pathology. Furthermore, both pain groups showed scores on measures of neuroticism and mood that were similar to those of a normal female population. They were not characteristic of groups of women with psychiatric disorders.

However some differences on psychological measures did emerge. Women experiencing pain in the absence of observed pathology were found to have higher disease conviction scores on the modified Illness Behaviour Questionnaire (Pilowsky & Spence, 1975). There was also a trend for the no-pathology group to have higher hypochondriasis scores than the pathology group. This suggests that women in the no-pathology group may be more concerned about their physical state and hence they may be monitoring bodily sensations more closely than the pathology group. It was also noted that women in the no-pathology group reported higher rates of serious illness and death of family members. It is clear that such exposure is not sufficient to *cause* unexplained pelvic pain (many of the illnesses and deaths had occurred several years before the onset of the pain). Direct and immediate modelling of pain or illness is therefore unlikely. Exposure to serious illness may however influence the development of attitudes towards pain and illness and result in closer monitoring of one's own bodily sensations and well-being. Given certain other conditions, this may lead to the report of pain. In the case of pelvic pain these 'other conditions' must include some process which explains why the pain has developed in the pelvis as opposed to any other part of the body. This has led to speculation about psychophysiological mechanisms. A similar model for other gynaecological disorders is discussed by Hunter (Chapter 9, p. 235).

# Psychophysiological theories

The possibility that there is a causative link between psyche and soma in women with pelvic congestion was discussed by Duncan and Taylor (1952). They suggested that changes in pelvic blood flow occur as part of the response to 'stress'. They used a thermal conductance measure to obtain continuous records of pelvic blood flow for 10 women during the course of an interview. All 10 showed marked variations in vaginal blood flow throughout the course of the interview and Duncan and Taylor concluded that these changes were related to the nature of the topics discussed. Emotionally laden topics appeared to cause increases in blood flow which returned to baseline levels when neutral topics were discussed.

Unfortunately, methodological problems with this study limit the conclusions that can be drawn about the aetiology of undiagnosed chronic pelvic pain. Firstly, because a no-pain control group was not used it is possible that these changes in vaginal blood flow represent normal responses to the discussion of anxiety provoking topics and are not specific to patients with pelvic pain. However, in support of Duncan and Taylor it should be noted that research on pelvic blood flow responses to sexual arousal suggests that normally orgasmic women show increases in vaginal blood flow only in response to sexual stimuli (Hoon, 1979). Other classes of stimuli, such as anxiety or anger, are not thought to elicit pelvic vascular change.

Most recently Beard *et al.* (1989) have hypothesized that the endocrine control of ovarian function may be disturbed by stress. This view is based on the observation that 54% of women with pelvic pain due to congestion have polycystic ovaries (Adams *et al.*, 1990). It is thought that these ovaries secrete more oestrogen due to the multiplicity of granulosa cells lining the cysts and it is suggested that the high local concentration of oestrogen and/or its metabolites leads to local venous stasis in the pelvis. This view is supported by the finding that suppression of ovarian function by medroxyprogesterone acetate significantly improves pelvic blood flow (Reginald *et al.*, 1989) and that oöphorectomy results in disappearance of pelvic pain in women who had demonstrable congestion (Beard & Reginald, 1990).

## A model of chronic pelvic pain

The model presented in Figure 10.1 is an attempt to draw together the findings from both the psychological and physiological studies.

In this model it is suggested that women who develop pain associated with pelvic congestion have a biological predisposition to pelvic blood flow responses to stress that are either greater in magnitude or take longer to

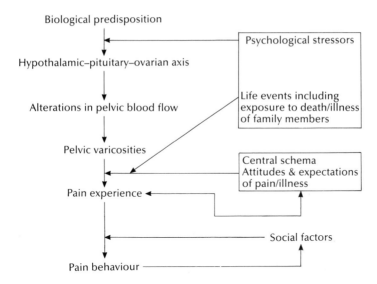

**Fig. 10.1.** Possible mode of interaction between psychological and somatic factors in pelvic pain associated with pelvic congestion.

return to baseline levels than normal. Hence, when exposed to psychological stressors, changes occur in the pelvic vasculature which lead over time to the development of chronically dilated pelvic veins. Although many women do have vascular congestion this is obviously not the only source of abnormal sensory afferent activity. The model suggests that any form of abnormal input, whether from adhesions, congestion or endometriosis, will be attended to and labelled as painful by those women who are closely monitoring their physiological state. This close monitoring may be a consequence of concern about illness in general or pelvic dysfunction in particular. The experience of pain and its associated distress then leads to 'pain behaviours' which are likely to be reinforced by concerned family members (Fordyce, 1982).

Feedback loops may arise at several of these levels of pain experience. In particular, being in pain is likely to direct further attention to the pelvis and strengthen the expectation and experience of pain. Such a model gives rise to a number of potential levels of intervention. These will be discussed in turn.

## Management

### Medical and surgical treatments

Many treatments have been used to treat chronic pelvic pain when no obvious physical cause has been identified. These include repeated prescriptions of antibiotics for supposed recurrent pelvic inflammatory disease, local anaesthetic injection of neurological trigger points (Slocumb, 1984), resection of pelvic varicosities (Rundqvist *et al.*, 1984), and hysterectomy (Mills, 1978). None of these treatments have been adequately tested so we cannot be confident of their efficacy.

The development of an effective form of treatment for the condition has been seriously hampered by the lack of understanding of specific physiological components of chronic pelvic pain. The demonstration that congestion is a common finding in women with this complaint (Beard *et al.*, 1984) suggests that alteration of venous flow may be a possible physical intervention. Reginald *et al.* (1987) studied the specific venoconstrictor dihydroergotamine (DHE) in a randomized controlled trial giving the drug or saline intravenously during an acute attack of pain. DHE was shown to reduce congestion by improving pelvic blood flow as a consequence of narrowing the pelvic veins to about one-third of their original diameter. Those who received the DHE had a significant reduction in pelvic pain compared with those receiving the saline. This demonstrates both that poor venous outflow can cause pelvic pain and that venoconstriction is an effective treatment.

Medroxyprogesterone acetate (Provera) also reduces pelvic blood flow by suppressing ovarian functions and has been reported to be effective in the short term (Luciano *et al.*, 1980).

Reginald *et al.* (1989) showed that suppression of ovarian function with 30 mg Provera resulted in amenorrhoea and a marked reduction in pain in women with pelvic pain due to congestion. The striking finding in this study was the return of the pelvic congestion and return of pain at the end of treatment. The therapeutic effect of Provera has been confirmed by Farquhar *et al.* (1989) in a randomized controlled trial using 50 mg of Provera a day. This study also compared the effects of psychological treatment and is discussed in more detail below.

Despite the warning by Taylor in 1949 against the indiscriminate use of surgery for chronic pelvic pain, it is logical to consider the possibility of a well directed surgical procedure if ovarian dysfunction plays an aetiological role in pelvic congestion. Hysterectomy with conservation of the ovaries as recommended by Mills (1978) has been disappointing, supporting the views of Taylor about poor results from this operation. Beard and Reginald (1990) have reported preliminary results on 15 women with pelvic congestion for whom medical treatment had failed. They underwent hysterectomy and bilateral oöphorectomy followed by hormone replacement therapy. At 6 months follow up 14 were pain free and appear to have experienced a major improvement in their quality of life. These results are important since they support the hypothesis that ovarian dysfunction may cause pelvic congestion. However, they should not be regarded as a recommendation that oöphorectomy should be resorted to when all other approaches have failed.

All these physical interventions have a number of disadvantages to women of childbearing age. Ovarian suppression by pharmacological means is only likely to be effective in the short term and the drawbacks of hysterectomy and oöphorectomy in women of reproductive age are obvious. Hence despite a clearer understanding of the physical aspects of pelvic congestion there is still considerable interest in psychological methods of pain control and the possible integration of these with physical interventions.

## Psychological interventions

### Contingency management methods

The development of contingency management methods for chronic pain derives from Fordyce's view of chronic pain as a behavioural or operant problem. Whatever the initial underlying cause of the pain problem, Fordyce considers that pain behaviours such as complaining of pain, inactivity or taking medication may come to be maintained by their reinforcing consequences. Pain behaviours may be either positively reinforced, for example by social factors such as concern from family members, or negatively reinforced, for example by avoidance of unwanted responsibilities.

The aim of operant programmes is to increase the frequency of well behaviours and decrease that of pain behaviours. Reduction in pain *intensity* is not specified as an aim. It is explained to patients that the goal of the programme is not to remove pain but rather to improve coping and to resume normal activities despite it. There is an underlying assumption that once the patient is active again and engaged in more distracting activities, attention to the pain sensations will be reduced and hence pain intensity will diminish. The methods used to achieve these aims are described in detail by Fordyce (1982). Briefly, patients are admitted to specialized inpatient programmes for periods of between 2 and 6 weeks. During this time staff give no attention to pain behaviours or requests for analgesics, but provide considerable social reinforcement for targeted well behaviours. Physical therapy programmes are developed to increase patient activity levels. Daily exercise quotas are determined on the basis of patients' initial tolerance levels. As the quota is increased each day the patient is able to manage significantly more than the initial level. Progress is charted graphically and staff attention or some other positive reinforcer is made contingent on successful daily completion of the quota.

A reduction in levels of medication is also an important aim of the

operant programmes. This is achieved by establishing initial drug requirements by placing the patient on a free operant schedule for a few days
immediately after admission. The amount of medication required is then
provided in a strong-tasting masking vehicle called the 'pain cocktail'. The
patient is unable to tell the strength of this concoction from its appearance or
taste. The pain cocktail is provided on a time-contingent rather than pain-
contingent basis; i.e. the patient has to take it every 4 hours whether in pain
or not. If it is refused, the patient must wait until the next interval before
medication becomes available again. In this way it is hoped to break the
association between pain and medication. The active ingredients of the pain
cocktail are reduced gradually so that by the end of the programme the
patient should be consuming only the inert vehicle.

Fordyce *et al.* (1973) reported the progress of 36 mixed diagnosis patients
who completed his programme. Patients showed a significant increase in
'uptime', (time either sitting, standing or walking) which was maintained at
follow-up, an average of 22 months later.

Linton (1986) has reviewed other studies which provided essentially
similar results. He concluded that operant programmes produce increases
in activity and decreases in consumption of medication, but less reliable
reductions in ratings of pain intensity.

We have adapted Fordyce's principles to interventions with selected outpatients, as the following case vignette shows:

> Mrs R, who was seen with her husband aged 54, had had pelvic pain
> for 5 years. It had started with an infection but continued after the
> infection had improved. Mrs R was now housebound, spending most of
> her time on the settee for fear that any activity would exacerbate the
> pain. It was explained to them both that Mrs R's inactivity may now be
> making the problem worse. The loss of her status and importance in
> the household was making her depressed. Her avoidance of social
> contacts and outings of all kinds was adding to her depression and her
> husband's considerable sympathy was no longer constructive.
>
> A simplified version of the model of pain outlined in Figure 10.1
> was discussed with her. She agreed to attempt daily exercise quotas
> which involved walking outside for 5 minutes each day, usually to post
> a letter. The length of these walking tasks was gradually increased by 3
> minutes per day until she was walking for 30 minutes. This exercise
> often involved social contacts, and she reported enjoying these despite
> the fact that she still felt the pain. In addition, her husband was advised
> to stop asking about her pain and fetching and carrying for her as if she
> were seriously ill. After 6 weeks she drew up a hierarchy of outings she
> would like to attempt, the most desirable of which was a trip to a shop-

ping centre. She achieved all these tasks and her mood and general level of activity increased substantially, although there was minimal reduction in her reports of pain intensity.

## Cognitive methods

These can be divided into two broad categories (Pearce, 1983). Firstly, those that are directly concerned with modifying pain-related cognitions, and secondly, those aimed at modifying cognitive responses to stress on the assumption that pain may be avoided or minimized if stress is dealt with better.

Cognitive methods aimed at altering the cognitive responses to pain have developed from laboratory studies. Some of the most commonly used strategies include the following:

*Imaginative inattention.* Here the subject's task is to imagine a scene generally considered incompatible with the experience of pain, for example, lying on a beach in the sun.

*Transformation of context.* Here the task is to imagine that the pain sensations experienced by the individual are actually occurring in another context. An example that is often cited is as follows: if one has a pain in the arm it may help to imagine that one is James Bond or some other brave person who has been shot in the arm and is running after an assailant. The aim is to enable the sensations to be imagined in a context in which they are appropriate and where they should assume a different meaning. The assumption is that if the sensations are associated with the affective state of courage rather than fear, anxiety and hence pain intensity will be reduced. Clinical experience suggests that this technique may have greater appeal to children than adults.

*Imaginative transformation.* The subject is instructed to 'relabel' the sensations as numbness or tightness, or some other experience that is easier to bear and less distressing than the pain itself. These may be elaborated to include, for example, asking the patient to imagine white cells surging to the site of the pain and devouring painful red cells, thereby reducing the pain area and intensity.

*Attention diversion.* This may involve either external diversion strategies, such as counting ceiling tiles, or internal ones such as counting backward from one thousand in threes or reciting poetry. This 'classification' of cognitive coping strategies is by no means definitive. In practice it is important not to adhere too rigidly to any classification system. Instead, certain strategies (which may be a combination of several of the above categories) can be used in individual patients.

Case vignette:

> A 35-year-old secretary with chronic pelvic pain made very effective use of relaxation and imaginative transformation. She had an image of her pain as a serpent eating her organs. She would relax, breath deeply and imagine the oxygen coming into her lungs, then into her blood to the site of her pain. In conjunction with the healing white cells of her body the oxygen would attack the serpent which was slowly consumed by the oxygen molecules and white cells. She found this strategy effective in reducing pain and distress.

### Relaxation

Relaxation training has been widely used in the treatment of chronic pain. For some conditions, such as tension headache, the rationale behind its use has been that the relaxation may produce a direct physiological change in the muscles thought to play a role in the aetiology of the pain. Relaxation may alter pelvic blood flow or prevent vascular responses to stressful stimuli. However, this is speculative and there are other reasons why relaxation may be effective apart from any direct effect on physiology. The relaxation procedure itself may serve a distracting function in that attention to exercises and relaxing mental imagery may reduce attention to unpleasant sensory input. Alternatively, it may act to increase the patients' perceived control over the pain. Many patients use it as a coping response and construe it as a strategy which helps them to control the pain rather than feel controlled by it, i.e. to use it as a means of increasing self-efficacy.

Linton (1986) has confirmed the efficacy of relaxation for chronic pain conditions other than headache. Turner (1982) showed that relaxation alone was more effective than no treatment and nearly as effective as cognitive therapy plus relaxation for patients with low back pain. Similarly, Linton and Gotestam (1984) showed that relaxation was nearly as effective as relaxation plus an operant programme conducted on an outpatient basis. However, these judgements of relative efficacy are dependent on the nature of the outcome measures used, and the different treatments produce different patterns of change on a range of measures. Operant programmes are better at reducing consumption of medication and increasing levels of activity, while relaxation seems better at reducing ratings of pain intensity. Hence it would be unwise to conclude that relaxation is as effective as either cognitive therapy or operant methods. All of these methods are of potential value in the management of pelvic pain. As yet however there have been few systematic attempts to apply such treatments to the specific problems of chronic pelvic pain.

Case vignette:

> Miss P aged 32 was a successful journalist who had been working only part time for the past 18 months on account of her pelvic pain which had increased in severity over the last 3 years. She was extremely anxious that the pain would affect her performance at work and a vicious circle seemed to have become established in which the pain caused her to be anxious and this anxiety triggered or exacerbated the pain. She responded well to progressive muscular relaxation. We made an individualized tape using her own therapist's voice of the relaxation instructions. She listened to this daily at home and adapted a version for her car to avoid becoming tense in situations such as traffic jams where she feared she would be late and her professional credibility jeopardized. She found that relaxation was useful not only for reduction of anxiety but also as a strategy to control the pain. Miss P was able to reduce the intensity and frequency of her pain episodes and this improvement was maintained 6 months after treatment.

### Evaluation of psychological treatments for chronic pelvic pain

Over the 30 years since Taylor's (1957) warning of the dangers of radical surgery for unexplained pelvic pain, there has been intermittent interest in the use of psychological methods for this group of patients. Despite this, there have been few attempts to evaluate them and those studies which have been conducted are generally methodologically inadequate and difficult to interpret. They have been reviewed by Pearce and Beard (1984).

Beard *et al.* (1977) were among the first to mention the use of psychological approaches to chronic pelvic pain. They found that some women responded well to relaxation training, but there was no formal evaluation of the efficacy of treatment. Most subsequent studies used inadequate control groups and unreliable measures and added little to our knowledge of psychological interventions for chronic pelvic pain (Petrucco & Harris, 1981; Pearce *et al.*, 1982). The results of a more adequately controlled trial of two different behavioural treatments does however provide some evidence that psychological interventions can be effective in the management of chronic pelvic pain. Pearce (1986) compared stress analysis and pain analysis (described below) with a minimal intervention control group. Women allocated to the 'stress analysis' group received a form of cognitive and behavioural stress management as well as relaxation training. Discussion of the pain was discouraged and the focus was directed towards identifying current worries and concerns apart from the pain. Treatment began with a semistructured interview to assess potential areas of stress such as difficulties with finance, marriage, housing. Specific problem areas were identified for each patient. The women were also asked to keep a daily record of their main concerns. The therapist's aim throughout was to identify cognitive strategies used by the women in response to identified stressors, and to discuss alternative responses. In addition, the use of Jacobsonian relaxation strategies in stressful situations was encouraged (Jacobson, 1938). The 'pain analysis' treatment involved the patient in close monitoring of her pain and its associated antecedent and consequent events. Therapy was aimed at identifying patterns associated with pain episodes and teaching alternative strategies for avoiding or reducing pain. These strategies were determined on an individual basis and included cognitive, behavioural and environmental manipulations. In addition, graded exercise programmes were instituted for each patient. Spouses were encouraged to prompt and reinforce 'well behaviours' and, whenever possible, were encouraged to become involved in the exercise programme. Patients allocated to the minimal intervention control group were given the same explanation as the treatment groups about the probable aetiology and frequency of their disorder, and were told that there was no proven medical or surgical treatment approach.

A range of measures was used to assess outcome. These included ratings of mood, pain intensity and behavioural disruption as well as 'blind' ratings by the gynaecologist of the extent to which the patient was affected by the pain. At 6 months follow-up both treatment groups were significantly better than the minimal intervention control group on all measures of outcome. Interestingly, there were no differences between the 3 groups at an earlier follow-up 3 months after treatment. This suggests the power of the investigation and explanation procedures which were common to all three groups including the minimal intervention group. The fact that by 6 months the two treatment groups were performing more effectively suggests that some active process of coping with stress and pain was assimilated and used to advantage in the follow-up period. Clearly, longer follow-up periods are required to assess the durability of these changes.

In one of the first studies to assess the interaction between a physical and psychological treatment, Farquhar *et al.* (1989) conducted a double-blind placebo controlled trial of medroxyprogesterone acetate or MHP (provera) and psychological treatment. All women had a history of pelvic pain for at least 6 months, no obvious pathology on laparoscopy, and abnormal venography.

Eighty-four patients were assigned to one of 4 groups: MPA alone, MPA plus psychotherapy, placebo alone, and placebo plus psychotherapy. Women allocated to the psychotherapy group attended for 6 sessions, each for 45 minutes in length, held at approximately fortnightly intervals. It included education about pain, stress management and guided exercise. The women kept detailed records of pain episodes and associated cognitive and behavioural responses to pain. They were treated for 4 months and thereafter followed up regularly for 9 months with pain assessment, pelvic ultrasound scanning, and hormone measurements.

At the end of treatment there was a significant reduction in pain in 73–74% of both MPA groups whether or not they also had psychological treatment. Only 33% of those treated with placebo reported improvement in pain. At 9 months after the end of therapy 71% of the MPA plus psycho-therapy group had reduced pain scores compared with only 43% of the MPA only group.

Farquhar and his colleagues suggested that provera led to a short term reduction in pain that allowed patients to benefit maximally from the stress and pain management techniques that had been taught during the psycho-logical treatment. As a consequence these patients did better in the long term than those who received either physical or psychological treatment alone.

## Conclusions

We propose an interactive model of chronic pelvic pain which involves pre-disposing biological factors (pelvic varicosities) as well as psychosocial factors. Prominent among the latter are a previous history of physical history in both the patient and her family, and experience of life stress. Child sexual abuse is one kind of previous life stress which may act as a predisposing factor, although it is probably not specific to pelvic pain. Somatic focusing on the pelvic area may aggravate the patient's experience of pain.

Optimum management includes a combination of both physical and psychological treatments. It seems likely that future advances in this area will occur as a result of careful integration of both psychological and physical methods of assessment and intervention.

## References

Adams, J., Reginald, P.W., Franks, S., Wadsworth, J. & Beard, B.W. (1990). Uterine size and endometrial thickness and the significance of cystic ovaries in women with pelvic pain due to congestion, *British Journal of Obstetrics & Gynaecology*, in press.

Beard, R.W. (1989). *Pelvic congestion as a cause of chronic pelvic pain*, presented at the 25th British Congress of Obstetrics and Gynaecology. London.

Beard, R.W., Belsey, E.N., Lieberman, B.M. & Wilkinson, J.C.M. (1977). Pelvic pain in women, *American Journal of Obstetrics and Gynaecology*, **128**, 566–570.

Beard, R.W., Highman, J.W., Pearce, S. & Reginald, P.W. (1984). Diagnosis of pelvic varicosities in women with chronic pelvic pain, *Lancet*, **ii**, 946–949.

Beard, R.W. & Reginald, P.W. (1990). Chronic pelvic pain, in *Gynaecology* (Ed. Shaw, R.), Churchill Livingstone, London (in press).

Beard, R.W., Reginald, P.W. & Pearce, S. (1989). Psychology and somatic factors in women with pain due to pelvic congestion, in *Mechanisms of Physical and Emotional Stress* (Eds. Chrousos, G.P., Loriaux, D.L. and Gold, P.W.), pp. 413–421, Plenum Press, New York.

Benson, R., Hanson, K. & Matarazzo, J. (1959). Atypical pelvic pain in women: Gynaecologic psychiatric considerations, *American Journal of Obstetrics and Gynaecology*, **77**, 806–823.

Castelnuovo-Tedesco, P. & Krout, B.M. (1970). Psychosomatic aspects of chronic pelvic pain, *International Journal of Psychiatric Medicine*, **1**, 109–126.

Duncan, C.H. & Taylor, H.C. (1952). A psychosomatic study of pelvic congestion, *American Journal of Obstetrics and Gynaecology*, **64**, 1–12.

Farquhar, C.M., Rogers, S., Franks, S., Pearce, S., Wadsworth, J. & Beard, R.W. (1989). A randomized controlled trial of medroxyprogesterone acetate and psychotherapy for the treatment of pelvic congestion, *British Journal of Obstetrics and Gynaecology*, **6**, 1152–1162.

Fordyce, W.E. (1982). A behavioural perspective on chronic pain, *British Journal of Clinical Psychology*, **21**, 1–12.

Fordyce, W.E., Fowler, R.S., Lehmann, J.F., Delateur, B.J., Sand, P.L. & Treischmann, R.B. (1973). Operant conditioning in the treatment of chronic pain, *Archives of Physical Medicine and Rehabilitation*, **54**, 399–408.

Gidro-Frank, L., Gordon, T. & Taylor, H.C. (1960). Pelvic pain and female identity, *American Journal of Obstetrics and Gynaecology*, **79**, 1184–1202.

Gillibrand, R.N. (1981). *The Investigation of Pelvic Pain*, Communication at the Scientific Meeting on 'Chronic Pelvic Pain — a Gynaecological Headache', Royal College of Obstetricians and Gynaecologists, London.

Gross, R.J., Doer, H., Calditola, D., Guzinski, G. & Ripley, H.S. (1980). Borderline syndrome and incest in chronic pain patients, *International Journal of Psychiatry in Medicine*, **10**, 79–86.

Harrop-Griffiths, J., Katon, W., Walker, E., Holm, L., Russo, J. & Hickok, L. (1988). The association between chronic pelvic pain, psychiatric diagnosis and childhood sexual abuse, *Obstetrics and Gynaecology*, **71**, 589–594.

Henker, F.O. (1979). Diagnosis and treatment of non organic pelvic pain, *Southern Medical Journal*, **72**, 1132–1134.

Hoon, P.W. (1979). The assessment of sexual arousal in women, in *Progress in Behaviour Modification*, Vol 7, pp. 41–61, Academic Press.

Jacobson, E. (1938). *Progressive Relaxation*, University of Chicago Press, Chicago.

Luciano, A.A., Turksey, R.N., Dlugi, A.M., Carleo, J.L. (1980). *Endocrine consequences of oral medroxyprogesterone acetate (MPA) in the treatment of endometriosis*, presentation at the 68th Annual Meeting of the Endocrine Society, Anaheim, California.

Linton, S.J. (1986). Behavioural remediation of chronic pain: A status report, *Pain*, **24**, 125–141.

Linton, S.J. & Gotestam, K.G. (1984). A controlled study of the effects of applied relaxation and applied relaxation plus aperant procedures in the regulation of chronic pain, *British Journal of Clinical Psychology*, **23**, 291–299.

Melzack, R. (1983). *The Challenge of Pain*, Penguin, London.

Mills, W.G. (1978). The enigma of pelvic pain, *Journal of the Royal Society of Medicine*, **71**, 257–260.

Morris, N. & O'Neill, D. (1958). Out-patient gynaecology, *British Medical Journal*, **1**, 1038–1039.

Pearce, S. (1983). A review of cognitive–behavioural methods for the treatment of chronic pain, *Journal of Psychosomatic Research*, **27**, 431–440.

Pearce, S. (1986). *A Psychological Investigation of Chronic Pelvic Pain in Women*, unpublished PhD thesis, University of London.

Pearce, S. (1988). The concepts of psychogenic pain, *Current Psychological Research & Reviews*, **6(3)**, 219–229.

Pearce, S. & Beard, R.W. (1984). Chronic pelvic pain, in *Psychology and Gynaecological Problems* (Ed. Broome, A. & Wallace, L.), Tavistock Press, London.

Pearce, S. & Erskine, A. (1989). Chronic pain, in *The Practice of Behavioural Medicine* (Eds. Pearce, S. & Wardle, J.), OUP/BPS.

Pearce, S., Knight, C. & Beard, R.W. (1982). Pelvic pain — a common gynaecological problem, *Journal of Psychosomatic Obstetrics and Gynaecology*, **1**, 12.

Petrucco, O.M. & Harris, R.D. (1982). *A Psychological and Venographic Study of Women Presenting with Non-organic Pelvic Pain*, 8th New Zealand Congress, Feb. 1982, Auckland, New Zealand.

Pilowsky, I. & Spence, N.D. (1975). Patterns of illness behaviour in patients with intractable pain, *Journal of Psychosomatic Research*, **19**, 279–287.

Rapkin, A.J. (1986). Adhesions & pelvic pain: A retrospective study, *Obstetrics and Gynaecology*, **68**, 13–15.

Reginald, P.W., Adams, J., Franks, S., Wadsworth, J. & Beard, R.W. (1989). Medroxyprogesterone acetate in the treatment of pelvic pain due to venous congestion, *British Journal of Obstetrics and Gynaecology*, **96**, 1148–1152.

Reginald, P.W., Beard, R.W., Kooner, J.S. *et al.* (1987). Intravenous dihydroergotamine to relieve pelvic congestion with pain in young women, *Lancet*, **ii**, 351–353.

Renaer, M. (1980). Chronic pelvic pain without obvious pathology in women, *European Journal of Obstetrics, Gynecology, and Reproductive Biology*, **10(6)**, 415–463.

Renaer, M., Vertommen, H., Nijs, P., Wagerians, L. & Van Hemelrijck, T. (1979). Psychological aspects of chronic pelvic pain in women, *American Journal of Obstetrics and Gynecology*, **134**, 75–80.

Rundqvist, E. & Sandholm, L.E. (1984). Treatment of pelvic varicosities causing lower abdominal pain with extraperitoneal resection of the left ovarian vein, *Annales de Chirurgiae et Gynaecologiae*, **73(6)**, 339–341.

Slocumb, J.C. (1984). Neurological factors in chronic pelvic pain: Trigger points and the abdominal pelvic pain syndrome, *American Journal of Obstetrics and Gynecology*, **149**, 536–543.

Sternbach, R.A. (1974). *Pain patients: Traits and treatments*, Academic Press, New York.

Taylor, H.C. (1949). Vascular congestion and hyperemia: I. Physiologic basis and history of the concept, *American Journal of Obstetrics and Gynecology*, **57**, 221–230.

Taylor, H.C. (1957). Chronic pelvic pain, in *Progress in Gynaecology* Vol. 3 (Eds. Meigs, J.V. and Sturgis, S.H.), Grune & Stratton, New York.

Theobald, G.W. (1951). Pelvic sympathetic syndrome, *Journal of Obstetrics and Gynaecology of the British Empire*, **58**, 733–761.

Turk, D.C. & Genest, M. (1979). Regulation of pain: The application of cognitive and behavioural techniques for prevention and remediation, in *Cognitive–Behavioural Interventions: Theory, Research and Procedures* (Eds. Kendall, P.C. and Hollon, S.D.), Academic Press, New York.

Turner, J.A. (1982). Comparison of group progressive–relaxation training and cognitive–behavioural group therapy for chronic low back pain, *Journal of Consulting & Clinical Psychology*, **50**, 757–765.

Weisenberg, M. (1977). Pain and pain control, *Psychological Bulletin*, **84**, 1008–1044.

# 11
# Dermatological Complaints

S.C. WESSELY

## Introduction

There can be little doubt of the importance of the skin to psychological well-being, and of the links between appearance and self esteem (Eller, 1974; Melli & Giorgini, 1984). Despite this, not all patients with skin disease will be psychologically disturbed. A leading textbook (Rook *et al.*, 1987) has estimated that approximately one-third of attenders at a skin clinic will have significant psychological distress. Methodologically sound studies have confirmed this: between 30 and 40% of patients seen in a skin clinic have psychological disturbance of sufficient severity to be classified as psychiatric 'cases' (Hughes *et al.*, 1983; Wessely & Lewis, 1989; Barth *et al.*, 1987). This is similar to the rates of psychiatric morbidity found in other general medical settings (Mayou & Hawton, 1986). Cassileth *et al.* (1984) studied five chronic diseases: diabetes, cancer, arthritis, renal and skin disease, and found no group differences on various measures of psychological ill health. However, these figures do not provide information about the aetiology of psychological morbidity, and it is clear that no single mechanism will be found. Before any specific links can be explored, it is first necessary to develop a logical classification for all the psychiatric problems encountered in the skin clinic.

In a random sample of new attenders to a dermatology clinic Wessely and Lewis (1989) used the results of standardized psychiatric interviews and measures of the impact made by skin disease for this purpose. They grouped patients in the following way:

1 *Pure dermatological disease.* That is, patients with skin disease only.

2 *Dermatological disease that has resulted in psychiatric distress.* These patients report that their life has changed since the onset of skin disease, perhaps due to disfigurement, social embarrassment etc., but their distress may be influenced by pre-existing attitudes and personality. In this study (Wessely & Lewis, 1989) they comprised 30% of the sample, and 70% of the psychiatric cases. An example would be a patient with severe skin disease

276

who is now significantly depressed, but another example might be a patient presenting with anxiety related to a trivial skin problem such as a wart, in modern parlance the 'worried well'.

**3** *Dermatological disease with coincidental psychiatric illness.* These patients will have standard dermatological disorders, and will be psychiatric cases, but will not report any behavioural changes as a result of skin disease. This group was characterized as those in whom skin disease had made no 'impact', and thus the observed psychopathology may have other causes. This group constituted 10% of the sample, and 25% of the psychiatric cases.

**4** *Psychiatric illness causing or mimicking skin disease.* The skin complaint, either real or imaginary, is the consequence of a psychiatric disorder. This group is the true somatic presentation of psychiatric disorder. In the above study such patients comprised only 5% of the sample, of whom just over half admitted to psychiatric symptoms. These are the 'true dermatoneuroses' of Obermayer (1955), or the 'dermatological non-disease' of some, but not all, authors (see later).

## Historical outline and review of terms

The history of the relationship between skin disease and psychiatry has two parallel strands. The first is the history and development of specific syndromes, the second the study of the overall relationship between skin and psyche. Significant changes have occurred in both. Recent developments in nosology and treatment have led to renewed interest in the area of specific syndromes, whilst the subject of the interaction between psyche and skin has turned full circle in recent years. The history of the psychology of skin disease has been elegantly reviewed by Whitlock (1976).

One of the features of previous work on the relation between psychiatry and skin disease has been an emphasis on a psychoanalytic approach. This developed as a reaction to the previous view that cutaneous diseases were related to mental illnesses simply by the under or overactivity of the nervous system linking brain and skin. Instead, the psychoanalytic approach tended to look at the relationship between personality and disease, exemplified by the works of Flanders Dunbar (1954). These theories in turn could not be substantiated for two reasons (MacAlpine, 1954). First, improved knowledge of the pathological basis of the common dermatoses highlighted the weaknesses of theories implicating a psychogenic aetiology, and secondly, the improved methodology in psychiatry exposed further flaws.

For example, alopecia areata (AA) was, and occasionally still is (Nadelson, 1987), listed as a psychosomatic disorder. However, Koo *et al.* (1987a) showed that 'The onset of AA is not associated with stressful life events in a great majority of patients. However, after the onset of AA, there is a higher pre-valence of serious psychiatric disorder among the AA patients than in the general population.'

Similarly, in atopic dermatitis, Koo *et al.* (1987b) demonstrated that the observed 'elevation in the serum of IgE, the presence of anergia, anxiety and possibly even the apparent personality deviations observed in the past may all represent state-dependent variables that reflect the severity of the skin involvement at the time of the observation.'

Further examples are to be found in the literature on psoriasis. Although originally classed as a psychosomatic complaint, improved research methods led to subsequent criticism (Baughman & Sobell, 1977) and eventual abandonment of this idea. More recent work concentrated on the relationship between precipitating factors and their impact on the individual rather than theories about aetiology; in other words, when but not why (Seville, 1978). In a current review (Rowland Payne, 1987) no mention was made of any psychological causes. Instead, attention has been directed towards the impact of psoriasis on the sufferer (Jobling, 1976; Hardy & Cotterill, 1982). Finally, psychiatrists have studied the psychological effects of all skin diseases, of which psoriasis is but one (Hughes *et al.*, 1983; Wessely & Lewis, 1989). Interestingly, these developments have not been reflected in the non-medical literature, as was demonstrated by Dennis Potter's acclaimed television series, 'The Singing Detective'. Commenting on the play, and the critical and journalistic reactions, Jobling (1987) wrote 'the overwhelming emphasis on stress, psychosomatic causes and personal responsibility is at variance with current professional consensus'.

## Terminology

The somatic presentations of psychiatric disorder can be grouped under two separate headings: (a) *visible lesions that are self-inflicted, which may or may not be denied;* and (b) *complaints of alteration in body image or sensation, which may or may not be part of a psychotic illness.* This division will be used throughout the rest of this chapter. For the purpose of this review the following terms will be used.

*Self-inflicted lesions*   This will include such categories as neurotic ex-coriations, deliberate self-harm, trichotillomania, dermatological patho-mimicry and dermatitis artefacta.

*Disorders of body image and body sensation.*   This will be further divided into two groups. The first are those conditions that are probably associated with a psychotic illness, such as delusional parasitosis, monosymptomatic hypochondriacal psychosis and other paranoid psychoses. The second are those more classically concerned with body image, and usually thought to be of non-psychotic origin, such as dysmorphophobia and other dissatisfactions with appearance or health.

At this stage it is worth discussing the term '*dermatological non-disease*', which has been used to describe those patients who report to dermatologists but have no visible skin disease. Unfortunately, this term has been used in several ways. Some have applied it to all the various skin disorders of strictly psychological origin (Sheppard *et al.*, 1986), whereas others (for example Cotterill, 1981) have excluded self-inflicted lesions, and restrict the term to include disorders of body image. Although the former broad usage has the advantage of grouping the various disparate conditions under one heading, it does not imply that similar psychopathological mechanisms are involved; far from it. The term is best used to describe patients in whom skin lesions are absent.

## Prevalence

Few studies (Table 11.1) enable even an estimate of prevalence to be made, as many of the conditions are rare, often undiagnosed, and subject to marked referral bias.

All such estimates are likely to be an underestimate of the true community prevalence of such disorders. For example, an uncertain number of cases of delusional parasitosis will be known only to pest control and public health departments (Edwards, 1977).

**Table 11.1.** Prevalence studies: specific psychiatric disorders (in dermatology clinics)

| | |
|---|---|
| All cases without visible skin disease | = 4.4% (Wessely & Lewis, 1988) |
| Delusional parasitosis (skin clinic) | = 0.3% (Skott, 1978) |
| Delusional parasitosis (community) | = 2.0% (Schwitzer *et al.*, 1987) |
| Dermatitis artefacta | = 0.3% (Gupta *et al.*, 1987a) |
| Neurotic excoriations | = 2.0% (Gupta *et al.*, 1987a) |

# Clinical features

### Self-inflicted lesions

There is a spectrum of self-inflicted lesions, grouped according to the degree of denial of the cause.

1 Perhaps the mildest is *neurotic excoriations*, also known as psycho-

genic pruritus (Musaph, 1967). The lesions are produced by repetitive self-excoriations, in the absence of underlying physical pathology, such as a recognized cause of pruritus. The patient is aware of, and can admit to, the source of the damage to the skin, but is unaware of the motives that lie behind it (Obermayer, 1955). The separation from lichen simplex and prurigo is difficult and of little practical relevance (Burton *et al.*, 1987).

The patient is usually middle-aged or elderly, with a peak in the mid-forties. In one series the disease had existed for an average of 10 years before presentation (Fruensgaard & Hjortshoj, 1982). Females are overrepresented in all published accounts. In general outpatient skin clinics the prevalence has been estimated at 2% (Gupta *et al.*, 1987a), whilst it was found in 9% of an inpatient series of patients with pruritus (Rajka, 1966).

2   This next degree of severity is deliberate, but admitted damage, occurring when the skin is damaged as part of *deliberate self-harm*. It is unusual for such cases to present to the dermatologist as the diagnosis is not often in doubt.

3   A non-scarring alopecia may result from self-inflicted damage, called *traction alopecia* or *trichotillomania*. It is seldom immediately admitted, but may not be denied on direct questioning. Often the hair is hidden, or even eaten (Obermayer, 1955). Characteristic features include the finding of hairs of different lengths over different areas of the scalp, with complete alopecia being very unusual. Although the scalp is the commonest site, occasionally eyebrows, axillary or even pubic hair may be involved (Eller, 1974; Krishnan *et al.*, 1985). Another variant, fortunately extremely rare, is an impulse to tear out the nails rather than the hair, termed onychotillomania. The only study citing prevalence found that 0.5% of children seen in a child psychiatric clinic were diagnosed as having trichotillomania (Mannino & Delgado, 1969).

4   An intermediate category includes those with known previous dermato-logical disease who reproduce their disease either directly or by interfering with therapy, described by Millard (1984) as *'dermatological pathomimicry'*. Lesions, which will be less bizarre than in true artefacta, may be exacerbations of dermatitis, repeated drug reactions, or non-healing ulcers.

5   The last category, and the most severe, is *dermatitis artefacta*, in which the damage is deliberate, but denied. This is an unsatisfactory term, as the lesions are not that of dermatitis, but it has gained widespread acceptance and will continue to be used. The vast array of clinical presentations of artefacta are best described by Lyell (1979). A variety of lesions may occur, including rashes, ulcers, blisters, excoriations, burns and bruises.

Cases of dermatitis artefacta show a marked female predominance (Fabisch, 1980; Sneddon & Sneddon, 1974; Sheppard *et al.*, 1986). Anecdotally, health service professionals have been identified less often among dermatitis artefacta patients than in other factitious diseases (Lyell, 1979). Perhaps arte-facta is too straightforward to execute, or perhaps patients feel dermatol-ogists are more alert to factitious disorders than other medical colleagues. Because this syndrome is characterized by difficulty in establishing satis-factory relationships with others, many sufferers will be single. In those who are not, other family members may be involved in the deception, as in *folie a deux* (Hubler & Hubler, 1980). Cases are described of similar lesions in a mother and her children (Stankler, 1977; Jones, 1983) — dermatitis artefacta coexisting with Munchausen's by proxy, a very serious situation (Meadow, 1985).

The diagnosis may be very difficult to establish: not all lesions are bizarre, some may even successfully mimic common skin conditions (Naish, 1979). To confirm the diagnosis it may be necessary to demonstrate that the lesions heal on total occlusion (if that can be guaranteed), or even to establish the lack of a primary disease process by biopsy (Halprin, 1967). In addition to a healthy degree of scepticism it cannot be overemphasized that the history is all important. A great deal of time needs to be spent with the telephone, contacting GPs and other hospitals, and considerable ingenuity may be needed. The purpose is to obtain the illness history of the patient (Chapter 3, p. 42), which usually extends back to childhood. A detailed history will also invariably reveal a disturbed developmental background in terms of personal and family psychopathology. This will be discussed further in the next section.

If the following cannot be established the diagnosis of artefactual illness should be questioned:
1  A history of abnormal illnesses and behaviour.
2  A disorder of personality.
3  Evidence of abnormal responses to stress in the past.

The status of bruising as a possible subgroup of artefacta has attracted considerable speculation, as it overlaps with the phenomenon of 'stigmata'. It is debated whether bruising can occur as part of a hysterical conversion in the so-called 'psychogenic purpura syndrome', or whether lesions are self-inflicted, consciously or otherwise. Research has not resolved the problem, but most authors consider it to be a form of artefact. It is evident that, whatever the mechanism, those involved (who are invariably female), show a high degree of psychopathology (Koblenzer, 1983). Agle and his colleagues have provided further details of this fascinating topic (e.g. Agle *et al.*, 1969).

Given that most patients with artefacta will have psychiatric disorders, and that some of them will have received previous treatment for affective disorder, it is worth emphasizing one particular pitfall. Many psychotropic drugs have dermatological side-effects which may be mistaken for artefacta, especially by the non-dermatologist. For example, lithium can cause a wide variety of skin diseases, including maculopapular eruptions, pustular psoriasis, folliculitis, a rash resembling dermatitis herpetiformis, and skin ulceration (Heng, 1982). Tricyclics are also associated with a variety of skin lesions (Gupta *et al.*, 1987b; Warnock & Knesvich, 1988).

### Disorders of body image or body sensation

The diseases in this section are those in which no lesions are visible to the trained eye, and, as has been discussed, are often grouped together as 'dermatological non-disease'. In this section a division will be made into psychotic and non-psychotic disorders.

Overall there are high rates of psychiatric morbidity. In direct interviews with all new cases without visible dermatological pathology, Wessely and Lewis (1989) found the incidence of psychiatric caseness to be 62%, using strict symptomatic criteria. Using different psychiatric instruments Owens and Millard (1987) reported a similar incidence. Because many of these patients minimize emotional distress but emphasize physical symptoms (Lloyd, 1983), this is likely to be an underestimate of psychopathology. Patients who present to a dermatologist without visible disease have a high risk of psychiatric disorder.

### *Psychotic conditions*

*Delusional parasitosis.* The classification of the psychotic conditions encountered in dermatology is complex, and there is no consensus. This is illustrated by the best known of these conditions, *delusional parasitosis.*

Although there is a lack of agreement concerning nosology, the clinical features of delusional parasitosis are clear cut. It has been defined by Skott (1978) as: 'A persistent condition in which the patient believes that small animals such as insects, lice, vermin or maggots are living and thriving on or within the skin. In spite of all negative evidence to the contrary, the patient has a firm conviction that he/she is infested. This belief is unshakable'.

The patient usually asserts that his or her skin is infested by an insect or parasite. Occasionally the patient claims that the organism is internal, or just under the skin, in which case it is often called a worm. Alternatively the patient may state that lumps or eggs have been deposited by the parasite under the skin.

Patients may present with scratches, marks or even burns, which reflect their efforts to remove the parasites (Lyell, 1983). This must not be confused with artefacta or excoriation. Patients may also often present with their own 'evidence' of infestation, in the form of collections of skin debris, usually brought in a container. This has been dubbed the 'matchbox sign' (Lancet, 1983). Such 'evidence' was provided in 39% of Skott's series.

Finally, other family members are frequently involved in the abnormal beliefs, and *folie a deux* was found in 25% of a large series (Skott, 1978).

The condition is rare, comprising 0.3% of attenders at a dermatology clinic (Skott, 1978). However, the community prevalence may be higher, as a survey of old people's homes reported that 2% showed delusions of parasitosis (Schwitzer *et al.*, 1987).

*Other psychotic conditions.*  Not all those who present to a dermatologist and are subsequently found to be psychotic believe themselves to be infested with parasites. Others present with the delusional belief that parts of the body are misshapen, or that they are giving rise to a foul odour, or express beliefs related to alleged abnormalities of appearance.

Because of a sex difference in age at presentation, (the average age of males at first contact (40 years) is considerably less than that of females (60 years)), Munro has speculated that there are at least two conditions that have similar presentations (Munro, 1980). However, he subsequently modified this view when it became evident there was a high incidence of substance abuse in male patients (Munro, 1982).

*Non-psychotic conditions*

*Body image and sensation.*  In the previous section it was noted that patients attend a skin clinic with a variety of odd beliefs. Many of these beliefs will not be held with delusional conviction, and may even have a basis in reality, but an objective observer will consider them to be exaggerated out of all proportion. Unusual complaints may include excessive sweating, having misshapen breasts and losing hair. Others may complain of a burning tongue, mouth or skin, or of facial redness. Such beliefs may be classified according to content, usually as dysmorphophobic concerns, or by intensity. In the latter case they are usually regarded as overvalued ideas (McKenna, 1984), which distinguishes them from the psychotic disorders mentioned above. However, in practice this distinction may be one of degree.

*Illness beliefs.*  A division that is easier to make in practice, and which has important treatment implications, is between parasitophobia and delusional parasitosis. Parasitophobia is one type of illness phobia; people who fear they have an illness despite all evidence to the contrary. When such fears become multiple and are associated with several body systems they are usually grouped as hypochondriasis (Marks, 1987). In parasitophobia the patient has no actual bodily sensations of having a parasite, but avoids all situations where there is the remotest possibility of encountering one. Such actions may bring temporary relief, but the anxiety will always return. Other types of illness phobia that may present to the dermatologist include a fear of syphilis ('venereophobia') (Macalpine, 1957), or, increasingly, misattributing trivial cutaneous blemishes to AIDS. Common to all illness phobias is the search for reassurance, which may become the most incapacitating feature of the condition (Marks, 1987; Chapter 3, p. 58).

# Pathophysiological mechanisms

The division between self-inflicted lesions and disorders of body image has been made on clinical grounds, but also has aetiological implications.

### The spectrum of self-harm

*Mild, admitted self-inflicted skin damage, often known as 'neurotic excoriations'.* Regrettably few studies have used reliable methods to assess psychopathology. One group found that 9 out of 10 cases of neurotic excoriation fulfilled DSM-III criteria for major depression (Koo *et al.*, 1987c). Other diagnoses have been made, and obsessional personality traits have been frequently emphasized (Gupta *et al.*, 1986a). Musaph has described a specific personality type, which can be summarized as an insecure, obsessional personality subjected to recent stress (Musaph, 1976).

The mechanism of symptom formation may be the desire to scratch at an abnormal perception, or a heightened awareness of a normal sensation. The act of excoriation may begin as a result of mood disorder, but may be perpetuated by obsessional traits.

Patients with neurotic excoriations and obsessional traits must be distinguished from those with hand irritation and paronychia. These result from the excessive hand-washing which is found in true obsessive–compulsive disorder.

*More severe cases of deliberate self-harm, but still admitted.* There are several characteristics common to most patients who deliberately injure themselves, although the extent to which the injury is admitted adds a further dimension. Simpson (1976) described the following characteristics in patients who habitually self-mutilate: low self-esteem, presenting as a dysphoric state; an abnormality of body image, with frequent evidence of an eating disorder; and a disordered developmental history, manifest as pervasive difficulties in social and sexual relationships. After the cutting there is an apparent temporary analgesic state, with a short-lived relief of tension and depression. Perhaps the most common psychiatric diagnosis is the borderline personality disorder (Schaffer *et al.*, 1982).

*Trichotillomania.*  Trichotillomania was described and named by Hallopeau (1889). Whitlock (1976) has pointed out that the term was introduced at a time when many other compulsive or repetitive acts were also classified as manias, for example kleptomania. He regarded this label as inappropriate, because it implied that trichotillomania was always associated with serious mental disorder, which it is not.

The psychopathology of trichotillomania varies with the age of presentation. Younger patients have a lower incidence of severe disturbance, and the condition is more benign when it occurs in younger children (Koblenzer, 1983; Medansky & Handler, 1981; Oguchi & Miura, 1977). In this age group it may have its origins in the same psychosocial and family stressors as enuresis, e.g. illness of a parent, fears of school, bullying, moving house etc. (Oranje *et al.*, 1986). However, it may rapidly develop into a habit. In older patients there are higher rates of serious coexisting psychiatric disturbance, the most common diagnoses being depression, borderline personality or schizophrenia (Greenberg & Sarner, 1965).

*Dermatitis artefacta.*  The variety of clinical presentations of artefacta may be grouped together for the purposes of discussing psychopathology, and may be included within the broader spectrum of factitious disorders (Lyell, 1979; Reich & Gottfried, 1983). This is because the choice of lesion in these disorders is often arbitrary. The fact that the skin is so often the target mainly reflects its accessibility, as it is far easier to fake symptoms on the skin than in other body organs.

As a general rule these patients have severe psychiatric disorder, and the combination of self-injury and denial reflects considerable personality disturbance (Fruensgaard, 1987). DSM-III (1980) states that factitious disorder is 'almost always superimposed upon a severe personality disorder'. In spite of this the patient may appear superficially normal until the nature of the complaint and details of past history are obtained. Extreme denial is characteristic of this disorder (Carney, 1980; Reich & Gottfried, 1983).

Dermatitis artefacta is best understood in terms of both cross-sectional and longitudinal data. Fabisch (1980) divided such cases equally between neurotic and personality disorders, but failed to identify any specific disorder. Only two had classic conversion symptoms which could be diagnosed as hysteria. Rarely, dermatitis artefacta may be associated with mental handicap or psychosis, but florid psychopathology other than the artefacta is unusual.

In a recent discussion of artefacta, Cossidente and Sarti (1984) include 'both conscious and deceitful pathomimesis' as well as 'the partially or completely unconscious forms of self-injury which can be considered fundamentally hysterical' — in other words dissociative states. This has links with the psychopathology of deliberate self-cutting without denial (Simpson, 1976). Finally, the thin line between dissociation and lying is indicated by a remarkable case of a patient with multiple personalities and artefacta whose lesions were only induced by one of her multiple personalities (Shelley, 1981). Regrettably, true malingering must always be kept in mind.

Fabisch (1980) remarked that a standard psychiatric diagnosis, though necessary, does not convey the complex psychosocial disturbances characteristics of artefacta. As with other cases of factitious illness it is important to look beyond the level of observable symptoms to the distortion of relationships and behaviour.

Doctors find it disturbing to be confronted by deception. However, it is important to keep in mind that the patient is attempting (consciously or unconsciously) to mislead the doctor. Thus abnormalities will be noted in the patient–doctor relationship, because the patient is trying to change the relationship for his/her own, non-therapeutic, ends. This is always maladaptive, and unless it is recognized (and often even when it is), it will ultimately lead to further despair and isolation.

Most patients with artefacta have difficulties in adult relationships. They are often socially isolated, have psychosexual problems and lack an adult confidant. An acute psychosocial stress may antedate the illness, but not invariably. Certainly, many patients will deny coexisting personal difficulties. It is tempting to hypothesize that the patient has used artefacta to avoid confronting these varied stressors. However, this does not explain the choice of a particular medical symptom.

The advantages of the sick role in terms of evasion of responsibilities, and attracting care and sympathy are well known. Furthermore, this choice is made easier by previous repetition and rehearsal, and many will have long histories of using illnesses for morbid purposes which extend into childhood. Early preoccupations with health and disease are common, and the history is replete with such terms as 'grumbling appendix', 'prone to viruses' etc. Indeed, it has been suggested that the reason many illness fabricators are employed in hospitals is not due to learning and availability of methods, but instead is a further 'manifestation of their life-long concerns with health' (Reich & Gottfried, 1983). The medical records of the parents may reveal similar illness patterns, and it is possible that the child has learnt at a very early stage to imitate such behaviours (Parker & Lipscombe, 1980).

In dermatological pathomimcry, i.e. those who interfere with the healing of organic skin lesions, a different pattern has been described. Characteristically, most patients are 'middle-aged women who are depressed, hypochondriacal, hostile, dissatisfied with their care and non-compliant' (Reich & Gottfried, 1983). These authors also found that 'all the patients had lives marked by personal losses, suffering and other chronic medical problems'.

## Disorders of body image and perception

These may be psychotic, or non-psychotic.

### *Delusional parasitosis*

Psychiatric taxonomies have always struggled to accommodate delusional parasitosis (see Chapter 2). Is it a symptom that is always part of another psychiatric syndrome, or a nosological entity in its own right? Both these possibilities will be discussed: first as a symptom, then as a syndrome.

As a symptom delusional parasitosis is found in many disorders, both medical and psychiatric. The symptom of delusional infestation coexists with many unusual physical illnesses (Berrios, 1985; Renvoize *et al.*, 1987), especially metabolic and endocrine. Unfortunately the rarity of the condition makes it difficult to ascertain whether or not these were chance occurrences. However, delusions of parasitosis that responded to the treatment of a coexisting illness have been reported with Vitamin $B_{12}$ deficiency (Pope, 1970).

Delusional parasitosis may also be a symptom of several psychiatric illnesses (Skott, 1978). The correct diagnosis may be made by the presence of additional features, which may suggest affective psychosis, schizophrenia or both acute and chronic organic brain syndromes. Toxic psychoses due to substance abuse, such as cocaine psychosis, have a particular tendency to produce the sensation of animals on or under the skin, known as formication or the 'cocaine bug'. Both visual and tactile hallucinations of animals on the skin may occur in delirium tremens (Lishman, 1987). In general, the presence of visual hallucinations of insects, rather than 'evidence' of infestation, should lead to an active search for the source of a toxic psychosis.

However, in many cases there are no further features which allow a psychiatric diagnosis to be made. The delusion of infestation may be the only evidence of psychopathology. In order to comprehend some of the complex arguments concerning the 'pure' syndrome, one must examine the history of the disease. Berrios (1985) provides an easily accessible historical account, but the definitive account is by Skott (1978). In an early account Perrin (1896) pointed out the poor prognosis, and grouped the condition with delusional rather than phobia disorders.

The opposing view, that it is a form of hallucinosis and not a delusion, was first articulated in the English literature by MacNamara (1928). Ekbom (1938) accepted both views, that it may be either a primary delusion or a hallucination, but it was Bers and Conrad (1954) who first linked the two concepts, introducing the term tactile-hallucinosis.

It is apparent that a number of conflicting views have emerged. Delusional parasitosis may be a delusional disorder, a hallucinatory disorder, or a mixture of the two. What is the current nosological status?

The disorder is regarded as a primary delusion in most English speaking countries. Arguments continue about its classification within the spectrum of the major psychoses, especially the relationship between delusional parasitosis, paranoid disorders and schizophrenia. This will be considered in the next section.

On the Continent delusional parasitosis is usually considered a disorder of perception to which a delusional explanation has been added, the so-called tactile-hallucinatory psychosis. It is thus a predominantly sensory abnormality, a disorder of perception as well as cognition. This is not widely accepted in the UK, perhaps because the best expositions of this view are to be found in the German literature. The work of Gross and Huber in particular deserves to be better known. They have written extensively on the topic of sensory experiences in many psychoses, including schizophrenia, and coined the term coenaesthesiae to describe the perceptual abnormalities commonly encountered. The concept has been further divided into an exaggeration of sensations of which the patient is not normally aware (perhaps because of increased vigilance and arousal), contrasted with a new sensation of entirely morbid origin. Although few British psychiatrists would use these perceptual concepts in relation to the major psychoses, it appears well suited to delusional parasitosis.

Although social factors are not directly implicated in the aetiology of delusional parasitosis, many authors report a significant association with variables loosely grouped as 'reduced sensory stimulation' (Skott, 1978) or 'contact deficiency paranoia' (Maier, 1987). These may include social isolation, deafness or visual impairment.

In summary, the symptom of infestation may occur in a variety of serious psychiatric illnesses. When it does not there remains a group in which the phenomenology is that of a tactile-hallucinatory psychosis. The current consensus is to classify these latter cases within the rubric of paranoid psychoses.

## Other psychotic conditions

These are a very mixed group that have also proved difficult to classify. Many of the arguments concerning the pathophysiological mechanisms underlying delusional parasitosis are equally applicable to the other isolated psychoses encountered in dermatology. Munro (1982) has argued that all these disorders should be grouped together as 'monosymptomatic hypochondriacal psychoses' (MHP). This has now been incorporated into DSM-III-R as *delusional (paranoid) disorder*, a term likely to gain wider acceptance. There is now persuasive evidence to suggest a symptomatic and genetic distinction between delusional disorder and schizophrenia (Munro, 1982; Kendler, 1987).

It is true that some patients originally diagnosed as 'delusional disorder' subsequently develop schizophrenia (Hay, 1970; Connolly & Gipson, 1978), but many develop other serious psychiatric illnesses. Such findings reflect the importance of a thorough search for evidence of other psychiatric diagnoses rather than specific evidence for the 'pure' syndrome. The separation of the secondary conditions resulting from other illnesses, and the true primary condition, is clinically and academically vital. Thomas (1984) has also highlighted the equally important distinction between the psychotic conditions reviewed in this section, and the non-psychotic conditions discussed below.

## Non-psychotic conditions

Many patients present with unusual morbid complaints concerning their appearance, but will not be considered psychotic. What are the possible origins of such symptoms?

Once again, it is vital to consider dysmorphophobia as a symptom before accepting it as a syndrome. It is found in many psychiatric disorders (Thomas, 1984), in particular depression. Using the Beck Depression Inventory, Hardy and Cotterill (1982) demonstrated an increased incidence of depressive symptoms in dysmorphophobia. In a series of women complaining of hair loss, the majority of those in whom there was no evidence of real hair loss were depressed, often as a result of marital or sexual problems (Eckert, 1976).

Other non-psychotic but unusual symptoms that are encountered in a dermatology clinic include the complaint of burning mouth ('glossodynia'). This is often regarded as a depressive 'equivalent' (Koblenzer, 1983; Cotterill, 1983), but in a recent systematic survey the multifactorial nature of the complaint was demonstrated (Lamey & Lamb, 1988). In addition to psychological causes, ill-fitting dentures, Vitamin $B_{12}$ deficiency and other metabolic abnormalities were reported.

It is worth emphasizing the difference between depressive 'equivalents', a term often applied to dysmorphophobic and hypochondriacal conditions, and true depressive illness. There is no evidence to support the notion of depressive 'equivalents' or 'masked' depression. The majority of depressive illnesses found in a skin clinic present in a conventional way and can be elicited if the appropriate questions are asked (Wessely & Lewis, 1989).

In the absence of affective disorder or psychosis, the literature on dysmorphophobia and related conditions suggests that the condition usually develops in the setting of an abnormal personality. This implies that such symptoms may begin during adolescence, when overvalued concerns about appearance are not infrequent. The persistence of such fears may be a consequence of, and contribute to, abnormal personality development. Thomas (1984) has pointed out the lack of an association with a single personality disorder, but that schizoid, narcissistic or obsessional traits are common. This is in keeping with clinical experience.

What mechanisms underly the choice of symptom? An anecdotal survey of patients undergoing plastic surgery (Harris, 1982a) included cases of 'developmental disproportion', many of whom resembled those with dysmorphophobia. The author confirmed that self-consciousness had developed in adolescence (compared with those with classic congenital malformations who became aware of their appearance at a much earlier stage), and was often triggered by a chance remark about appearance, rather than enhanced self-awareness. The symptom was then maintained by a variety of reinforcing factors, such as teasing, but of particular interest was the frequent mention of an awareness of being stared at, or remarks made behind the subject's back, similar to ideas of reference (see Chapter 2, p. 19). Finally, severe behavioural avoidance and restriction of lifestyle developed, which further compounded the situation. This will have relevance when treatment is discussed. Harris (1982b) has also argued that innate sensitivities to appearance and aesthetic perception may determine whether a person becomes excessively self-conscious about what may not be a morbid abnormality.

## Reliefs about appearance and all skin diseases

The preceding paragraphs have shown the importance of personality in determining perceived appearance. This is relevant in a number of conditions, which range from dysmorphophobia, to patients with exaggerated reactions to subtle blemishes, and others with genuine skin lesions but of a trivial and perhaps long standing nature.

Wessely and Lewis (1989) found that none of the conventional measures of the severity of skin disease, such as the amount of skin affected, the visibility of the lesion, or any particular diagnosis, correlated with psychological distress in a sample of general dermatology patients. Instead, both the self-report of the impact made by skin disease, and the attitude of the patient towards appearance, correlated with distress. This provides empirical evidence to support the statement that the 'magnitude of the effect [disfigurement] will be related to the subject's self-image and how he relates to others. Any blemish, no matter how small, may be the focus of severe emotional problems in a given patient' (Eller, 1974). Attitudes to appearance provide a link between the 'abnormal' reactions to appearance, as in dysmorphophobia (Harris, 1982b), and 'normal' reactions to skin disease (Wessely & Lewis, 1989).

## Management strategies

It is very difficult to separate the common minor psychiatric conditions encountered in a skin clinic from the effects of skin disease itself, and there is now evidence that in the majority of cases the two are closely related (Wessely & Lewis, 1989). The management of such conditions does not require psychiatric expertise, and should be the responsibility of the dermatologist or general practitioner. The rest of this section will be devoted to the more complex management strategies that may require more skilled psychological assistance.

In general, treatments may be divided into the pharmacological and the psychological, the latter including the various forms of behavioural therapy.

Whatever the condition being treated, the possibility of a concurrent mood disorder must always be remembered. If evidence of depression is found, it should be treated appropriately regardless of whether the clinician considers it to be aetiologically relevant or a consequence of the skin disease. Treatment decisions in psychiatry are still symptom-driven rather than related to diagnosis (Williams, 1979), and the presence of the symptoms of depression is a powerful indication for therapy.

### Treatment of specific syndromes

Once again, it is important to separate the conditions encountered into distinct groups.

**1** *Self-inflicted lesions of minor or moderate severity ('Neurotic excoriations').* Koo *et al.* (1987c) used antidepressants to treat patients with chronic, severe psychogenic excoriations. The results were encouraging. However, all the sample fulfilled criteria for major depression. With regard to non-depressed patients, there is now intriguing evidence that tricyclics may have specific antipruritic activity independent of their mood-elevating effects. This may be a consequence of their antihistaminic properties (Gupta *et al.*, 1987b).

**2** *Trichotillomania.* It has already been noted that trichotillomania is rarely as serious as its name suggests. Some cases may not need direct intervention, or respond to a 'gentle exploration by the physician of changes at home' of the sort required to support a child through a difficult but transient period (Koblenzer, 1983). A variety of approaches are available in more serious cases. Previous enthusiasm for psychoanalytically orientated treatments (Greenberg & Sarner, 1965) has waned and modern therapies using behavioural techniques such as self-monitoring, positive and negative reinforcement and anxiety management are now the treatment of choice (Horne, 1977). These may be carried out by a psychologist or behaviour nurse therapist. The prognosis is related to the severity of the underlying disorder (Krishnan *et al.*, 1985).

**3** *Self-inflicted lesions of greater severity.* Before embarking on any plan of management the physician must decide whether to inform the patient that he/she is aware of the self-inflicted nature of the lesions. This involves confrontation. Opinion is divided as to the propriety of such action.

Many authors, including the dermatologists who take an interest in this condition, advise against confrontation (Lyell, 1979; Cotterill, 1983; Sneddon & Sneddon, 1975; Gomez, 1987). However, Reich and Gottfried (1983) pointed out that the dangers of non-confrontation, such as alienation of the nursing and medical staff, may outweigh those of confrontation. They adopted this strategy in 39 patients and, although only 13 admitted the deception, none subsequently harmed themselves or left the hospital. Millard (1984) also advises against non-confrontation, stating that 'in none of the cases did a benign, empathic supportive role produce any reduction in symptoms; indeed, it was clear that there was reinforcement of the maladjustment', emphasizing the risks of collusion. Millard suggests only one exception, that elderly isolated patients are probably best treated 'without confrontation and allowed their sickness role'.

Who is the most appropriate person to carry out this intervention? As lack of psychological insight is characteristic of the condition, direct psychiatric intervention is liable to be met with tacit or overt hostility, at least initially. The best strategy is a joint medical–psychiatric management, during which a non-challenging supportive role is adopted. It is axiomatic that although the patient should not be encouraged in deception, he or she should still be allowed the status of illness. However, this should be directed towards real rather than fake problems. This may be carried out by either the psychiatrist, or by a physician in close liaison with the psychiatrist. The process does not need to be immediate, and may be performed 'in instalments'. Initial gentle suggestion that the doctor is aware of the deception may be followed later by a more unambiguous confrontation.

A variety of further psychological approaches have been attempted. There is some evidence that insight orientated psychotherapy may produce an exacerbation of symptoms (Seitz, 1953). Given the setting in which most patients present, and the often severe personality disorder in patients with artefacta, this is not surprising. In general, patients who present with skin diseases as a manifestation of psychiatric disorder are likely to deny emotional problems, to lack psychological mindedness, and to be prone to abnormal illness behaviour. These characteristics make them unsuitable for dynamic psychotherapy. The difficulty that many of these patients experience in personal relationships is apparent in their interactions with doctors, no matter how psychotherapeutically skilled.

In the most extreme cases of self-mutilation the lesions themselves may rarely require surgery (Hollender & Abram, 1973), although far more often the task of the doctor is to protect the patient from 'further unnecessary medical and surgical procedures' (Koblenzer, 1983). Whatever management plan is adopted, it is essential to inform the general practitioner.

Published results of treatment in this field are sparse. This is partly a result of the absence of reliable information concerning the natural history of these conditions without treatment; the nature of the disorder determines that many are lost to follow-up. There are no sound outcome studies with the exception of one 2 year study of 12 patients with dermatological patho-mimicry, who were treated with supportive psychotherapy after confrontation. Two-thirds had a good outcome, but one-third relapsed with further self-injury, denied or admitted (Millard, 1987). In classic dermatitis artefacta the prognosis is probably very poor. In one study (Sneddon & Sneddon, 1974; 1975) many patients developed other factitious or conversion symptoms. A recent report of factitious anaemia emphasizes the poor outcome and the failure of psychotherapeutic interventions (Fey & Radvilla, 1988).

## Dysmorphophobic or hypochondriacal beliefs of nondelusional intensity

Two promising lines of behavioural treatment have recently been proposed for both hypochondriacal and dysmorphophobic fears. In the former Warwick and Marks (1988) used a cognitive–behavioural treatment which involved a ban on reassurance, allowing the patient to become exposed to his/her own fears of illness (see Chapter 3, p. 65). In the related condition of dysmor- phophobia a similar emphasis is placed on the maintaining role of avoidance behaviour, noting how patients avoid feared situations because of beliefs about abnormal appearance (Marks & Mishan, 1988). Before treatment, patients were asked which anxiety-evoking situations they avoided because of their dysmophophobic beliefs. Patients were then encouraged to re-enter the avoided situations, to stay there for long periods until the ensuing dis- comfort slowly subsided and to record exposure homework in a daily diary. Measures of particular anxieties and avoidance showed that they reduced as relevant exposure tasks were executed.

Such studies highlight the importance of paying close attention to actual activities, or lack of them, as well as the reported symptoms. However, such treatments would be unlikely to be successful (or even feasible) in patients with an abnormal belief but no associated avoidance behaviour.

There is no evidence that major tranquillizers are effective in dysmopho- phobia when it is not associated with psychosis. However, the distinction can be very difficult in practice, and a trial of therapy may be required to clarify this issue (Birtchnell, 1988).

Finally, the role of plastic surgery in the treatment of disorders of body image remains controversial. Birtchnell (1988) has reviewed the arguments, pointing out that a very careful psychological assessment is needed before surgery can be recommended.


*Psychosis*

*General.*   Before embarking on any treatment of a psychotic condition every effort must be made to establish the diagnosis of either a primary physical illness, or a primary psychiatric disorder, such as affective disorder, schizo- phrenia or paraphrenia. Because many affected patients are old there may be both a physical and psychiatric diagnosis. In those with a major psychiatric illness, the prognosis is better when delusions are part of an affective rather than a paranoid psychosis (Skott, 1978). Vigorous treatment of mood disorder results in symptom resolution even in very elderly patients (Morris & Jolley, 1987). The rest of this section will deal with the treatment of patients with a single isolated delusion.

Not all cases will require treatment. Although delusional parasitosis is regarded as having a poor prognosis if untreated, this may not be so. Macaskill (1987) and Wessely (1987) have reported cases of spontaneous remission, suggesting that the gloomy natural history reported by psychiatrists may partly reflect patterns of referral by dermatologists. In a postal survey of UK dermatologists (Batchelor & Reilly, 1986), one-third of cases had a duration less than 1 year, whilst self-limiting periods of illness were reported in approximately one-quarter of Skott's series. However, this must not be taken as an endorsement of the misguided advice of Zaidens (1951) that patients are best left with their delusions because they serve a protective function. If the delusion persists for more than a few weeks most patients will require treatment.

*Pharmacotherapy.*  Neuroleptics are the drugs of choice. Uncontrolled studies suggest that pimozide, a major tranquillizer of the diphenylbutyl-piperidine class, is effective in delusional parasitosis and other related psychoses (Reilly *et al.*, 1978; Riding & Munro, 1975; Munro, 1982). One study of 11 patients has compared pimozide with placebo in a crossover design, and demonstrated the superiority of the drug over the placebo (Hamann & Avnstrop, 1982). However, there is no study comparing pimozide with other phenothiazines, and given the rarity of the condition and the necessary size of the trial it is unlikely that one will ever be undertaken. Indeed, no acceptable double-blind placebo controlled study of the treatment of any of the disorders such as paranoia, paranoid psychosis or MHP exists (Kendler, personal communication). Instead, the choice of drug is likely to be influenced by personal preference and the range of side-effects. One advantage of pimozide is that it can be given once daily, which aids compliance. The dosage range is 2–12 mg daily. Occasionally drowsiness will be a problem, in which case the drug may be given at night.

All experts acknowledge that persuading patients to take antipsychotic medication is a daunting task. Treatment usually causes a general improvement (Munro, 1988), but some will remain deluded despite treatment with adequate doses (e.g. Hunt & Blacker, 1987).

## Acknowledgements

I thank David Batchelor of Janssen Pharmaceuticals for help with literature, and Mr R. Wessely for help with the German translation.

## References

Agle, D., Ratnoff, O. & Wasman, M. (1969). Conversion reactions in autoerythrocyte sensitisation, *Archives of General Psychiatry*, **20**, 438–447.

Barth, J., Catalan, J., Day, A. & Cherry, C. (1987). Psychological aspects of acne and hirsutes, in *Proceedings of the International Symposium on Dermatology and Psychiatry*, Vienna, May 31–June 2, 1987.

Batchelor, D. & Reilly, T. (1986). Epidemiological aspects of delusional parasitosis in the United

Kingdom, in *Proceedings of the 15th European Conference on Psychosomatic Research* (Eds. Lacey, J. and Sturgeon, D.), John Libby & Co.

Baughman, R. & Sobell, R. (1977). Emotional factors in psoriasis, in *Psoriasis; Proceedings of the 2nd International Symposium*, New York Medical Books, New York, pp. 180–188.

Berrios, G. (1985). Delusional parasitosis and physical disease, *Comprehensive Psychiatry*, **26**, 395–403.

Bers, N. & Conrad, K. (1954). Die chronische taktile halluzinose, *Fortschritte der Neurologie-Psychiatrie*, **22**, 254–270.

Birtchnell, S. (1988). Dysmorphophobia — a centenary discussion, *British Journal of Psychiatry*, **153** (suppl. 2), 41–43.

Burton, J., Rook, A. & Wilkinson, D. (1987). Eczema, lichen simplex and prurigo, in *Textbook of Dermatology* Vol. 3 (Eds. Rook, A., Wilkinson, D., Ebling, F., Champion, R. and Burton, J.) (4th edn.), Blackwell Scientific Publications, Oxford.

Carney, M. (1980). Artefactual illness to attract medical attention, *British Journal of Psychiatry*, **136**, 542–547.

Cassileth, B., Lusk, E., Strouse, T. *et al.* (1984). Psychosocial status in chronic illness: a comparative analysis of six diagnostic groups, *New England Journal of Medicine*, **311**, 506–511.

Connolly, F. & Gipson, M. (1978). Dysmorphophobia — a longterm study, *British Journal of Psychiatry*, **132**, 568–570.

Cossidente, A. & Sarti, M. (1984). Dermatologically expressed psychiatric syndromes, *Clinics in Dermatology*, **2**, 201–220.

Cotterill, J. (1981). Dermatological non-disease: a common and potentially fatal disturbance of cutaneous body image, *British Journal of Dermatology*, **104**, 611–619.

Cotterill, J. (1983). Psychiatry and skin disease, in *Recent Advances in Dermatology* (Eds. Rook, A. and Maibach, H.), Churchill Livingston, Bath.

Dunbar, F. (1954). *Emotions and Bodily Change*, Columbia University Press, New York.

Eckert, J. (1976). Diffuse hair loss in women: the psychopathology of those who complain, *Acta Psychiatrica Scandinavica*, **53**, 321–327.

Edwards, R. (1977). Delusions of parasitosis, *British Medical Journal*, **i**, 1219.

Ekbom, K. (1938). Der presenile dermatozoenwahn, *Acta Psychiatrica et Neurologica Scandinavica*, **13**, 227–259.

Eller, J. (1974). Skin disorders and the psyche, *Cutis*, **13**, 395–416.

Fabisch, W. (1980). Psychiatric aspects of dermatitis artefacta, *British Journal of Dermatology*, **102**, 29–34.

Fey, M. & Radvilla, A. (1988). Long-term followup of factitious anaemia, *British Medical Journal*, **296**, 1504–1505.

Fruensgaard, K. (1987). Disease patterns seen in dermatological cases of factitious illness, in *Proceedings of the International Symposium on Dermatology and Psychiatry*, Vienna, May 31–June 2, 1987.

Fruensgaard, K. & Hjortshoj, A. (1982). Diagnosis of neurotic excoriation, *International Journal of Dermatology*, **21**, 148–151.

Gomez, J. (1987). *Liaison Psychiatry: Mental Health Problems in the General Hospital*, Croom Helm, London.

Greenberg, R. & Sarner, C. (1965). Trichotillomania: symptom and syndrome, *Archives of General Psychiatry*, **12**, 482–489.

Gupta, M., Gupta, A. & Haberman, H. (1986a). Neurotic excoriations: a review and some new perspectives, *Comprehensive Psychiatry*, **27**, 381–386.

Gupta, M., Gupta, A. & Haberman, H. (1986b). Psychotropic drugs in dermatology: A review and guidelines for use, *Journal of the American Academy of Dermatology*, **14**, 633–645.

Gupta, M., Gupta, A. & Haberman, H. (1987a). The self-inflicted dermatoses: a critical review, *General Hospital Psychiatry*, **9**, 45–52.

Gupta, M., Gupta, A. & Ellis, C. (1987b). Antidepressant drugs in dermatology: an update, *Archives of Dermatology*, **123**, 647–652.

Hallopeau, X. (1889). Alopecia par grottage (Trichomania on trichotillomania), *Annales de Dermatologie et Syphilographie*, **10**, 440.

Halprin, K. (1967). The art of self-mutilation. III. Factitial dermatitis or dermatitis artefacta? *Journal of the American Medical Association*, **199**, 155.

Hamann, K. & Avnstrop, C. (1982). Delusions of infestation treated by pimozide: a double-blind cross-over clinical study, *Acta Dermato-Venereologica* (Stockholm), **62**, 55–58.

Hardy, G. & Cotterill, J. (1982). A study of depression and obsessionality in dysmorphophobic and psoriatic patients, *British Journal of Psychiatry*, **140**, 19–22.

Harris, D. (1982a). The symptomatology of abnormal appearance: an anecdotal survey, *British Journal of Plastic Surgery*, **35**, 312–323.

Harris, D. (1982b). Cosmetic surgery: Where does it begin? *British Journal of Plastic Surgery*, **35**, 281.

Hay, G. (1970). Dysmorphophobia, *British Journal of Psychiatry*, **116**, 399–406.

Heng, M. (1982). Lithium carbonate toxicity: acneiform eruption and other manifestations, *Archives of Dermatology*, **118**, 246–248.

Hollender, M. & Abram, H. (1973). Dermatitis factitia, *Southern Medical Journal*, **66**, 1279–1285.

Horne, D. (1977). Behaviour therapy for trichotillomania, *Behaviour Research and Therapy*, **15**, 192–195.

Hubler, W. & Hubler, W. (1980). Folie a deux, *Archives of Dermatology*, **116**, 1303–1304.

Hughes, J., Barraclough, B., Hamblin, L. & White, J. (1983). Psychiatric symptoms in dermatology patients, *British Journal of Psychiatry*, **143**, 51–54.

Hunt, N. & Blacker, V. (1987). Delusional parasitosis (letter), *British Journal of Psychiatry*, **150**, 713–714.

Jobling, R. (1976). Psoriasis — a preliminary questionnaire study of sufferers. Subjective experiences, *Clinical and Experimental Dermatology*, **1**, 233–236.

Jobling, R. (1987). Medicine and the media, *British Medical Journal*, **295**, 1054–1055.

Jones, D. (1983). Dermatitis artefacta in mother and baby as child abuse, *British Journal of Psychiatry*, **143**, 199–200.

Kendler, K. (1987). Paranoid disorders in DSM-III, in *Diagnosis and Classification in Psychiatry: A Critical Appraisal of DSM-III* (Ed. Tischler, G.), Cambridge University Press, Cambridge.

Koblenzer, C. (1983). Psychosomatic concepts in dermatology. A dermatologist-psychoanalyst's viewpoint, *Archives of Dermatology*, **119**, 501–512.

Koo, J., Shellow, W. & Yager, J. (1987a). Psychiatric, immunological and atopic aspects of alopecia areata; an epidemiologic study of 321 patients, in *Proceedings of the International Symposium on Dermatology and Psychiatry*, Vienna, May 31–June 2 1987.

Koo, J., Weiner, H. & Kaplan, R. (1987b). Psychiatric, immunological and psychoimmunological study of atopic dermatitis, in *Proceedings of the International Symposium on Dermatology and Psychiatry*, Vienna, May 31–June 2 1987.

Koo, J., Wintroub, B. & Odom, R. (1987c). Chronic psychogenic excoriation as a manifestation of major depression: a preliminary report of the efficacy of psychopharmacologic treatment, in *Proceedings of the International Symposium on Dermatology and Psychiatry*, Vienna, May 31–June 2 1987.

Krishnan, K., Davidson, J. & Guajardo, C. (1985). Trichotillomania — a review, *Comprehensive Psychiatry*, **26**, 123–128.

Krishnan, R., Davidson, J. & Miller, R. (1984). MAO inhibitors in the treatment of trichotillomania associated with depression, *Journal of Clinical Psychiatry*, **45**, 267–268.

Lamey, P.-J. & Lamb, A. (1988). Prospective study of aetiological factors in the burning mouth syndrome, *British Medical Journal*, **296**, 1243–1246.

Lancet, Leading Article (1983). The matchbox sign, *Lancet*, **ii**, 261.

Lishman, A. (1987). *Organic Psychiatry*, Blackwell Scientific Publications, Oxford.

Lloyd, G. (1983). Medicine without signs, *British Medical Journal*, **287**, 539–542.

Lyell, A. (1979). Cutaneous artefactual disease, *Journal of the American Academy of Dermatology*,

**1**, 391–407.

Lyell, A. (1983). Delusions of parasitosis, *British Journal of Dermatology*, **108**, 485–499.

Macalpine, I. (1954). A critical evaluation of psychosomatic research in relation to dermatology, in *Modern trends in dermatology* (Ed. Mckenna, R.), Butterworth, London.

Macalpine, I. (1957). Syphilophobia, *British Journal of Venereal Diseases*, **33**, 92–99.

Macaskill, N. (1987). Delusion parasitosis: successful non-pharmacological treatment of a folie-a-deux, *British Journal of Psychiatry*, **150**, 261–263.

McKenna, P. (1984). Disorders with overvalued ideas, *British Journal of Psychiatry*, **145**, 579–585.

MacNamara, E. (1928). A note on cutaneous and visual hallucinations in the chronic hallucinatory psychosis, *Lancet*, **i**, 807–808.

Maier, C. (1987). Zum problem des dermatozoenwahnsyndroms, *Nervenarzt*, **58**, 107–115.

Mannino, F. & Delgado, R. (1969). Trichotillomania in children: a review, *American Journal of Psychiatry*, **126**, 505–511.

Marks, I. (1987). *Fears, Phobias and Rituals*, Oxford University Press.

Marks, I. & Mishan, J. (1988). Dysmorphophobic avoidance with disturbed bodily perception: a pilot study of exposure therapy, *British Journal of Psychiatry*, **152**, 674–678.

Mayou, R. & Hawton, K. (1986). Psychiatric disorder in the general hospital, *British Journal of Psychiatry*, **149**, 172–190.

Meadow, R. (1985). Management of Munchausen syndrome by proxy, *Archives of Disease in Childhood*, **60**, 385–393.

Medansky, R. & Handler, R. (1981). Dermatopsychosomatics: classification, physiology and therapeutic approaches, *Journal of the American Academy of Dermatology*, **5**, 125–136.

Melli, C. & Giorgini, S. (1984). Aesthetics in psychosomatic dermatology. 1. Cosmetics, self-image, attractiveness, *Clinics in Dermatology*, **2**, 180–187.

Millard, L. (1984). Dermatological pathomimicry: a form of patient maladjustment, *Lancet*, **ii**, 969–971.

Millard, L. (1987). Dermatological Pathomimicry—a Follow-up Study, *Proceedings of the International Symposium on Dermatology and Psychiatry*, Vienna, May 31–June 2 1987.

Morris, M. & Jolley, D. (1987). Delusional infestation in late life, *British Journal of Psychiatry*, **151**, 272 (correspondence).

Munro, A. (1980). Monosymptomatic hypochondriacal psychosis, *British Journal of Hospital Medicine*, **24**, 34–38.

Munro, A. (1982). *Delusional hypochondriasis: a description of monosymptomatic hypochondriacal psychosis (MHP)*, Clarke Institute of Psychiatry Monograph Series, No 5. University of Toronto.

Munro, A. (1988). Monosymptomatic hypochondriacal psychosis, *British Journal of Psychiatry*, **153** (Suppl. 2), 37–40.

Musaph, H. (1967). Psychogenic pruritus, *Dermatologica*, **135**, 126–136.

Musaph, H. (1976). Psychodermatology, in *Modern Trends in Psychosomatic Medicine* (Ed. Hill, O.), Butterworths, London.

Nadelson, T. (1987). Psychological understanding and management of cutaneous disease, in *Dermatology in General Medicine* (3rd edn.) (Eds. Fitzpatrick, T., Eisen, A., Wolff, K., Freedberg, I. and Austen, K.F.), Macgraw Hill, New York.

Naish, J. (1979). Problems of deception in medical practice, *Lancet*, **ii**, 139–142.

Obermayer, M. (1955). *Psychocutaneous Medicine*, Charles Thomas, Springfield.

Oguchi, T. & Miura, S. (1977). Trichotillomania: its psychopathological aspect, *Comprehensive Psychiatry*, **18**, 177–182.

Oranje, A., Peereboom-Wynia, J. & De Raeymaecker, D. (1986). Trichotillomania in childhood, *Journal of the American Academy of Dermatology*, **15**, 614–619.

Owens, D. & Millard, L. (1987). Psychiatric assessment in dermatological non-disease, in *Proceedings of the International Symposium on Dermatology and Psychiatry*, Vienna, May 31–June 2 1987.

Parker, G. & Lipscombe, P. (1980). The relevance of early learning experiences to adult dependency, hypochondriasis and utilisation of primary physicians, *British Journal of Medical Psychology*, **53**, 355–363.

Perrin, L. (1896). Des nevrodermies parasitophobiques, *Annales de Dermatologie et Syphilographie*, **7**, 129–138.

Pope, F. (1970). Parasitophobia as the presenting symptom of Vitamin $B_{12}$ deficiency, *Practioner*, **204**, 421–422.

Rajka, G. (1966). Investigation of patients suffering from generalised pruritus, *Acta Dermato-Venereologica* (Stockholm), **46**, 190–194.

Reich, P. & Gottfried, L. (1983). Factitious disorders in a teaching hospital, *Annals of Internal Medicine*, **99**, 240–247.

Reilly, T., Jopling, W. & Beard, A. (1978). Successful treatment with pimozide of delusional parasitosis, *British Journal of Dermatology*, **98**, 457–459.

Renvoize, E., Kent, J. & Klar, H. (1987). Delusional infestation and dementia, *British Journal of Psychiatry*, **150**, 403–405.

Riding, J. & Munro, A. (1975). Pimozide in the treatment of monosymptomatic hypochondriacal psychosis, *Acta Psychiatrica Scandinavica*, **52**, 23–30.

Rook, A., Savin, J. & Wilkinson, D. (1987). Psychocutaneous disorders, in *Textbook of Dermatology* Vol. 3 (4th edn.) (Eds. Rook, A., Wilkinson, D., Ebling, F., Champion, R. and Burton, J.), Blackwell Scientific Publications, Oxford.

Rowland Payne, C. (1987). Psoriatic science, *British Medical Journal*, **295**, 1158–1160.

Schaffer, C., Carroll, J. & Abramowitz, S. (1982). Self-mutilation and the borderline personality, *Journal Nervous Mental Disease*, **170**, 468–473.

Schwitzer, J., Meise, U., Gunther, V., Neumann, R. & Schifferle, I. (1987). Etiopathology of Acarophobia, in *Proceedings of the International Symposium on Dermatology and Psychiatry*, Vienna, May 31–June 2 1987.

Seitz, P. (1953). Dynamically-oriented brief psychotherapy: psychocutaneous excoriation syndromes, *Psychosomatic Medicine*, **15**, 200–213.

Seville, R. (1978). Psoriasis and stress II, *British Journal of Dermatology*, **98**, 151–154.

Shelley, W. (1981). Dermatitis artefacta induced in a patient by one of her multiple personalities, *British Journal of Dermatology*, **105**, 587–589.

Sheppard, N., O'Loughlin, S. & Malone, J. (1986). Psychogenic skin disease: a review of 35 cases, *British Journal of Psychiatry*, **149**, 636–643.

Simpson, M. (1976). Self-mutilation, *British Journal of Hospital Medicine*, **16**, 430–438.

Skott, A. (1978). *Delusions of Infestation: Dermatozoenwahn-Ekbom's Syndrome*, Reports from the Psychiatric Research Centre, St. Jorgen Hospital, University of Goteborg, Sweden.

Sneddon, I. & Sneddon, J. (1974). What happens to patients with artefacts? *British Journal of Dermatology*, **91** (Suppl. 10), 29.

Sneddon, I. & Sneddon, J. (1975). Self-inflicted injury. A follow-up study of 43 patients, *British Medical Journal*, **iii**, 527–530.

Snyder, S. (1980). Trichotillomania treated with amitriptyline, *Journal of Nervous and Mental Disease*, **168**, 505–507.

Stankler, L. (1977). Factitious skin disease in a mother and her two sons, *British Journal of Dermatology*, **97**, 217–219.

Thomas, C. (1984). Dysmorphophobia: a question of definition, *British Journal of Psychiatry*, **144**, 513–516.

Warnock, J. & Knesvich, J. (1988). Adverse cutaneous reactions to antidepressants, *American Journal of Psychiatry*, **145**, 425–430.

Warwick, H. & Marks, I. (1988). Behavioural treatment of illness phobia and hypochondriasis: a pilot study of 17 cases, *British Journal of Psychiatry*, **152**, 239–241.

Wessely, S. (1987). Delusional parasitosis (letter), *British Journal of Psychiatry*, **151**, 560–561.

Wessely, S. & Lewis, G. (1989). The classification of psychiatric morbidity in attenders at the dermatology clinic, *British Journal of Psychiatry*, **155**, 686–691.

Whitlock, F. (1976). *Psychophysiological Aspects of Skin Disease*, W.B. Saunders, London.
Williams, P. (1979). Deciding how to treat — the relevance of psychiatric diagnosis, *Psychological Medicine*, **9**, 179–186.
Zaidens, S. (1951). Self-inflicted dermatoses and their psychodynamics, *Journal of Nervous and Mental Disease*, **113**, 395–404.

# 12

## Somatization Disorder: Critique of the Concept and Suggestions for Future Research

C.M. BASS AND M.R. MURPHY

## Introduction

The DSM-III definition of somatization disorder (SD) has evolved from earlier concepts of hysteria and Briquet's syndrome (BS) (Guze & Perley, 1963). All three of these terms denote a chronic relapsing disorder in which patients report multiple, recurrent symptoms that cannot be adequately explained in organic terms. The diagnosis is said to have a high degree of reliability, good validity, stability over time (Guze, 1975), and to be very rare in men (Smith *et al.*, 1986a).

In this chapter we examine the concept of SD and explore some of the reasons for USA/UK differences in prevalence and diagnostic practices. We are currently studying patients with SD, and have experience of managing them in a general hospital setting. We draw on this data and experience to illustrate the points and support arguments raised in this chapter. Finally, we suggest ways in which patients with chronic somatization can be characterized in a more comprehensive and systematic fashion.

### Brief historical review

The development of the concept of somatization disorder in the USA between 1951 and 1980 has been briefly described in Chapter 2 p. 20. Before Purtell and colleagues published their influential descriptive study of 'hysteria' in 1951, most articles and reports in the USA were psychoanalytically orientated. Having started the basic groundwork for a 'medical model' of hysteria these authors urged that further studies should be 'scientific' and not based on 'pure discussion, speculation and the use of psychodynamic concepts'. Purtell thus advocated that 'hysteria' be used as a descriptive term for a polysymptomatic disorder in which physical disease has an insignificant role, but for which the aetiology is obscure.

This move away from psychodynamics to an 'atheoretical' descriptive approach to psychopathology has become a dominant trend in psychiatry in the USA, and in 1980 it was enshrined in DSM-III (see Chapter 2, p. 10). The work which followed Purtell's recommendations for extending the medical model of hysteria reflects this trend. In 1962 Perley and Guze of the Washington University Department of Psychiatry in St Louis proposed a set of operational criteria for the diagnosis of hysteria. These were later incorporated in the Feighner criteria (FC), which were developed in the same department.

These are:

**1**  a chronic or recurrent illness beginning before age 30, presenting with a dramatic, vague, or complicated medical history;

**2**  the patient must report at least 25 medically unexplained symptoms (from a list of 60) for a 'definite' diagnosis and 20 for a 'probable' diagnosis. The 60 symptoms are listed in 10 groups, 9 of which must be represented before a diagnosis can be made (Feighner *et al.*, 1972).

These symptom groups are shown in Table 12.1. In FC the criteria for women and men are identical although one of the ten groups of symptoms (female reproductive symptoms) cannot be endorsed by men.

In 1970 Guze suggested that the term hysteria be replaced by the less pejorative term Briquet's syndrome. When the Research Diagnostic Criteria (RDC) (Spitzer *et al.*, 1978) were developed, Briquet's syndrome was included in the 25 main diagnostic categories but the criteria were further modified. The number of symptom groups was reduced to six — general sickliness, conversion symptoms, gastrointestinal symptoms, female reproductive, sexual dysfunction, and musculoskeletal symptoms. For an RDC diagnosis men must endorse symptoms in four of five groups (1 group is female reproductive symptoms) and women five of six groups. The RDC does not require a minimum symptom count for the diagnosis but age of onset must be before 25.

In 1980, the Task Force on Nomenclature and Statistics of the American Psychiatric Association further modified the concept, called it somatization disorder and distinguished it from conversion disorder, psychogenic pain, and hypochondriasis. The 60-item symptom list used in the diagnosis of hysteria (Briquet's syndrome or BS) was shortened to 37 on the basis of statistical analysis by Guze on his original sample (see Cloninger, 1987, pp. 254–5 for a fuller description of how this was carried out). The purpose of this analysis was to simplify the diagnostic criteria for SD for inclusion in DSM-III. The criteria for SD represented the first major revision of BS and were as follows:

**1**  the total symptom list was reduced from 60 to 37 symptoms (Table 12.2) and all depressive symptoms were eliminated;

**Table 12.1.** The Perley–Guze (1962) criteria for hysteria[*]

Group 1
  Headaches
  Sickly most of life

Group 2
  Blindness
  Paralysis
  Anaesthesia
  Aphonia
  Fits or convulsions
  Unconsciousness
  Amnesia
  Deafness
  Hallucinations
  Urinary retention
  Ataxia
  Other conversion symptoms

Group 3
  Fatigue
  Lump in throat
  Fainting spells
  Visual blurring
  Weakness
  Dysuria

Group 4
  Breathing difficulty
  Palpitation
  Anxiety attacks
  Chest pain
  Dizziness

Group 5
  Anorexia
  Weight loss
  Marked fluctuations in weight
  Nausea
  Abdominal bloating
  Food intolerances
  Diarrhoea
  Constipation

Group 6
  Abdominal pain
  Vomiting

Group 7
  Dysmenorrhoea
  Menstrual irregularity
  Amenorrhoea
  Excessive bleeding

Group 8
  Sexual indifference
  Frigidity
  Dyspareunia
  Other sexual difficulties
  Vomiting 9 months pregnancy or
    hospitalized for hyperemesis
    gravidarum

Group 9
  Back pain
  Joint pain
  Extremity pain
  Burning pains of the sexual
    organs, mouth or rectum
  Other bodily pains

Group 10
  Nervousness
  Depressed feelings
  Need to quit working or inability
    to carry on regular duties
    because of feeling sick
  Crying easily
  Feeling life was hopeless
  Thinking a good deal about dying
  Wanting to die
  Thinking of suicide
  Suicide attempts

[*] Perley and Guze, 1962
(later incorporated in the Feighner criteria, 1972)

**Table 12.2.**   37 Somatization symptoms identified by diagnostic interview schedule (DIS)

| | |
|---|---|
| Pain | Gastrointestinal symptoms |
|   Chest pain |   Excessive gas |
|   Abdominal pain |   Nausea |
|   Back pain |   Diarrhoea |
|   Arm or leg pain |   Food intolerance |
|   Joint pain |   Vomiting (other than during pregnancy) |
|   Painful urination | |
|   Mouth or genital pain | Cardiovascular symptoms |
|   Pain elsewhere |   Heart palpitations |
| |   Dizziness |
| Female reproductive symptoms |   Shortness of breath |
|   Painful periods |   Weakness |
|   Excessive bleeding during periods | |
|   Irregular periods | Psychosexual symptoms |
|   Vomiting throughout pregnancy |   Sexual indifference |
| |   Lack of sexual pleasure |
| Conversion or pseudoneurological symptoms |   Pain during intercourse |
|   Fainting | |
|   Lump in throat | |
|   Blurred vision | |
|   Trouble walking | |
|   Lost voice | |
|   Blindness | |
|   Unusual spells | |
|   Loss of consciousness | |
|   Seizure | |
|   Paralyzed | |
|   Amnesia | |
|   Deafness | |
|   Urinary retention | |

**Table 12.3.**   Comparison of symptom groups of Briquet's syndrome with somatization disorder

| 10 groups of Briquet's syndrome (PDI)* | Number of symptoms | 7 groups of somatization disorder (DSM-III) | Number of symptoms |
|---|---|---|---|
| Conversion | 12 | Conversion | 13 |
| Conversion | 6 | — | — |
| Pain | 4 | Pain | 6 |
| Gastrointestinal (GI) | 2 | GI | 6 |
| Cardiopulmonary | 5 | Cardiopulmonary | 4 |
| GI | 9 | — | — |
| Female reproductive | 4 | Female reproductive | 4 |
| Psychosexual | 6 | Psychosexual | 3 |
| Sickly | 2 | Sickly | 1 |
| Depression | 10 | — | — |
| *Total* | 60 | — | 37 |

* PDI  Indicates psychiatric diagnostic interview.

**2** 10 symptom groups were reduced to 7 (Table 12.3), and the requirement that the symptoms be distributed over groups was dropped;
**3** the total number of symptoms required for a positive diagnosis was reduced from 25 to 14 symptoms in women and 12 symptoms in men.

De Souza and Othmer (1984) attempted to validate these new criteria in a sample of female psychiatric outpatients who reported having multiple unexplained physical problems before age 30. They found that 90% of patients who satisfied criteria did so for both SD and BS, indicating a high concordance between the two sets of criteria. The authors concluded that the new DSM-III criteria were as valid as the Feighner criteria for identification of patients with SD. Because the symptoms list for SD is almost half that of BS the authors argued that the newer criteria made assessment more practical. However, in a more recent study Cloninger *et al.* (1986) demonstrated overlap in only 71% of cases and the authors came to quite different conclusions (see Chapter 2, p. 20).

### Diagnosis of somatization disorder

Because the essence of SD is the presence of multiple unexplained somatic symptoms, establishing a definite diagnosis can be a long and arduous procedure. Several groups of investigators have therefore attempted to develop a short screening index. Othmer and De Souza (1985) showed that the assessment of seven specified symptoms identified 80–90% of cases diagnosed by DSM-III criteria (Table 12.4). Swartz *et al.* (1986b) developed a screening index for use with the DIS — the diagnostic interview schedule used to generate DSM-III diagnoses — in the National Institute of Mental Health sponsored Epidemiological Catchment Area programme (NIMH-ECA) (Regier *et al.*, 1984). They used 11 symptoms and found that the presence of any five correctly identified 97.6% of the patients with DIS/DSM-III SD, while correctly classifying 99% without the disorder (Table 12.5). The authors suggested that the screening index could be used for clinical and community studies of SD.

In the 1987 revised edition of the DSM-III (DSM III-R) the criteria for SD were further slightly modified. The symptom list was reduced to 35 items and the number of symptoms required for the disorder was made the same for males and females (thirteen). On this basis of Othmer and De Souza's findings, seven of the symptoms have been highlighted to serve as a screening test with the suggestion that the presence of any two gives a high probability of the disorder. These seven symptoms are shown in Table 12.4.

Numerous studies of SD have relied exclusively on structured interviews to make the diagnosis — a technique of doubtful reliability. The most widely

**Table 12.4.** Seven symptom screening test for somatization disorder

| Mnemonic | Symptom | Organ system |
| --- | --- | --- |
| **S** omatization | Shortness of breath | Respiratory |
| **D** isorder | Dysmenorrhoea | Female reproductive |
| **B** esets | Burning in sex organs | Psychosexual |
| **L** adies | Lump in throat | Pseudoneurological |
| **A** nd | Amnesia | Pseudoneurological |
| **V** exes | Vomiting | Gastrointestinal |
| **P** hysicians | Painful extremities | Skeletal muscle |

(Reproduced with permission from De Souza & Othmer, 1984, copyright 1984, American Psychiatric Association.)

**Table 12.5.** Distinguishing symptoms in Piedmont Health Survey respondents with DIS/DSM-III somatization disorder (n=3798) (unweighted %)

| | Percentage reporting symptom | | |
| --- | --- | --- | --- |
| Symptom | Somatization disorder positive | Somatization disorder negative | Difference |
| --- | --- | --- | --- |
| Abdominal gas | 90.9 | 13.4 | 77.5 |
| Nausea | 77.3 | 6.2 | 71.1 |
| Diarrhoea | 68.2 | 5.0 | 63.2 |
| Feels sickly | 63.6 | 4.2 | 59.4 |
| Abdominal pain | 68.2 | 9.2 | 59.0 |
| Dizziness | 68.2 | 9.3 | 58.9 |
| Chest pain | 68.2 | 11.6 | 56.6 |
| Fainting spells | 63.6 | 8.0 | 55.6 |
| Pain in extremities | 59.1 | 7.2 | 51.9 |
| Vomiting | 54.6 | 3.7 | 50.9 |
| Weakness | 54.6 | 4.6 | 50.0 |

(Reproduced with permission from Swartz *et al.*, 1986b).

used interview schedule, the DIS, is designed for use by *lay workers*, yet the interviewer has to decide whether each symptom has an organic cause or not. The enquiry covers the patient's entire lifetime and may involve asking about episodes that occurred many decades previously. Our conclusion after using the DIS and comparing responses to data from medical records is that this technique, used alone, is unreliable. Patients often label episodes with spurious diagnostic terms, for example gastrointestinal symptoms are confidently attributed by the patient to her Crohn's disease when medical records indicate that the patient has been investigated for, but does not have, Crohn's disease.

Furthermore, it has been shown that there is significant discordance

(Kappa value of 0.5) between lay interviewers and psychiatrists for the diagnosis of SD using the DIS. In the same study sensitivity was only 41% — the lowest sensitivity of all DSM-III diagnoses (Robins *et al.*, 1982).

A second source of unreliability in making the diagnosis of SD at interview is the tendency of patients with chronic somatization to endorse any question which implies great suffering. In many of our patients this tendency is restricted to physical complaints but in others includes psychiatric symptomatology as well. Thirdly, patients with SD have often been told that their problems are psychological and not physical and that there is no need for further physical investigations. This can lead to patients concealing previous consultations and investigations in the fear that the physician will not take current symptoms 'seriously'. In our own unit we routinely request the general practitioner's casenotes and all previous hospital records before making a diagnosis. We are often surprised by the amount of information that this simple measure brings to light; these notes usually contain information which did not emerge from interviews with the patient and informants.

## Epidemiology

Varying prevalence rates of SD have been reported for different populations (Table 12.6). Rates of 1–2% were cited in early reports, but these were based on small samples of postpartum women. Three studies were conducted at the St Louis Maternity Hospital: Majerus *et al.* (1960) found two cases among 66 women; Murphy *et al.* (1962) identified one case in a sample of 101; and Farley *et al.* (1968) found one (or possibly two) in 100 women. Thus four to five cases of hysteria were found in 267 postpartum women, giving the often quoted figure of 1–2%. But by selecting women in the puerperium the authors were probably inflating their prevalence figures, since this period can be a time of emotional distress and somatic symptoms.

In a questionnaire study of university students, Spalt (1980) found rates of 23.5% in women and 13% in men—extraordinarily high rates which must certainly be a consequence of invalid questionnaire methodology.

In psychiatric outpatient populations prevalence rates of 6% have been reported (De Souza and Othmer, 1984). Similar high prevalence was found at the Washington University Medical Centre, where rates of 10% were recorded in psychiatric inpatients (Bibb & Guze, 1972) and 11% in psychiatric outpatients (Woodruff *et al.*, 1971). More recently Orenstein (1989) found definite Briquet's syndrome in 9% of 188 consecutive female psychiatric patients. (In this study patients were excluded if they had a history of psychosis, were currently suffering from an organic mental disorder or involved in legal or disability evaluations.) Purtell *et al.* (1951) reported rates of 12% in

**Table 12.6.**   Prevalence of somatization disorder

| Authors | Year | Rate (%) |
|---|---|---|
| *Non-psychiatric population-based studies* | | |
| Majerus *et al.*[1] | 1960 ⎤ | |
| Murphy *et al.*[1] | 1962 ⎬ | 1–2 |
| Farley *et al.*[1] | 1968 ⎦ | |
| Weissman *et al.*[2] | 1978 | 0.40 |
| Deighton & Nicol[3] | 1985 | 0.20 |
| Swartz *et al.*[4] | 1986 | 0.38 |
| Spalt *et al.*[5] | 1980 | ⎧ 23.5 (F) ⎨ 13.0 (M) |
| Swartz *et al.*[6] | 1987 | 0.67 |
| *Psychiatric populations* | | |
| Purtell *et al.*[7] | 1951 | 12.0 |
| Woodruff *et al.*[8] | 1971 | 11.0 |
| De Souza & Othmer[8] | 1984 | 5.7 |
| Orenstein[8] | 1989 | 9.0 |
| Bibb & Guze[9] | 1972 | 10.0 |

[1] Studies of small samples of women in the puerperium.
[2] Study included whole population, including males; used SADS-S and RDC criteria.
[3] UK study of women aged 16–25.
[4] NIMH-ECA study; used DIS and DSM-III criteria.
[5] Questionnaire-based study of university students.
[6] See text.
[7] Medical and surgical inpatients referred for psychiatric opinion.
[8] Psychiatric outpatients.
[9] Psychiatric inpatients.

a medical/surgical inpatient population referred for psychiatric assessment.

In a household survey of adults over 18 in an urban community Weissman *et al.* (1978) found a prevalence of 0.4% for SD. In the NIMH-ECA study, five sites geographically distributed throughout the USA (New Haven, East Baltimore, St Louis, the Piedmont region of North Carolina, and East Los Angeles) were randomly sampled. The highest rate of SD — 0.38% — was found in North Carolina (Swartz *et al.*, 1986b), but considerably lower rates (0.03% to 0.1%) were found at other sites (Escobar *et al.*, 1987; Myers *et al.*, 1984). Two-thirds of the cases of SD in North Carolina were from rural counties, a finding that suggests SD is more common in southern rural communities.

In a recent study that used three sets of diagnostic criteria (Feighner criteria, Research Diagnostic Criteria, and DSM-III criteria), Swartz *et al.* (1987) found a prevalence rate of SD of 0.67%. Cases were identified if they satisfied any one of the three sets of criteria. Feighner criteria identified the fewest cases, followed by DSM-III criteria and the RDC criteria. Like De Souza and Othmer (1984), Swartz *et al.* (1987) found that diagnostic concordance was highest for Feighner criteria vs. DSM-III criteria (79%).

In the only UK prevalence study, Deighton and Nicol (1985) reported a rate of 0.2% in women aged 16–25 drawn from one large family practice. This figure is not comparable with US findings because of the young age group studied.

In summary, the commonly cited prevalence rates of 1–2% are almost certainly overestimates. More recent community studies using better methodology have found rates of between 0.4 and 0.7%.

## USA/UK differences in diagnosis (and clinical interest)

It is surprising that a clinical syndrome with a reported prevalence approaching 1% in the USA is seldom mentioned in UK journals and textbooks. There are two possible explanations. Either the disorder is very uncommon in the UK, or UK psychiatrists see patients with similar characteristics but call it something else. We suspect that both are true.

The UK prevalence study mentioned above requires careful interpretation: its authors stated that many patients with high consultation rates had features characteristic of Briquet's syndrome but failed to satisfy its stringent diagnostic criteria. They considered the criteria to be unduly restrictive because they excluded a substantial number of patients with abnormal illness behaviour, multiple functional complaints and other psychosocial characteristics associated with Briquet's syndrome. Their findings suggest that the disorder is not the discrete syndrome claimed by Guze *et al.* (1986).

Other evidence that the disorder is more common in the USA comes from studies carried out in general hospitals. Lloyd (1986) studied 85 referrals to a liaison service with 'somatization' and compared psychiatric diagnoses in his sample with two similarly ascertained USA samples. The somatoform disorders were diagnosed more frequently in the USA and they formed the largest group in studies by Slavney and Teitelbaum (1985) and Katon *et al.* (1984); more specifically there was only one UK patient with somatization disorder compared with 6% in Katon's series and 8% in Slavney and Teitelbaum's series.

The reasons for a greater prevalence of this syndrome in the USA could be related to cultural factors or to health care delivery. It is possible that differences between USA and UK health care systems contribute to the higher prevalence of this disorder in the USA. For example, widespread medical insurance makes it easier for patients to gain direct access to hospital specialists without being initially 'screened' by the family doctor. In Britain the family practitioner serves an important 'gatekeeper' function which might protect patients from needless overinvestigation in hospital (Bass & Murphy, 1990).

The second possibility — that a disorder with the characteristics of SD is called something else in the UK, e.g. affective disorder or personality disorder — is also likely. It is not difficult to make an alternative diagnosis in most cases of SD: more than three-quarters of patients satisfy criteria for an additional DSM-III diagnosis if exclusion criteria (see Chapter 2, p. 22) are not used (Swartz *et al.*, 1986a). A study of the sort that compared USA/UK diagnostic practices in schizophrenia would be required to establish these facts. However, virtually all the cases that we have diagnosed as having SD have received alternative diagnoses when a previous psychiatric assessment has taken place.

UK psychiatrists tend to be reluctant to diagnose 'hysteria'. This can, in part, be traced to two influential papers by Slater (1961, 1965), who criticized the American view that hysteria was a unitary syndrome. He did not support the view that these patients comprised a sufficiently homogeneous group to warrant the term and commented that the stability of the diagnosis over time was supplied by the criteria for selection. That is to say, patients who have been ill for long enough to satisfy the criteria for hysteria or Briquet's syndrome are likely to remain ill when studied some years later. Slater's own follow-up study of 85 patients given a diagnosis of hysteria in a neurological hospital confirmed his belief that the concept of hysteria 'fragments as we touch it'. A mean period of 9 years after the diagnosis one-third of Slater's patients were found to have an organic disorder. A residual group comprising only 14 patients (16%) had a disorder satisfying the criteria proposed by Guze.

Slater's conclusions can be criticized on two counts. First, in two-thirds of the patients the diagnosis of hysteria was made in a tertiary referral hospital for neurological diseases. The sample studied is likely to have been biased towards atypical cases in whom diagnosis had proved difficult. Second, Slater's series contained a higher proportion of patients with acute conversion reactions than those with the chronic polysymptomatic disorder. Nevertheless, others share Slater's view that hysteria is a spurious entity. Noting that most of the research studies on SD are from four centres (St Louis, Kansas City, Arkansas, and Iowa City) in the mid-Western USA (Fig. 12.1) Vaillant (1984) has cynically remarked that SD is 'as regional as Kuru', and that 'the diagnosis lies in the eyes of the beholder'.

One interesting recent development has been the inclusion in the ICD-10 draft (WHO, 1987) of a less stringently defined version of SD. This disorder (multiple somatization disorder or MSD) has been defined as follows:

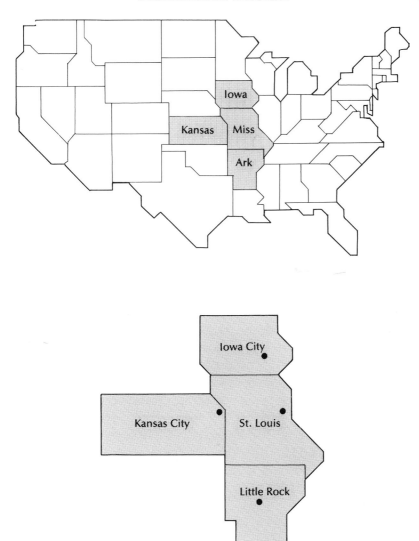

**Fig. 12.1.** Map of the USA showing the four states (Kansas, Iowa, Missouri and Arkansas) from which over 95% of research reports on somatization disorder (Briquet's syndrome) have been published.

**1** At least 2 years of multiple and variable physical symptoms for which no adequate physical explanation has been found;

**2** Persistent refusal to accept advice or reassurance of several different doctors that there is no physical explanation for the symptoms;

**3** Some degree of impairment of social and family functioning attributable to the nature of the symptoms and resulting behaviour.

To date there have been few systematic studies of chronic somatization in Britain. Perhaps publication of ICD-10 will provide the necessary impetus.

## Clinical features of patients with somatization disorder (SD)

### Sociodemographic characteristics

The investigators responsible for the Epidemiologic Catchment Area programme of the NIMH reported that SD was found almost exclusively among women, and was more common among Black people and the less educated. Sufferers were more often separated from a spouse or partner and used the health services more than the rest of the community (Swartz *et al.*, 1988). The authors also remarked that SD appeared to be more common in the southern rural communities of the USA than in northern and industrial areas.

In another important study of a community sample of mixed ethnicity in Los Angeles, Escobar *et al.* (1987) found that Mexican-American women over the age of 40 somatized more than other groups regardless of diagnostic status. Furthermore, those Mexican-American women who had largely assimilated the values of the host culture somatized *less* than those who had not. These findings support previous cross-cultural observations (Kirmayer, 1984).

### Psychiatric diagnoses (Axis I)

The diagnosis of SD (DSM-III-R criteria, 1987) requires a complicated and dramatic medical history beginning before the age of 30. In addition, 13 of 35 medically unexplained symptoms must have occurred. *No mental state symptoms need to be elicited for the diagnosis.* The associated psychopathology in SD has been relatively neglected, and it is fair to say that 'symptom counts' have preoccupied clinicians and researchers at the expense of methodical descriptions of psychopathology.

It is particularly surprising, for example, that so little attention has been paid to the occurrence of phobic disorders in patients with SD. Many of the somatic symptoms listed for SD occur with anxiety disorders, yet not all studies have reported a high prevalence of concurrent anxiety disorders in SD patients. One reason for this might be that when Feighner criteria were employed (Feighner *et al.*, 1972) the diagnosis of anxiety neurosis (approximately equivalent to DSM-III panic disorder) could not be made 'in the presence of other psychiatric illness' unless symptoms of anxiety neurosis 'antedate the onset of the other psychiatric illness by at least two years'. It is also explicitly stated that 'patients with another definable psychiatric illness should not receive the additional diagnosis of phobic neurosis'. Therefore, with the Feighner criteria, symptoms of anxiety were regarded as part of Briquet's syndrome (see below).

There have been few studies of concurrent psychiatric syndromes in patients with SD. But the consensus from studies published since 1980 is that SD has heterogeneous psychopathology and that the diagnosis of Briquet's syndrome or SD should not rule out the possibility of other psychiatric diagnoses. It is not clear how SD and coexisting psychopathological syndromes interact to affect the course, prognosis, and treatment of either the SD or coexisting disorders.

One consistent finding is that patients with SD have a high lifetime prevalence of affective disorders. In a study of 78 female outpatients who met the diagnostic criteria for Briquet's syndrome, only one had no other psychiatric diagnosis in addition to Briquet's syndrome (Liskow *et al.*, 1986a). Using a structured interview (the Psychiatric Diagnostic Interview) based on that devised by Feighner *et al.* (1972), the authors calculated the lifetime prevalence of 15 basic syndromes among these 78 patients (Table 12.7). The high rates for depression, panic disorder and phobic disorder might not be surprising, but the high percentage of mania and schizophrenia were unexpected. How can these findings be explained? First, we have already remarked that SD patients may endorse a great number of psychiatric symptoms, just as they report a great number of medical symptoms, and thus appear spuriously to have a multitude of psychiatric syndromes. This possibility has not been discounted (Liskow *et al.*, 1986b). Second, Briquet's syndrome is inherently associated with a broad spectrum of heterogeneous psychiatric symptomatology so that a variety of other syndromes can be diagnosed. A fuller understanding of the pathogenesis and psychopathology of SD might be achieved if the onset, course and duration of these concurrent syndromes were studied in relation to each other. Similarly, other factors such as personality and psychophysiological variables which might influence the clinical picture need to be considered (see below).

Further evidence of heterogeneity was provided by Zoccolillo and Cloninger (1986) in a retrospective case note study of 50 women who satisfied the criteria for both Briquet's syndrome (Feighner criteria) and SD (DSM-III). They found that 60% of cases had at least one other diagnosis, the most frequent being major depression (52%). Twenty-four per cent had a psychiatric diagnosis other than major depression, most often drug or alcohol abuse or panic disorder (Table 12.7).

Persuasive evidence suggests that SD is probably also confounded with panic disorder (PD) (Katon, 1984). For example, Sheehan and Sheehan (1982) found that 71% of agoraphobic patients met the criteria for Briquet's syn-

**Table 12.7.** Prevalence of additional psychiatric syndromes in patients with somatization disorder (SD)

| Study | Liskow et al. (1986a)[1] (%) | Swartz et al. (1986a)[2] (%) | Zoccolillo & Cloninger (1986)[3] (%) | Liskow et al. (1986b)[4] (%) |
|---|---|---|---|---|
| Major depression | 87 | 65 | 52 | 94 |
| Agoraphobia | — | 64 | 2 | — |
| Panic disorder | 45 | 43 | 10 | 31 |
| Phobic disorder[5] | 39 | — | — | 25 |
| Social phobia | — | 30 | — | — |
| Obsessive compulsive disorder | 27 | 52 | — | 50 |
| Drug dependence | 23 | — | | 31 |
| Alcohol dependence | 17 | 18 | | 31 |
| Atypical bipolar disorder | — | 35 | — | — |
| Mania | 40 | — | — | 38 |
| Anorexia nervosa | 6 | — | 2 | 0 |
| Antisocial personality disorder | 17 | — | 6 | 25 |
| Schizophrenia | 27 | 38 | 0 | 38 |

[1] 78 female psychiatric outpatients with Briquet's syndrome; diagnosis with Psychiatric Interview or PDI (lifetime prevalence).
[2] 15 patients with SD, diagnosed in community survey using DIS (weighted % given).
[3] Retrospective case note survey of 50 women who met Feighner criteria for Briquet's syndrome and DSM-III criteria for SD. Schizophrenics *excluded*; no patient interviewed.
[4] 16 female psychiatric inpatients with Briquet's syndrome; diagnosis with PDI. Note similarity in prevalence rates to column 1 (study also used PDI).
[5] In the Swartz *et al.* study (column 2) there was a prevalence rate of 70% for 'simple phobia'.

drome. The NIMH-ECA study also points to the confusion between the diagnoses of panic disorder and somatization disorder (Boyd *et al.*, 1984). The data from this large psychiatric epidemiological survey of five American cities demonstrated that patients who met DSM-III criteria for SD were 96 times more likely also to meet criteria for PD than if they did not meet criteria for SD.

In another study King *et al.* (1986) compared 44 patients with PD with 27 non-anxious controls. They found that the PD patients had more somatic symptoms as well as greater awareness of cardiovascular and gastrointestinal sensations than controls. Moreover, more than a quarter of the 44 panic patients also qualified for a DSM-III diagnosis of SD, i.e. they reported more than 14 of the requisite 37 symptoms. Somatization was furthermore associated with higher levels of phobic avoidance and with reported visceral sensitivity. The authors concluded that the factors underlying the relationship between panic attacks and somatization require further study.

Our own findings are consistent with these latter studies. One-half of our patients with SD have either a previous history or current evidence of agoraphobia with extensive avoidance, and measures of phobic avoidance on both the Fear Questionnaire (Marks & Mathews, 1979) and SCL-90 (Derogatis *et al.*, 1973) are significantly higher than in controls. Thus, panic disorder (with or without phobic avoidance) appears to be the most frequent con-current Axis I diagnosis in our sample.

Orenstein (1989) found that patients with Briquet's syndrome were more likely to have a lifetime history of major depression and either panic disorder or agoraphobia than with major depression or panic disorder/agoraphobia alone. These findings suggest that somatization disorder involves the complex aggregation of both psychiatric and physical symptoms. It is also worth noting that agoraphobic patients have elevated rates of alcoholism (Smail *et al.*, 1984; Stockwell *et al.*, 1984), which is also common among the first degree relatives of patients with Briquet's syndrome.

This co-occurrence of Axis I disturbances may be an important deter-minant of chronic somatization. But disorders classified on other Axes may also be relevant to its development. These may include personality disorder; a coexisting medical disorder (which may be iatrogenic); or a psychophysio-logical disorder such as hyperventilation. In patients with SD several of these factors may be identified as significant in the aetiology through their inter-actions with each other and with the patient's environment.

**Personality disorder in Briquet's syndrome (Axis II)**

There has often been a tendency for psychiatrists to regard patients as suffering from *either* a psychiatric illness *or* a personality disorder. More recently as-sessment of personality has been regarded as a separate axis of classification. Tyrer (1989) has remarked that the population can be divided into four diag-nostic groups: (i) those with no mental illness and a personality disorder; (ii) those with a mental state disorder and a normal personality; (iii) those with no mental illness and no personality disorder; and (iv) those with both a mental state disorder and a personality disorder.

Most of the literature that deals with the relationship between personality and chronic hysteria is either psychoanalytical or concerned with the category of hysterical (histrionic) personality disorder. There is however, little sys-tematic descriptive research on the personalities of patients who chronically somatize. This neglect may be related to the uncertain nosological status of personality disorder and the lack of reliable methods of assessment. The diagnosis of personality disorder can also have pejorative connotations and some psychiatrists regard it as a way of blaming the patient for failing to respond to treatment. An additional problem arises in patients who are chronically ill for whom the development of personality and development of illness are inextricably linked. Nevertheless, it should be possible to assess personality traits systematically in chronically ill patients and in some instances obtain information about personality functioning before the onset of the somatizing illness.

Kaminsky and Slavney (1976) have suggested that a disease model is inappropriate to our understanding of the aetiology and mechanisms involved in somatization disorder. They also suggested that personality characteristics were likely to give the condition both its stability and its recalcitrance to treatment, and that SD could be meaningfully understood not as an illness but as a set of behaviours arising from an abnormal personality.

In a subsequent study of 20 patients meeting criteria for Briquet's syndrome and another 20 with hysterical personality disorder they found that Briquet patients, though manifesting similar hysterical traits, had more obsessional features than the patients with hysterical personality disorder (Kaminsky & Slavney, 1983). That is to say, Briquet patients exhibit traits of emotional lability and self-dramatization *in addition to* perfectionism and a tendency to monitor bodily sensations carefully. Presumably this obsessionality contributes to the complaint behaviour that is so characteristic of these patients.

The DSM-III's adoption of a multiaxial approach offers a framework for empirical study of the relationship between illness (Axis I) and personality (Axis II). Several schedules have been designed to identify the criteria of operationally defined personality disorders. Two schedules have been devised by UK authors, both of which make use of an informant other than the patient. One generates DSM-III axis II diagnoses (Mann *et al.*, 1981) and the other, the Personality Assessment Schedule or PAS, derives computer-coded categories of personality disorder very similar to the ICD-10 classification of personality disorders (Tyrer *et al.*, 1979; Tyrer & Alexander, 1987; Chapter 3).

### Physical disorders (Axis III)

There is little doubt that the presence of coexisting medical disorders makes the assessment of patients with SD more complicated. As with personality, medical disorders have received little attention in SD. Data from a study of acute somatization in primary care shows that physical illness often coexists with somatic presentations of psychiatric disorder (Bridges & Goldberg, 1985). Indeed, somatization in this setting is more likely to occur with physical illness than without it (Chapter 4, pp. 81–2).

**Table 12.8.** Physical illness in patients with somatization disorder

| Diagnoses | Number (%) of patients |
|---|---|
| Hypertension | 9 (22) |
| Adult-onset diabetes mellitus | 6 (15) |
| Musculoskeletal disorders, including degenerative disc disease, degenerative joint disease, and herniated disc disease | 11 (27) |
| Haemorrhoids | 4 (10) |
| Hiatus hernia | 2 (5) |
| Upper respiratory tract infection: | |
|    Chronic obstructive pulmonary disease | 5 (12) |
|    Bronchitis | 4 (10) |
| Pregnancy without complication | 2 (5) |
| Hypothyroidism | 2 (5) |
| Urticaria | 2 (5) |
| Mitral valve prolapse | 2 (5) |
| Iron-deficiency anaemia | 3 (7) |

(Reproduced with permission from Smith *et al.*, 1986a, copyright 1986, American Medical Association.)

It is our impression that patients with SD, who make frequent visits to specialized hospital units, are also more likely to be suffering from chronic diseases, such as diabetes mellitus. There is very little published data on this relationship, and only one recent study has provided details of physical illness in patients with SD (Smith *et al.*, 1986a; Table 12.8).

We have previously argued that the doctor's role in the genesis of SD has been neglected (Bass & Murphy, 1990). Somatization disorder cannot evolve without the unwitting complicity of the doctor. Patients who somatize may be prescribed unnecessary medication, undergo invasive investigations and may be the victims of iatrogenic illness. Steel *et al.* (1981) found that over one-third of patients admitted to the general service of a university hospital in the USA developed an iatrogenic illness (adverse drug reactions being the most common). In 9% of all admissions the iatrogenic event had threatened life or produced considerable disability. These figures suggest that patients with SD are exposed to a considerable risk of iatrogenic disease.

Patients with SD are often subjected to unnecessary surgery (Cohen *et al.*, 1953; Martin *et al.*, 1977) which, in addition to exposing the patient to unnecessary medical risks, may aggravate the functional disability associated with SD. To illustrate this point, one of our patients with SD developed a femoral artery thrombosis after her *third* normal coronary angiogram. After repeated ileo-femoral surgery she developed an hysterical paresis of both legs and became wheelchair-bound. Although her new illness is non-organic it can be considered iatrogenic.

Medical illness in childhood may also contribute to the development of chronic somatization, as may a family environment which encourages the somatic manifestation of distress (see Chapter 3, p. 42 for further discussion). Our own clinical impression is that lengthy hospitalization for conditions such as rheumatic fever, especially in cases where the family environment has been hostile or emotionally impoverished, can shape subsequent illness behaviour. This suggests that somatization can be a form of 'care-eliciting' behaviour (Henderson, 1974). For example, one of our patients with SD had numerous hospital admissions between 2 to 5 years for diabetes and, according to her mother, called the ward sister 'Mommy' throughout most of that period.

### Abnormal psychosocial stressors and situations (Axis IV)

There has been little systematic research in this field. However, the relationship between adverse life events and somatization, referred to elsewhere in this book, suggests that these are of great importance in patients with SD. The relationship between SD and abnormal psychosocial situations is likely to be complex: marital, occupational and family problems are commonplace and are likely to be both a consequence and a cause of further psychosocial impairment.

Not surprisingly, indices of poor parenting, as measured by child abuse or the removal of the child from home, are more common in women with SD than in age-matched depressed controls (Zoccolillo & Cloninger, 1985). This latter point is demonstrated in the following case example:

> A 57-year-old woman was the fifth of six children who was reared by an uncaring and rejecting mother. Her father died when she was 15 and following this she had a depressive illness with fatigue as a prominent symptom. Subsequently she developed panics and agoraphobia which remain to this day. She contracted an early and unhappy marriage, and after giving birth to two sons her husband deserted her. She began drinking heavily, had a succession of male friends and neglected her children. When her youngest son was 14 he ran away from home and was not seen for 10 years. As an adult he has ambivalent feelings about his mother and this is reflected in alternately abusive and submissive behaviour. Arguments with him lead to aggravation of her physical symptoms. Her older son became delinquent, spent his adolescence in an institution, and as an adult refuses to see his mother, although he abuses her on the telephone. Having neglected her own children, this solitary woman now suffers relapses (which present somatically to general hospitals) whenever she comes into conflict with her sons.

Women with SD are likely to marry men with alcohol problems, and, like the woman described, are more likely than depressed controls to marry anti-social men (Zoccolillo & Cloninger, 1986). In the British study previously referred to, patients with 'high functional complaints' were more likely than controls to be separated or divorced, to be unemployed, to have relatives with chronic recurrent hospitalizations and to admit to drinking problems (Deighton & Nicol, 1985).

## Disabilities (Axis V)

Many patients with SD are unemployed and in receipt of disability benefits. Zoccolillo and Cloninger (1986) found that women with SD were more likely than depressed controls to have left work for medical/psychiatric reasons and to be 'socially disabled'. In the months before diagnosis, Smith *et al.* (1986a) found that patients with SD reported a mean of seven (SD=8.8) days that ill health kept them in bed most or all of the day (range 0–30). This compared with only 0.48 days in bed per month for a general population group. The functional disability of this sample was further demonstrated by their report that 83% had stopped work because of their health. Our own findings support these high rates of disability in patients with SD: 10% of our sample are confined to wheelchairs.

# The origin of symptoms in SD

Before a symptom can count towards the requisite 13 necessary for a diagnosis of SD it must satisfy the criterion that *no* 'pathophysiologic mechanism' accounts for its production. It is not specified in the criteria for SD that increased autonomic activity or musculoskeletal tension are included in this term. (This is a peculiar omission, given that the examples of 'pathophysiological mechanisms' listed are less likely to be a source of confusion: 'e.g. a physical disorder or the effects of injury, medication, drugs, or alcohol'). Yet many of the 35 listed symptoms of SD are commonly autonomically mediated, for example palpitations.

This ambiguity is made worse by two further statements. First, it is specified that symptoms that occur during a panic attack cannot be counted unless they occur at other times as well. For example, if a patient experiences palpitations, and at the same time has 3 other physical symptoms (criteria for panic attack) then the symptom does not count. If, however, the patient then has palpitations without sufficient other symptoms for the diagnosis of a panic attack, then palpitations can count as a symptom of SD. The inference here is that somatic manifestations of anxiety (short of panic) can be counted.

This conclusion, however, is contradicted in the introduction to the chapter on Somatoform Disorders which states that: 'Although the symptoms of somatoform disorders are "physical", the specific pathophysiologic processes involved are not demonstrable or understandable by existing laboratory procedures and are conceptualized most clearly by means of psychological constructs'. But symptoms such as palpitations, diarrhoea, irregular menstrual periods and dizziness (all symptoms of SD) have often been shown to result from pathophysiological processes accompanying anxiety and stress. Increased sympathetic nervous system activity and catecholamine release, increased gastrointestinal motility, hypothalamo–pituitary–gonadal axis disturbance and hyperventilation could account for each of these symptoms respectively. But as the diagnosis of SD usually relies on eliciting a past history of these symptoms it is very difficult to know whether these 'specific pathophysiologic processes' were involved or not.

**Psychophysiological studies**

Interest in this topic was stimulated by Meares and Horvath (1972), who compared 6 patients with short-lived conversion symptoms with a 'chronic polysymptomatic group of 11 patients who had sought treatment over an extended period for symptoms in most organ systems'. This latter group presumably resembled patients with SD. The authors measured skin resistance, resting heart rate, frontalis EMG and habituation to an auditory stimulus, in addition to psychometric data. The patients were easily divisible on physiological grounds: none of the patients in the 'chronic' group habituated to a stimulus that was presented 20 times, whereas all the patients with the transient conversion symptoms habituated at a rate which was similar to normals (Chapter 8, p. 222). Furthermore, the chronic group had significantly higher rates of spontaneous fluctuation of skin conductance per minute, higher mean resting heart rate, and higher mean frontalis EMG activity than the acute group. Interestingly, these patients with evidence of physiological arousal also had high scores on measures of neuroticism and state anxiety, yet despite this their 'manner belied their emotional state'. This suggests that although anxiety may have been experienced, it was neither reported by the patients nor apparent to observers.

In a subsequent study Horvath *et al.* (1980) concluded that this failure to habituate was *not* a function of abnormally high levels of arousal; rather, they suggested that these patients may have an impaired ability to filter out or not attend to irrelevant afferent stimuli. This latter hypothesis was investigated by Gordon *et al.* (1986) who compared 15 patients with SD with age and sex matched normal controls. Evoked response potentials (ERPs) were used to assess cognitive processing of relevant and comparatively irrelevant auditory afferent stimuli, and the authors hypothesized that if SD is associated with impairments in stimulus processing and/or attention, then this will be manifest as an abnormality of P3 responses, a component which to some extent reflects both processes. They found that subjects with SD showed normal P3 auditory evoked potentials, as compared with anxiety state patients and normal controls. However, the amplitude of their N1 component responses to background tones, which they had been told to ignore, was significantly greater than for other groups (Gordon *et al.*, 1986), and their N1 responses to background and target tones did not differ. These preliminary findings suggest that in SD there is an impaired ability to filter out and *not* respond to meaningless stimuli.

### Hyperventilation and chronic somatization

There is another possible pathophysiological explanation for the high lifetime rates of symptoms reported by patients with SD. Chronic hyperventilation (HV) is common in general hospital outpatient clinics and has been extensively studied during the last 30 years (Lewis, 1954; Lum, 1976; Gardner & Bass, 1989). Accounts of this disorder are usually published in medical rather than psychiatric journals. It has been estimated to occur in 5–10% of medical outpatients (Lum, 1981), although rates vary according to the medical specialty. For example, rates are likely to be much higher in cardiac than dermatology clinics. The symptoms produced by HV are not only diverse but also have the potential to become chronic. It is not clear how or why this happens, but it may be the consequence of either an abnormality in the central control of

**Table 12.9.** The most frequently reported symptoms in patients with somatization disorder

| Symptom | Number (%) of patients |
|---|---|
| Chest pain | 37 (90) |
| Palpitations | 35 (85) |
| Abdominal bloating | 35 (85) |
| Depressed feelings | 34 (83) |
| Dizziness | 34 (83) |
| Weakness | 34 (83) |
| Quitting work because of health | 34 (83) |
| Shortness of breath | 33 (81) |
| Headache | 32 (78) |
| Fatigue | 31 (76) |

(Reproduced with permission from Smith *et al.*, 1986a, copyright 1986, American Medical Association.)

breathing (Gardner *et al.*, 1986), or the result of 'habit' (Lum, 1976; Magarian, 1982). But once chronic HV has become established the patient has the potential to develop multiple and diverse somatic complaints, which may or may not be associated with conspicuous psychiatric symptoms.

It is possible that chronic HV could generate symptoms in some patients with SD. To our knowledge this question has not been studied in a systematic manner but there is circumstantial evidence to support this view. Smith *et al.* (1986a) studied 41 patients with SD and noted that the most common somatic complaints were chest pain, palpitations, abdominal bloating, dizziness, weakness and shortness of breath (Table 12.9). These symptoms have a striking resemblance to HV, and suggest that future studies of patients with SD should include measures of respiratory variables such as end-tidal $P_{CO_2}$, respiratory rate, and breath-holding time. We are currently studying these variables in patients with SD in our unit.

## Management

There have been few systematic intervention studies in SD. Effective intervention might have a considerable economic impact given the high prevalence of SD in general hospitals. Perhaps investigators have been deterred from embarking on treatment studies because these patients are so difficult to treat psychiatrically. In fact, refusal to accept a psychiatric approach to their condition appears to be characteristic of patients with this disorder. Nearly 30 years ago Guze and Purley (1963) noted that very few patients with this diagnosis (hysteria) were interested in psychotherapy, and most rejected a psychiatric approach to their complaints.

Our account of treatment will be discussed from the perspective of the psychiatrist working in the outpatient department of a general hospital. Although these patients can be managed by family doctors, their demanding and occasionally disruptive behaviour and need for numerous prolonged consultations may be better managed by a psychiatrist experienced with such patients.

Treatment of SD must be directed towards controlling the demands on medical care as well as the treatment of the symptoms and social disability. In essence it involves long term supportive psychotherapy and our approach is based on the writings of Wahl (1963), Brown and Vaillant (1981), Smith (1985), and Bloch (1986).

Establishing the diagnosis is an important first step. This usually takes time because a considerable amount of information has to be collected from a variety of sources, including a reliable informant, previous hospital notes, and discussion with the patient's general practitioner.

Secondly, it is important for one person to take overall responsibility for the management of the patient. The responsibility should not be taken lightly, because organizing and maintaining a management plan for these patients can be a very taxing job. By establishing a long term supportive relationship, the opportunities and need for repeated 'doctor-shopping' can be reduced and unnecessary diagnostic procedures may be avoided. The psychiatrist in overall charge should communicate with other agencies, for example Social Services, health visitors, general practitioner, in order to prevent the treatment plan being sabotaged by other health care professionals involved with the patient.

Thirdly, patients should not be seen 'on demand' but be given regular appointments. These patients have often learnt that they can see doctors if they present new crops of symptoms that require urgent attention. By responding to new symptoms or exacerbations of existing complaints with offers of earlier appointments, the doctor may inadvertently reinforce the patient's illness behaviour and encourage the use of symptoms as currency in the doctor–patient relationship.

Fourthly, it is important to understand the patient's physical complaints as a form of communication rather than as evidence of disease. Because many have difficulty in recognizing and talking about emotional issues, patients may only be able to communicate distress in the form of somatic symptoms. A psychodynamic understanding of the patient's complaint behaviour can help the doctor to make sense of the case and respond appropriately to difficult demands. Some patients with SD give a history of having been abused, neglected, scapegoated, or severely maltreated during childhood. These individuals often bring with them into adult life unacceptable aggressive and angry impulses which do not find a satisfactory outlet. As a consequence, covert anger and feelings of persecution may be represented firstly in the form of self-reproach or criticism (as in depression), but also in reproachful complaints to others of bodily pains or somatic illness. A doctor who feels persecuted by such patients is the recipient of the anger and persecution that the patient experienced during childhood. Many of our patients attribute their problems to medical neglect or to previous invasive medical procedures. Some have become litigious and complained to hospital administrators or even the Minister of Health.

In a thoughtful review of this topic Brown and Vaillant (1981) remarked that 'in lieu of openly complaining that others have ignored or hurt him, the patient settles on belabouring those present with his genuinely felt, but misplaced, bodily pains or discomforts'.

But changing the agenda from talking about the patient's bodily pain to emotional pain can be difficult. It can be facilitated by taking a complete psychosocial history, empathizing with the patient's past experiences of distress, and gradually building on a relationship of mutual trust in which the patient comes to believe that his/her complaints (emotional and physical) are taken seriously. We have found that many of these patients are willing to discuss their miserable and traumatic childhoods, often showing considerable affect and anguish when they do. This only seems to take place after a reasonable rapport has been established with the psychiatrist. It may take several appointments before the psychiatrist gets past the barrier of physical complaints and is able to sense the enormity of the patient's anguish and suffering.

Brown and Vaillant (1981) also suggest a paradoxical approach to the endless physical complaints, which involves making empathic statements designed to exaggerate the patient's suffering such as: 'I don't know how you stand so much pain,' or 'it must be awful to endure such terrible pain all the time'. Merely requesting the patient to provide a list of somatic symptoms experienced since his/her previous outpatient visit serves little purpose.

The patient will of course continue to complain of somatic symptoms during this treatment process. The physician should reassure the patient that he/she recognizes that the symptoms are important, but believes that the best course of action is to observe them over time rather than embark on unnecessary, possibly dangerous, diagnostic procedures.

The place of the physical examination in patients with SD is controversial, and depends to a large extent on the setting in which the patient is seen. For example, some authors advise that the family doctor should conduct at least a partial physical examination at each visit (Smith, 1990). This should involve the organ system in which the patient has complaints. Such an approach may be appropriate for the family doctor, but we do not routinely examine the patient at each visit. However, when new symptoms appear which suggest the presence of disease, the physician should take them seriously and examine the patient thoroughly. Judicious referral to a consultant colleague to assess the importance of new physical complaints may be helpful, but the referral note should include a comment about the dangers of injudicious remarks concerning disease made in front of these patients.

Fifthly, it is important to minimize the use of psychotropic and/or analgesic medication. If, however, a psychiatric syndrome that is normally responsive to drug treatment is present, e.g. panic disorder or depressive illness, a carefully monitored trial of treatment is worthwhile. It is important to explain to the patient that the drug will not cure the illness but may have a modest effect on the symptoms being targeted. Most patients with SD are peculiarly sensitive to side-effects. It is best therefore to commence with low doses, to increase the dose slowly, and to see the patient frequently. The patient should be encouraged to persevere until the effect of the drug can be fully evaluated.

**Table 12.10.** Management of chronic somatization (general principles)

---

Establish diagnosis
Discuss and agree management plan with the family doctor
Arrange regular spaced visits (e.g. every 4–6 weeks)
Do not see the patient 'on demand'
During these visits aim to:
    (a) 'change the agenda', i.e. help the patient to make links between
       events and bodily symptoms
    (b) reduce unnecessary medications and avoid unnecessary tests
    (c) perform at least a partial physical examination of the organ
       system in which the patient has complaints[*]
    (d) involve other family members
    (e) treat any coexisting anxiety or depressive symptoms
Damage limitation is a more realistic goal than cure
Arrange support for yourself

---

[*] This is controversial. Some psychiatrists may prefer to depute this task to
the family practitioner.

Finally, it is important to obtain permission to contact the patient's family. The patient's spouse or partner should be made aware of the treatment plan at the outset, the rationale and details of which should be fully explained. A summary of the important components of management is shown in Table 12.10.

In a controlled study of patients with chronic somatization which used some of these simple treatment techniques, Smith *et al.* (1986b) showed that both health care charges and the mean number of days spent in hospital were reduced significantly in those patients who received psychiatric consultation. In this study 38 patients were randomly assigned to treatment or control. The treatment group received education about their disorder and recommendations to the physician, who was encouraged to serve as the primary physician of the patient with the disorder. All physicians were advised to make regular scheduled appointments for each patient (possibly every 4 or 6 weeks) and not to see the patient on demand. Other recommendations were for each patient to receive a physical examination at each visit, and physicians were advised to avoid hospitalization, diagnostic procedures, surgery, and the use of laboratory assessments, unless they were clearly indicated. The 38 patients were studied prospectively for 18 months. After 9 months, the control group was crossed over to receive treatment with the same intervention. The results were impressive: after the psychiatric consultation, the quarterly health care charges in the treatment group declined by 53%, but there was no change in the controls. After the control group were crossed over to receive treatment, their quarterly charges declined by 49%. The reductions in expenditure in both groups were due largely to decreases in hospitalization.

This study demonstrated that intervention in SD brings about substantial reduction in medical and health care charges. It is unclear how many patients felt subjectively improved but the authors believe that providing more appropriate medical care may lead to a reduction in symptoms and associated handicaps.

There is an obvious need for studies of this kind to be carried out on a UK sample. We have had no difficulty in recruiting a sample of patients with SD in a London teaching hospital. Like USA samples, our patients have had innumerable costly, invasive and unnecessary investigations and hospital admissions. And we have anecdotal evidence that intervention is effective.

Lipowski (1988) has described an inpatient treatment programme for persistent somatizers that involves a multidisciplinary approach. Comprehensive assessment by social workers, occupational therapists, psychologists and psychiatrists is supplemented by a work history and data about the patient's level of functioning in daily activities. The treatment programme involves an individually tailored combination of individual and group psychotherapy, family therapy, occupational therapy, physiotherapy, relaxation training, biofeedback, psychotropic drugs, and vocational counselling. Not all of these treatment modalities are applied in every case. In frequent group meetings patients are encouraged to become self-assertive and to set their own goals for the future after leaving hospital. The results of such a comprehensive approach to treatment have yet to be published.

Lipowski has remarked that the greatest challenge is to identify susceptibility to chronic somatization early and to treat these patients actively in order to *prevent* chronicity. This will involve physicians referring patients at a relatively early stage in the development of the illness in the hope that the correct diagnosis can be made and the patient's psychosocial difficulties dealt with.

## Conclusions

The evidence from clinical studies supports the view that SD, as defined in DSM-III, is heterogeneous with respect to psychopathology. Furthermore, it is doubtful whether SD is best viewed as a discrete categorical disorder. Many patients fall 'just short' of the designated number of symptoms needed for a DSM-III-R diagnosis but are not qualitatively different from 'cases' of SD. SD may merely be a severe, persistent and intractable form of a process ubiquitous in most cultures.

In our own sample we have not recognized SD as a unitary disorder. Although all patients were diagnosed as 'cases' using the DIS, i.e. reported the requisite number of lifetime symptoms (>13 out of a possible 35), they do not comprise a homogeneous group. All are of necessity polysymptomatic, but for different reasons. For example, some have a phobic diathesis with co-occurring depressive episodes and intermittent hyperventilation; others have histrionic personalities accompanied by a tendency to dissimulate and mislead doctors; still others appear to be driven by a 'disease conviction' more characteristic of hypochondriacal patients, but which involves so many different systems that the patient qualifies for SD. Among our sample are patients with additional factitious and hypochondriacal complaints, and it is clear that hypochondriasis and factitious disorders overlap with SD. This calls into question the classification of the somatoform disorders, a topic that is discussed more fully elsewhere (Chapter 2).

'Somatization' is best conceived as a *process* rather than as a discrete disease entity (Kleinman *et al.*, 1978). Acute and subacute forms of somatization are seen most frequently in primary care settings (Chapter 4, p. 80), whereas chronic somatization is a process that is maintained over many years and is more likely to be encountered in general hospital settings. To a large extent this process is dependent on doctors, who are often instrumental in initiating further consultations, investigations, medications and surgery. Regrettably, by the time the diagnosis of SD is established, this mutually unrewarding interactive process is very difficult to halt.

Because the doctor is so important in the genesis of this disorder, we believe that the prevalence of SD in a given population partly reflects the organization of its healthcare system. This issue has been discussed in more detail elsewhere (Bass & Murphy, 1990).

We believe that a multiaxial diagnostic approach is most applicable to these patients. This will ensure that mental state, personality, medical illnesses, current stressors and functional impairment are all given equal consideration. Furthermore, exploration of abnormalities in mental state must take into account the importance of illness beliefs and attitudes to bodily sensations; these beliefs are of central importance in these patients and often determine the 'doctor-shopping' that characterizes the disorder. Our clinical experience of these patients suggests that anxiety is a core factor in SD and that a multitude of other push factors (e.g. co-morbidity with other mental state disorder, personality disorders and psychophysiological abnormalities) as well as pull factors (doctors' reliance on biomedical explanations, the 're-wards' of the sick role) give the disorder its final colouring.

There is a need for controlled intervention studies in this group of patients, who have been ignored by physicians and psychiatrists alike. These patients inhabit a no man's land between medicine and psychiatry, and it is not surprising that many are now attracted to alternative practitioners. The economic benefits of intervention have already been demonstrated in an American sample, and in these cost-conscious times, studies of this nature should be given priority. Two questions need to be addressed: first, how can physicians be helped to develop the skills required to identify these patients early in the course of illness? second, which therapeutic intervention(s) will prevent patients with complex psychosocial problems from developing chronic and intractable somatoform disorders? Studies of this nature might have considerable financial implications for the National Health Service.

Finally, the disorder has important implications for the education of both medical students and psychiatrists. Somatizing patients attend general hospitals, and in the UK students often learn psychiatry in mental hospital settings. As a consequence they have little exposure to these patients and do not acquire any expertise in their assessment and management. There is a case, therefore, for more of the psychiatry clerkship to be spent in the general hospital.

But it is not only medical students who are unlikely to be educated about chronic somatization. Many psychiatric trainees receive no experience of general hospital psychiatry and feel ill-equipped to assess and manage these patients when they are referred. Many will offer oversimplified explanations of the patient's behaviour and make a diagnosis of depression or personality disorder, often accompanied by inappropriate prescription of psychotropic drugs. This is usually a clumsy and futile attempt to 'persuade' the patient that the problem is psychological. What we have rarely seen is *liaison* with other doctors. Without this the psychiatric clinic becomes merely another resource for the patient to utilize rather than a place where a full psychosocial assessment can be carried out and management co-ordinated. Patients with chronic somatization are among the most emotionally taxing that doctors encounter (thus 'heartsink'), but they provide the psychiatrist with an opportunity to exercise his or her clinical skills.

# References

American Psychiatric Association (1980), *Diagnostic and Statistical Manual of Mental Disorders* 3rd edn. (DSM-III), Washington DC.
American Psychiatric Association (1987). *Diagnostic and Statistical Manual of Mental Disorders* 3rd edn., revised, (DSM III-R), Washington DC.
Bass, C. & Murphy, M. (1990). The chronic somatiser and the Government White Paper, *Journal of the Royal Society of Medicine*, **83**, 203–205.
Benjamin, S. (1988). Illness behaviour and neurosis, *Current Opinion in Psychiatry*, **1(2)**, 142–149.
Bibb, R.C. & Guze, S.B. (1972). Hysteria (Briquet's syndrome) in a psychiatric hospital: the significance of secondary depression, *American Journal of Psychiatry*, **129**, 224–228.
Bloch, S. (1986). Supportive psychotherapy, in *An Introduction to the Psychotherapies*, (Ed.

Bloch, S.) Oxford University Press, Oxford.

Boyd, J.H., Burke, J.D., Gruenberg, E. *et al.* (1984). Exclusion criteria of DSM-III, *Archives of General Psychiatry*, **41**, 983–989.

Bridges, K.W. & Goldberg, D.P. (1985). Somatic presentation of DSM-III — psychiatric disorders in primary care, *Journal of Psychosomatic Research*, **29**, 563–569.

Briquet, P. (1859). *Traite Clinique et Therapeutique de L'Hysterie*, J.B. Balliere & Fils, Paris.

Brown, H.N. & Vaillant, G.E. (1981). Hypochondriasis, *Archives of Internal Medicine*, **141**, 723–726.

Cloninger, C.R. (1987). Diagnosis of somatoform disorders. A critique of DSM-III, in *Diagnosis and Classification in Psychiatry* (Ed. Tischler, G.L.) Oxford University Press, Oxford.

Cloninger, C.R., Martin, R.L., Guze, S.B. & Clayton, P.J. (1986). A prospective follow-up and family study of somatization in man and woman, *American Journal of Psychiatry*, **143**, 873–878.

Cohen, M.E, Robins, E., Purtell, J.J., Altmann, M.W. & Reid, D.E. (1953). Excessive surgery in hysteria, *Journal of the American Medical Association*, **151**, 977–986.

Deighton, C.M. & Nicol, A.R. (1985). Abnormal illness behaviour in young women in a primary care setting: is Briquet's syndrome a useful category? *Psychological Medicine*, **15**, 515–520.

Derogatis, L.R., Lipman, R.S. & Covi, L. (1973). The SCL-90: an out-patient psychiatric rating scale, *Psychopharmacology Bulletin*, **9**, 13–28.

De Souza, C. & Othmer, E. (1984). Somatization disorder and Briquet's syndrome. An assessment of their diagnostic concordance, *Archives of General Psychiatry*, **41**, 334–336.

Escobar, J.I., Burnam, A., Karno, M., Forsythe, A. & Golding, J.M. (1987). Somatisation in the community, *Archives of General Psychiatry*, **44**, 713–718.

Farley, J., Woodruff, R.A. & Guze, S.B. (1968). The prevalence of hysteria and conversion symptoms, *British Journal of Psychiatry*, **114**, 1121–1125.

Feighner, R.A., Robins, E. & Guze, S.B. *et al.* (1972). Diagnostic criteria for use in psychiatric research, *Archives of General Psychiatry*, **26**, 57–63.

Gardner, W.N. & Bass, C. (1989). Hyperventilation in clinical practice, *British Journal of Hospital Medicine*, **41**, 73–81.

Gardner, W.N., Meah, M. & Bass, C. (1986). Controlled study of respiratory responses during prolonged measurement in patients with chronic hyperventilation, *Lancet*, **ii**, 826–830.

Gordon, E., Kraiuhin, C., Kelly, P., Meares, R. & Howson, A. (1986). A neurophysiological study of somatization disorder, *Comprehensive Psychiatry*, **27**, 295–301.

Guze, S.B. (1975). The validity and significance of the clinical diagnosis of hysteria (Briquet's syndrome), *American Journal of Psychiatry*, **132**, 138–141.

Guze, S.B., Cloninger, C.R., Martin, R.L. & Clayton, P.J. (1986). A follow-up and family study of Briquet's syndrome, *British Journal of Psychiatry*, **149**, 17–23.

Guze, S.B. & Perley, M.J. (1963). Observations on the natural history of hysteria, *American Journal of Psychiatry*, **119**, 960–965.

Henderson, S. (1974). Care-eliciting behaviour in man, *Journal of Nervous and Mental Disease*, **159**, 172–181.

Horvath, T., Friedman, J. & Meares, R. (1980). Attention in Hysteria: a study of Janet's Hypothesis by means of habituation and arousal methods, *American Journal of Psychiatry*, **137**, 217–221.

Kaminsky, M.J. & Slavney, P.R. (1976). Methodology and personality in Briquet's syndrome: a reappraisal, *American Journal of Psychiatry*, **133**, 85–88.

Kaminsky, M.J. & Slavney, P.R. (1983). Hysterical and obsessional features in patients with Briquet's syndrome (somatisation disorder), *Psychological Medicine*, **13**, 111–120.

Katon, W. (1984). Panic disorder and somatization, *American Journal of Medicine*, **77**, 101–106.

Katon, W., Ries, R.K. & Kleinman, A. (1984). Prospective DSM-III study of 100 consecutive somatisation patients, *Comprehensive Psychiatry*, **25**, 305–314.

King, R., Margraf, J., Ehlers, A. & Maddock, R. (1986). Panic disorder — overlap with symptoms of somatisation disorder, in *Panic and Phobias* (Eds. Hand I., and Wittchen, H.V.) Springer-Verlag, Berlin.

Kirmayer, L.J. (1984). Culture, affect and somatization, *Transcultural Psychiatry Research*, **21**, 159–188.

Kleinman, A., Eisenberg, L. & Good, B. (1978). Culture, illness, and care, *Annals of Internal Medicine*, **88**, 251–258.

Lewis, B.I. (1954). Chronic hyperventilation syndrome, *Journal of the American Medical Association*, **155**, 1204–1208.

Lipowksi, Z.J. (1988). An in-patient programme for persistent somatizers, *Canadian Journal of Psychiatry*, **33**, 275–278.

Liskow, B., Othmer, E., Penick, E.C., De Souza C. & Gabrielli, W. (1986a), Is Briquet's syndrome a heterogeneous disorder? *American Journal of Psychiatry*, **143**, 626–629.

Liskow, B., Penick, E.C., Powell, B.J., Haefele, W.F. & Campbell, J.L. (1986b). In-patients with Briquet's syndrome: presence of additional psychiatric syndromes and MMPI results, *Comprehensive Psychiatry*, **27**, 461–470.

Lloyd, G.G. (1986). Psychiatric syndromes with a somatic presentation, *Journal of Psychosomatic Research*, **30**, 113–120.

Lum, L.C. (1976). The syndrome of habitual chronic hyperventilation, in *Modern Trends in Psychosomatic Medicine* (Ed. Hill, O.) Butterworth, London.

Lum, L.C. (1981). Hyperventilation and anxiety state, *Journal of Royal Society of Medicine*, **74**, 1–4.

Magarian, G.J. (1982). Hyperventilation syndromes: infrequently recognised common expressions of anxiety and stress, *Medicine*, **61**, 219–236.

Majerus, P.W., Guze, S.B., Delong, W.B. & Robins, E. (1960). Psychologic factors and psychiatric disease in hyperemesis gravidarum: a follow-up study of 69 vomiters and 66 controls, *American Journal of Psychiatry*, **117**, 421–428.

Mann, A.H., Jenkins, R., Cutting, J.C. & Cowen, P.J. (1981). The development and use of a standardised assessment of personality, *Psychological Medicine*, **11**, 839–847.

Marks, I.M. & Matthews, A.M. (1979). Brief standard self-rating for phobic patients, *Behaviour Research and Therapy*, **17**, 263–267.

Martin, R.L., Roberts, W.V., Clayton, P.J. & Wetzel, R. (1977). Psychiatric illness and non-cancer hysterectomy, *Diseases of the Nervous System*, **00**, 974–980.

Meares, R. & Horvath, T. (1972). 'Acute' and 'chronic' hysteria, *British Journal of Psychiatry*, **121**, 653–657.

Murphy, G.E., Robins, E., Kuhn, N. & Christensen, R.F. (1962). Stress, sickness and psychiatric disorder in a 'normal' population: a study of 101 young women, *Journal of Nervous and Mental Diseases*, **134**, 228–236.

Myers, J.K., Weisman M.M., Tischsler G.L. *et al.* (1984). Six month prevalence of psychiatric disorders in three communities: 1980 to 1982, *Archives of General Psychiatry*, **44**, 959–967.

Orenstein, H. (1989). Briquet's syndrome in association with depression and panic: a reconceptualisation of Briquet's syndrome, *American Journal of Psychiatry*, **146**, 334–338.

Othmer, E. & De Souza, C. (1985). A screening test for somatization disorder (hysteria), *American Journal of Psychiatry*, **142**, 1146–1149.

Perley, M.J. & Guze, S.B. (1962). Hysteria — the stability and usefulness of clinical criteria. A quantitative study based on a follow-up period of 6–8 years in 39 patients, *New England Journal of Medicine*, **266**, 421–426.

Purtell, J.J., Robins, E. & Cohen, M.E. (1951). Observations on clinical aspects of hysteria. A quantitative study of 50 hysteria patients and 156 control subjects, *Journal of the American Medical Association*, **146**, 902–909.

Regier, D.A., Myers, J.K., Kramer M. *et al.* (1984). The NIMH epidemiological catchment area project: historical context, major objectives, and study population characteristics, *Archives of General Psychiatry*, **41**, 934–941.

Robins, L.N., Helzer, J.E., Ratcliff, K.S. & Seyfried, W. (1982). Validity of the diagnostic interview schedule, version II: DSM-III diagnoses, *Psychological Medicine*, **12**, 855–870.

Sheehan, D.V. & Sheehan, K.H. (1982). The classification of anxiety and hysterical states. Part I. Historical review and empirical delineation, *Journal of Clinical Psychopharmacology*, **2**, 235–244.

Slater, E. (1961). 'Hysteria 311', *Journal of Mental Science*, **107**, 359–381.

Slater, E. (1965). Diagnosis of 'hysteria', *British Medical Journal*, i, 1395–1399.

Slavney, P.R. & Teitelbaum, M.L. (1985). Patients with medically unexplained symptoms: DSM-III diagnoses and demographic characteristics, *General Hospital Psychiatry*, **7**, 21–25.

Smail, P., Stockwell, T., Canter, S. & Hodgson, R. (1984). Alcohol dependence and phobic anxiety states. I-A prevalence study, *British Journal of Psychiatry*, **144**, 53–57.

Smith, G.R. (1990). *Somatization Disorder in the Medical Setting*, National Institute of Mental Health. DHHS Publication No. (ADM) 89–1631, Washington D.C.

Smith, G.R., Monson, R.A. & Ray, D.C. (1986a). Patients with multiple unexplained symptoms, *Archives of Internal Medicine*, **146**, 69–72.

Smith, G.R., Monson, R.A. & Ray, D.C. (1986b). Psychiatric consultation in somatization disorder. A randomized controlled study, *New England Journal of Medicine*, **314**, 1407–1413.

Smith, R.C. (1985). A clinical approach to the somatizing patient, *Journal of Family Practice*, **21**, 294–301.

Spalt, L. (1980). Hysteria and anti-social personality — a single disorder? *Journal of Nervous and Mental Disease*, **168**, 456–464.

Spitzer, R.L., Endicott, J. & Robins, E. (1978). Research diagnostic criteria: rationale and reliability, *Archives of General Psychiatry*, **35**, 773–782.

Steel, K., Gertman, P.M., Cresenzi, C. & Anderson, J. (1981). Iatrogenic illness on a general medical service at a university hospital, *New England Journal of Medicine*, **304**, 638–642.

Stockwell, T., Smail, P., Hodgson, R. & Canter, S. (1984). Alcohol dependence and phobic anxiety states. II-A retrospective study, *British Journal of Psychiatry*, **144**, 58–63.

Swartz, M., Blazer, D., George, L. & Landerman, R. (1986a). Somatization disorder in a community population, *American Journal of Psychiatry*, **143**, 1403–1408.

Swartz, M., Blazer, D., George, L. & Landerman, R. (1988). Somatization disorder in a southern community, *Psychiatric Annals*, **18**, 335–339.

Swartz, M., Hughes, D., George, L., Blazer, D., Landerman, R. & Bucholz, K. (1986b). Developing a screening index for community studies of somatization disorder, *Journal of Psychiatric Research*, **20**, 335–343.

Swartz, M., Hughes, D., Blazer, D. & George, L. (1987). Somatization disorder in the community. A study of diagnostic concordance among three diagnostic systems, *Journal of Nervous and Mental Disease*, **175**, 26–33.

Tyrer, P. (1989). Clinical importance of personality disorder, *Current Opinion in Psychiatry*, **2**, 240–243.

Tyrer, P. & Alexander, M.S. (1987). Personality assessment schedule, in *Personality Disorders: Diagnosis, Management and Course* (Ed. Tyrer, P.) Wright, Bristol.

Tyrer, P., Alexander, M.S., Cichetti, D.V., Cohen, M.S. & Remington, M.C. (1979). Reliability of a schedule for rating personality disorders. *British Journal of Psychiatry*, **135**, 168–174.

Vaillant, G. (1984). The disadvantages of DSM-III outweigh its advantages, *American Journal of Psychiatry*, **141**, 542–545.

Wahl, C.W. (1963). Unconscious factors in the psychodynamics of the hypochondriacal patient, *Psychosomatics*, **4**, 9–14.

Weissman, M.M., Myers, J.K. & Harding, P.S. (1978). Psychiatric disorders in a US urban community: 1975–76, *American Journal of Psychiatry*, **135**, 459–462.

Woodruff, R.A., Clayton, P.J. & Guze, S.B. (1971). Hysteria: studies of diagnosis, outcome, and prevalence, *Journal of the American Medical Association*, **215**, 425–428.

World Health Organization (1987). Mental, behavioural and developmental disorders, in *Inter-

*national Classification of Diseases* (10th revision) Draft Chapter V (F). Division of Mental Health, World Health Organization, Geneva (copyright reserved).

Zoccolillo, M. & Cloninger, C.R. (1985). Parental breakdown associated with somatisation disorder (hysteria), *British Journal of Psychiatry*, **147**, 443–446.

Zoccolillo, M. & Cloninger, C.R. (1986). Somatization disorder: psychologic symptoms, social disability, and diagnosis, *Comprehensive Psychiatry*, **27**, 65–73.

# Index

333